DO WE CARE?

'Sujatha Rao is a longtime leader in public health who has decided she has nothing to lose from telling the truth. The result is this definitive book on the Indian health system—the tangled way it came about, how it works, where it is serving citizens well, and where it has thoroughly failed them. *Do We Care?* is a fearless book. Rao speaks from the heart. And she has solutions. This is a voice worth listening to.'

—Atul Gawande, Professor, Harvard Chan School of Public Health, and author of *Being Mortal*

'*Do We Care?* is a passionate account of government failure in ensuring basic healthcare to people. Sujatha Rao brings out the glaring inadequacies of the system vividly with the anguish of denial of this basic human right. The book reflects her long years of experience, unflinching commitment, and deep analytical approach and is a must read for all health policy analysts and policymakers.'

—M. Govinda Rao, Member, Fourteenth Finance Commission, Government of India, and Emeritus Professor, National Institute of Public Finance and Policy, New Delhi, India.

'Despite recent progress, health systems in developing countries must still contend with various challenges: promoting healthy lifestyles, preventing disease, delivering high-quality care to everyone who needs it, protecting families from the financial consequences of ill health and, underlying all of the above, closing the unacceptable gaps that so unequally allocate opportunities along gender, racial, ethnic, and socio-economic lines. Few countries better exemplify the trials that health systems in low- and middle-income countries are facing than India. For this reason, the study of this case is always revealing and enriching. *Do We Care?* provides a fresh and rigorous look at the past and current evolution of a national health system that offers valuable lessons for the developing world. It is a must read for scholars and decision makers interested in India, in particular, and in global health, in general.'

—Julio Frenk, President, University of Miami, Florida, USA, and former Minister of Health, Mexico

DO WE CARE?
India's Health System

K. Sujatha Rao

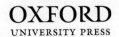
OXFORD
UNIVERSITY PRESS

OXFORD
UNIVERSITY PRESS

Oxford University Press is a department of the University of Oxford.
It furthers the University's objective of excellence in research, scholarship,
and education by publishing worldwide. Oxford is a registered trademark of
Oxford University Press in the UK and in certain other countries.

Published in India by
Oxford University Press
2/11 Ground Floor, Ansari Road, Daryaganj, New Delhi 110 002, India

© Oxford University Press 2017

The moral rights of the author have been asserted.

First Edition published in 2017
Fifth impression 2018

All rights reserved. No part of this publication may be reproduced, stored in
a retrieval system, or transmitted, in any form or by any means, without the
prior permission in writing of Oxford University Press, or as expressly permitted
by law, by licence, or under terms agreed with the appropriate reprographics
rights organization. Enquiries concerning reproduction outside the scope of the
above should be sent to the Rights Department, Oxford University Press, at the
address above.

You must not circulate this work in any other form
and you must impose this same condition on any acquirer.

ISBN-13: 978-0-19-946954-3
ISBN-10: 0-19-946954-7

Typeset in Bembo Std 11/14
by Tranistics Data Technologies, New Delhi 110044
Printed in India by Replika Press Pvt. Ltd

*For my parents and my sister Nirmala, who suffered needlessly
for want of good-quality care, and the thousands of health professionals
and caregivers saving lives in India*

Contents

List of Tables, Figures, and Boxes	vii
Preface	ix
Acknowledgements	xxiv
List of Acronyms	xxvi

Part I: India's Health System: Challenges and Constraints — 1

1. Evolution of India's Health System — 7
2. Health Financing — 38
3. Governance: Impacting the Health System — 111

Part II: Implementing Policy: Successes, Failures, and the Road Ahead — 197

4. Scaling Up to Reverse the HIV/AIDS Epidemic — 201
5. Revitalizing Rural Primary Healthcare: The National Rural Health Mission — 298
6. Making Our Future — 388

Select Bibliography	425
Index	434
About the Author	447

Tables, Figures, and Boxes

Tables

2.1	Interstate Comparison of Average Per Capita Spending in 19 Major States: 2004–5 and 2011–12 (in 2004–5 Prices)	61
2.2	Allocative Efficiencies in Spending in 19 Major States during 2007–8 and 2011–12 (Rs Crores)	63
2.3	Interstate Comparison of Spending by Component: 2007–8 and 2011–12 (Rs Crores)	70
2.4a	Government-sponsored Health Insurance Schemes	87
2.4b	Other Health Insurance Schemes in the Country	90
3.1	Social Determinants of U5MR among the Top-three and Bottom-three States	142
4.1	Prevalence Levels of HIV Infection among Different Key Population Groups (in Percentage Points)	212
4.2	Categories of Districts, 2007	213
4.3	Comparison of HIV Testing for TB Patients and Treatment for HIV-Positive TB Patients: Global versus Indian Averages	241
4.4	Releases for HIV/AIDS during the Twelfth Plan: 2012–17 (Rs Crores)	285
4.5	Achievements under the NACP (End Phases I, II, and III)	291
5.1	Maternal Mortality Ratio per 100,000 Live Births, 2001–12	335

5.2	Comparative Table of Indicators Impacting Maternal Mortality: Some States	336
5.3	Rates of Decline among Key Indicators Pre- and Post-NRHM (%)	357
5.4	Budget Allocations for NRHM: 2007 to 2016–17 (Rs Crores)	370

Figures

2.1	Financial Resource Flows	78
3.1	System of Health Governance in India	119
3.2	Problems of Poor Data in Decision-making	178
4.1	Scaling up ART	240
4.2	Scaling up of the ART Programme Guidelines	244

Boxes

3.1	Policy for Creating a Cadre of Doctor–Assistants	123
3.2	NEET	130
3.3	Regulations Required in the Health Sector	163
4.1	Lack of Experience	203
4.2	Early Years of the Epidemic	208
4.3	Kamathipura, Mumbai, 1992	250
4.4	Ashodaya, 2006	258
4.5	Society for Community Intervention and Rehabilitation (SCIR), Kolkata, 2006	269
5.1	Health Workers in Ethiopia	347
6.1	Current Status of Primary Healthcare in India	396
6.2	Reorganization of the Primary Healthcare System	397

Preface

The Preamble and the Directive Principles of India's Constitution provide a direction that must underscore India's policies and governance. Under Article 38(1), the Constitution refers to the Indian state as a welfare state,[1] and in Article 41, it exhorts the state to strive towards extending public assistance in 'cases of unemployment, old age, sickness and disablement, and in other cases of undeserved want'. It provides for 'maternity relief' in Article 42; under Article 47, it states 'the level of nutrition and the standard of living of its people and the improvement of public health as among its primary duties'; and, above all, under Article 14, all citizens have an equal right to life. However, nowhere does India's Constitution explicitly state health as a human right.

With the years rolling by, India has gone further away from the letter and spirit of the Constitution, resulting in wide disparities and inequalities in the living standards of the people, with the rich getting richer while the vast majority of the poor continues to struggle to meet their essential needs. The state is rapidly trending towards becoming a minor player in most fields of economic and social significance. The divide between the rich and the poor could not be starker.

In other parts of the world, arguments and debates on what constitutes development, poverty, and equity has been a subject of constant reflection. During the late 1980s, the World Bank categorized countries into high-, middle-, and low-income, based on their gross domestic product (GDP). This was mainly to help decide its lending policies. In the early 1990s, a composite human development index (HDI) was developed that placed the longevity of life, female literacy, infant mortality rate (IMR), and under-five mortality rate (U5MR) alongside the GDP in order to rank countries. To some extent, the inclusion of such indicators did help in assessing the impact of GDP-measured growth on human development. But while the HDI was a useful index for advocacy purposes and raising awareness of policymakers on what should, and must, define development, it still fell short. These efforts were followed by further refinements like the inequality-adjusted HDI, gender inequality index, gender development index, and so on.

Of late, scholars are measuring poverty and equity by associating other factors to develop a multidimensional poverty index (MPI). The MPI seeks to capture poverty in terms of the consequential deprivation or the 'clustered disadvantage' that a poor person faces in accessing basic goods like education, healthcare, safe water, nutrition, environmental hygiene, and such related elements that are required to enhance one's capability to live life to the optimum and also, in a more utilitarian sense, access opportunities for one's betterment.[2] A further refinement of indices to categorize countries in terms of disease and well-being is now being attempted for channelizing development aid and financial flows. Such a redefinition has been necessitated since 70 per cent of disease and health inequity is concentrated in the low-income and middle-income countries, challenging the notion that incomes do not, by themselves, ensure the health and well-being of a people. Thus, while there are several studies that show strong correlations between economic growth and poverty reduction, there are not many to show the correlation between growth and non-income related indicators.

It is in this context that the report of the Commission on Macroeconomics and Health (CMH) published in 2000 by the World Health Organization (WHO) was a landmark of sorts for clearly establishing the link between health and wealth, between the development of a society and economic prosperity. The CMH report[3] argued that healthy people generate wealth, and ill health and disease significantly impact the growth momentum. In an ageing world, India's 40 per cent young and productive population can be, and is, an enviable advantage, but only if they are healthy. Sick people do not produce wealth.

Thus, notwithstanding the constitutional provisions and guidance; international discourse on issues related to development, poverty, and equity; and despite being home to one of the largest numbers of the poor and sick in the world, public discourse in India does not focus on health or education in its growth story and continues to pursue a perfunctory understanding of the values of equity and fairness. Clearly, India's tragedy has been its failure to forge a national consensus and a political system founded on the principle of a social contract where ensuring access to fundamental public (basic) goods—clean air, safe water, sanitation, hygiene, nutritious food, and basic healthcare—and ensuring security to vulnerable populations from health expenditure shocks are visualized as its primary obligations, not options.

Likewise, India still does not define poverty in all its multidimensional aspects. Instead, it continues to define poverty in terms of an income level rather than a state of being that induces low self-esteem, and when combined with illiteracy, hunger, and sickness, becomes a morass from which it is almost impossible to pull oneself out. Similarly, in trapping the notion of equity in the endless squabbling over quotas and reservations in admissions to educational institutions and government jobs, the narratives about equity continue to ignore the more important need to ensure conditions that enable every citizen—irrespective of their social or economic status—to live with dignity and without any discrimination.

While the absence of an understanding of equity and fairness, for instance, seriously impeded and impacted our work for HIV/AIDS patients and population groups most vulnerable to this infection, the absence of data sets required to evaluate the urban–rural or gender or social differentials and continuing to measure progress in aggregate terms reflect the extent to which the system of governance really cares for the welfare of the marginalized or the deprived. As argued by Timothy Evans and others, this happens despite knowing that 'risk factors change but tend to cluster disproportionately within the lower end of the social hierarchy'[4] and regardless of the fact that between the individual and biological dispositions there are social circumstances and the policy environment that determine the severity of the impact on health and well-being.[5]

In fact, India seems stuck. In a deeply stratified society like ours, the state has to be proactive and lead from the front in creating a fairer and more equal environment. But such state leadership has been elusive—so elusive that even after nearly seven decades of Independence and a 9 per cent growth rate in the recent past, two-thirds of Indians do not have access to tap water and a clean toilet, over a third are malnourished, while a million-and-a-half children die before they turn five. Millions continue to die or suffer from communicable diseases such as tuberculosis, malaria, and other infectious diseases that are not only treatable but also at an incredibly low cost. Why? One might ask. Similarly, being born a woman in a particular caste or religious denomination, and living in a village or an urban slum create barriers that are not easy to overcome by individual effort. Such systemic inequities necessitate the negotiating presence of a strong and assertive state.

This book attempts to highlight my understanding of India's health system from an insider's perspective,[6] having been an active participant in the field of policymaking. My experience of having worked for two decades in the health sector in various capacities at the central Ministry of Health & Family Welfare (MOHFW) and in the state of united Andhra Pradesh gives me a specific vantage point. The story of India's health system, as recounted in this book, is based on my perception as an active actor in policy formulation and implementation. In order to reduce bias, I have relied upon documentary evidence as well as interviewed some key players. At the end of the day, this is a personal analysis and interpretation but also one that is based, to the extent possible, on facts and experience.

This book seeks to analyse India's health policy seen through the prism of a development process that appears to have gone awry, where discrimination and deprivation continue to be issues of wide concern. It is divided into two parts: Part I has three chapters that discuss the evolution of India's health policy, followed by a comprehensive discussion on financing and governance in health—the two determinants of health outcomes and well-being.

Chapter 1 traces the evolution of India's health system in the context of the shifting role of the state. The state that was once characterized as following the tenets of Fabian socialism now seems to have swung to the other extreme of a liberal state expounding 'minimum government and maximum governance'. Due to a lack of clarity about what that means, there is apprehension that it may entail a further deepening of privatization and reduction of public investment. There is also a concern about a more rapid withdrawal of the state from discharging its obligations of supplying public goods and leaving them to the markets. The cavalier manner in which health budgets were reduced by the central government during the three years of the Twelfth Five Year Plan (2012–17) exacerbates such apprehensions. Reduced public spending and the aggressive pushing of public–private partnerships can be a dangerous cocktail. The deafening silence regarding the strengthening of the state's regulatory capacities required to ensure the private sector's adherence to standards and protection of patients' interests is also worrisome.

Chapter 2 discusses the need to recognize the interface between politics and economics to understand why India's health sector has faced chronic underfunding over the years since Independence. India is one of the fifteen countries with the ignominious distinction of public spending of less than or about 1 per cent of the GDP on health—other similarly placed countries spend twice the amount while the developed ones spend ten times more. Low public spending means that the burden of financing is borne by individual households, resulting in their impoverishment and a denial of care on grounds of unaffordability. Since the turn of the century, there has been a growing demand for a threefold increase in public spending from the abysmal 1 per cent of the GDP but with little impact on the policymakers.

Inter and intra-state differentials in India are wide. Seventy per cent of maternal, infant, and child mortality is concentrated in the poorer states that have the least institutional capacity to deliver even essential services. Yet the centre that has access to financial resources is unable to bring in any modicum of equalization between these backward states and the ones that are better off. To start with, tax-to-GDP ratio is low and spending priorities seem skewed in favour of the more vocal sections of society than being guided by welfare. Within the residual fiscal space, health competes with education, nutrition, social services, environment, urban development, tourism, and so on. Therefore, unless there is a widening of the tax base and a serious reprioritization of spending, the prospect of enhancing health allocations within the existing structures of public finance is limited, if not impossible. Similar is the position in the states as well.

Besides, the manner in which funds are allocated, released, and spent by public authorities is archaic and calls for systemic reforms. The 'accounting–auditing' model served the British well but is inherently inefficient for a developing country. The funds should be released in accordance with an 'outcome assessment' and the achievement of health benefits should be the justification for the same. The processes, procedures, and systems for releasing funds in India are so complex that more often than not, the implementing agencies never get funds on time. These are important issues because in an environment of scarcity, 'low' utilization determines future allocation despite the fact that allocated budgets have not been released in the first instance. For example, during the Eleventh Five Year Plan (2007–12), states constituted autonomous health societies at the state and district levels to which the central government directly released funds by way of electronic transfers. Speedy releases enabled the implementing agencies to utilize the funds quickly. Under the Twelfth Five Year Plan, this procedure was reversed and central funds are now routed through the state's finance department, without introducing concomitant reforms to ensure timely releases. With the main focus of the finance departments being on managing the 'ways-and-means' position of the state budget rather than ensuring health outcomes, funds are not released, or are withheld, diverted, or provided in small instalments that are inadequate to provide all the inputs in a synchronized manner. The accruing savings or unspent balances are then termed as 'poor utilization', implying an inability to spend and justifying lower allocations. This self-perpetuating cycle needs to be addressed.

There is a growing trend towards government-sponsored social health insurance schemes under which the entire risk is borne by the government. Under such schemes, the government provides to the implementing agency—an insurance company or a trust constituted for the purpose—the entire premium in one or two instalments on behalf of the proposed target population. This money is then spent by the agency in procuring services availed of by the people in public or private hospitals in accordance with the guidelines laid down. Undertaken within restricted budgets, such insurance schemes have substituted other essential expenditures such as preventive services and primary healthcare. Substituting prevention with treatment is a more costly and unsustainable option. Besides, such financing has also strengthened private hospitals without putting in place regulations to monitor them for price and quality. Thus, as per the 71st household survey by the National Sample Survey Office (NSSO), despite the expansion of insurance coverage, there has been no appreciable reduction in out-of-pocket expenditures, particularly between the last two quintiles.

India's health policy is often described as good on paper but weak in implementation with wide gaps between what the policy documents state and the actual achievement on the ground. Many scholars find this baffling. While health advocates blame low public funding for health as the primary cause, economists blame it on poor governance, questioning the persistence of huge absenteeism and non-accountability in public facilities. Why are hospitals dirty? Why do children continue to die of diarrhoea or respiratory infections or are left unimmunized even when the required funds have been provided? These are legitimate questions but have no simple answers. Clearly, since money is only a vector, good governance, implying carefully evaluated policies and their effective implementation, has to be in tandem for optimizing impact.

Governance in India is based on the principles of a participatory democracy through the institutional architecture established by the Constitution. To ensure the effective inclusion of diverse opinions and voices, and to avoid the concentration of power in any one of the pillars of democratic functioning—political executive, parliament, judiciary, or the media—institutional checks and balances have been provided. But this model is not without risks. Multiple institutions have often duplicated, stalled, or delayed the decision-making process—a factor that often comes up in discussions comparing India and China.[7]

Additionally, the policy environment is confusing and inconsistent. For example, while the Constitution has demarcated the functional responsibilities of the centre and the states, it is the central government that sets the agenda on areas that fall under the domain of the states. Or, say, in the case of the policy related to physician practice, where doctors are permitted to do private practice even while working in the public sector with no regulatory oversight to minimize potential conflicts of interest. Yet another example of such policy inconsistency is clearly discernible in the realm of medical education that is being aggressively privatized but the regulatory authority is left weak and incapable of enforcing the quality and standards of education. Such policy inconsistencies reflect the lack of will to govern, with the political executive failing to carry out their responsibilities, namely institute laws, reform and revamp the institutional architecture to suit the changing scenario, build systems to guarantee transparency and accountability, and ensure implementation of policies with professional oversight. In a highly contested arena such as health, with different stakeholders pulling in opposite directions, a clear strategy based on a long-term vision of what we want and where we want to be 30 years hence is the business of the polity and not of bureaucrats, no matter how able or willing.

If policymaking is the business of politicians, the administrative and technical bureaucracies have the responsibility of forming rules and regulations, instituting processes, implementing policies, and managing the contradictions. India's record in this aspect has been woeful. We still formulate strategies on questionable data and mismanagement is a common thread running through the health system, be it at the level of policy articulation or at the floor level in a hospital. Yet there is still scope to do what needs to be done within the existing architecture, despite all its imperfections and inadequacies. There is still a lot of latitude available for instituting evidence-based and data-driven processes and ensure outcomes with better supervision, close monitoring, and good management practices as our experience with eradicating polio or reducing HIV incidence has so convincingly demonstrated. There is no excuse, for example, for a *10-day-old* infant in the intensive care unit (ICU) of a teaching hospital to die from rodent bites, or for snakes to wander around the operation theatre, or for the sharp spike in dengue cases and deaths. Such instances are disturbingly routine and a reflection of a major management failure and collapse of accountability.

Chapter 3 reflects on such governance deficits in the wide range of issues it is concerned with—the price being paid for regulatory failure; centralization of policy; absence of human resource policies related to recruiting, training, and deployment; the need for systematizing uninterrupted supply of drugs; establishing supervisory and monitoring processes; inter-sectoral coordination; laying down laws, rules, and regulations for ensuring accountability; monitoring; and finally, sharing responsibility and providing space for participation of individuals and communities.

Besides managing public systems, governance in health also implies oversight of the private sector. The government alone cannot provide health services wholly and fully. It never has. India has always had the ubiquitous private providers taking care of minor ailments. Now with technological advances and the rise of modern medicine, healthcare delivery is more organized and institutionalized, calling for sophisticated management and larger financial outlays. Stagnant budgets and poor governance have inhibited public hospitals from keeping pace, resulting in the rapid growth of the private sector to meet the increasing demand for services. The dominant provider of care today is the private sector, as it provides 70 per cent of outpatient care and 60 per cent of inpatient treatment and has 80 per cent of the specialists and modern technology. In such a scenario, partnering with the private sector seems inevitable, calling for new expertise and capacities that are currently non-existent in the public system. In other words, the governance challenge is how to engage with the private sector, more particularly the non-commercialized arm—social enterprises, not-for-profit trusts, non-governmental organizations (NGOs)—and also how to use their resources for public welfare and not get short-changed in the process. Navigating such stormy waters calls for evidence, understanding of health economics and the way markets work and people behave, as well as ensuring a stable professional leadership.

The health sector is but a reflection of the governance model set up by the political system. Think about it. Why is it that a system that is able to produce an atom bomb, send an unmanned spacecraft to Mars at an incredibly low cost, execute the Delhi Metro Rail within record time, develop an IT industry, and create a host of other such success stories, fails to efficiently run a hospital or a high school? These questions trouble me, and I simply cannot accept the fact that this is so because our system of governance does not see any value in these goods.

India has four sensitive points of social conflict—caste, religion, language, and class. But the connecting thread underlying these fissures is class—the rich class and the poor class. Opting out of the public hospitals and government schools that they once used and benefited from, the privileged rich and middle classes have made their own arrangements to meet their daily needs by setting up private hospitals, private insurance, and private schools. So much so that several state governments are unable to make private hospitals comply with the conditions for providing free treatment to a proportion of the patients they treat in lieu of the land provided to them at highly subsidized rates or waiving custom duties on imported equipment. Nor can the states make private schools earmark a proportion of their services and seats for the poor as required under the Right to Education Act, 2010.

The worn-down conditions of the public facilities, utilized by the most vulnerable and the poorest, are a stark reflection of the inequities and disparities that characterize India's development story in general and the health system in particular. Such conditions are often explained away by citing a lack of resources, indifference of caregivers, or an apathetic bureaucracy. This is not true. India failed to introduce a system of social security based on the principle of universalism in the initial years of Independence. It is inexplicable as to why Nehru, who was committed to welfarism, did not pay any attention to education and health. After all, the UK, which was the source of most of our ideas of equality and democracy, had introduced its National Health Service (NHS) in the midst of economic collapse as a result of World War II. The logic was known, where William Beveridge had justified introducing the NHS stating, 'Social insurance fully developed may provide income security; it is an attack upon Want. But Want is one only of five giants on the road to reconstruction and in some ways the easiest to attack. The others are Disease, Ignorance, Squalor and Idleness.'[8] Goods that are universally and fairly available to all benefit all. In this way everyone develops a stake in protecting the system.[9] We failed to understand this simple logic. The migration of the middle classes to the private sector and their reluctance to bear the increase in taxes for building a public health system explain why the health concerns of the poor are not a political priority and why those in power just do not care.

A third factor contributing to the health crisis is the absence of sustained leadership at the political, administrative, and technical levels and an erosion of values. No ship can sail without a captain and no wars can be fought without a general. Every sector in our development story that has succeeded has had a leader or mentor one can name. Finding a champion who has steered the health sector through the rough and tumble of political vicissitudes has been a challenge. We have never had a minister resign for preventable deaths or a secretary in government sacked for failing to achieve the targets that have been laid down. There is no evidence of Parliament being stalled for the whole season because 1.5 million children below the age of five die every year due to the lack of adequate healthcare. We have never witnessed strikes or processions to stop the privatization of health and handing over of medical education to profiteers. We have never seen doctors use their political power and influence to revamp the Medical Council of India (MCI) and ensure standards in medical education. Leadership is invaluable, more so since the landscape is an untidy mess with several players and stakeholders working at cross purposes.

Notwithstanding this remarkable failure of leadership at the top, some gains continue to be witnessed with doctors and health workers working on the front lines, seizing opportunities that come their way, and providing leadership on issues that are important for their survival. The success of eliminating polio and reversing HIV/AIDS are examples of leadership at the decentralized levels. The local vaccinators' commitment to duty in the first case and the sex workers who promote the use of condoms throughout their network to stop the transmission of the virus demonstrate how individuals working at the edge can, and do, make a difference. In fact, waiting for our elected leaders to provide leadership to the health sector appears to be futile. Ultimately, it is the people who will have to assume responsibility. And in this context, greater awareness, the formal and social media, the right to information (RTI), and social audits are encouraging developments in India today. They have the power to make the system more accountable and flag health as an election issue. Only then will the government act and respond to address this crisis.

However, there is a more disturbing aspect of the quality of India's leadership than just indifference. The absence of guilt or the loss of values that Joseph Stiglitz refers to in *The Price of Inequality* (2013) is, in my opinion, an even more critical factor. Society as a whole seems to have lost its soul in its blind pursuit of making money. The floods that inundate our cities and towns are explained away as the result of climate change and 'unprecedented' rains. This is partly true. But it is also because governments have failed to protect the tank bunds, riverbeds, irrigation canals, or drainage channels from being occupied by the privileged or by their vote banks, choking the water off to run on to roads and into houses. It is the same 'indifference' that characterizes India's health policy, where the health sector has been reduced to profiteering, be it in the area of medical education or providing services. That the injustice and unfairness of it all does not seem to bother us is, in my opinion, the fault line. The state of our public health and hospitals is as much a strong indictment of ourselves as a society as of the current government.

Part II of the book seeks to document and recount the two remarkable stories of how HIV incidence was reduced by more than half, the highest in the world, and how access to essential services was scaled up in the rural areas of the country in a manner not witnessed ever before in India. Chapters 4 and 5 recount the National AIDS Control Organisation's (NACO) strategy to reduce HIV/AIDS and the National Rural Health Mission's (NRHM) efforts to revitalize rural primary care.

The scaling up of the HIV/AIDS programme and access to rural healthcare under the NRHM were flagship programmes launched under the UPA I (United Progressive Alliance I) that provided an unprecedented level of leadership that, however, was not sustained under UPA II. These two stories reveal how, and in what manner, financing, governance, and leadership at various levels—assumed by different stakeholders at different times—impacted the policy as it unfolded during the course of implementation. They illustrate how politics played out, how agendas were set, policies made and implemented in the real world, and why and how—within the same political context, same environment for governance, and similar constraints—the outcomes were different. They also show how with the withdrawal of political leadership, most noticeably under the NDA (National Democratic Alliance) government in power since May 2014, both have since plateaued and stagnated.

It is difficult not to conclude that health policymaking in India has lacked imagination. Even as India struggles to consolidate its few gains, it is now faced with the challenge of a dual burden of disease. Alongside communicable diseases that account for nearly 36 per cent of morbidity, there is an emergence of non-communicable diseases such as hypertension, diabetes, vascular diseases, and cancers. Besides, deaths and morbidities due to injuries account for 10 per cent of the total mortality in the country. There is growing concern about the re-emergence of vector-borne diseases in a more virulent form as seen in 2015, when the dengue outbreak in Delhi threatened the political legitimacy of the popularly elected government, and as now feared with the impending threat of Zika, caused by similar conditions that are responsible for dengue, opening its account in India. Even as India continues to battle with the backlash of leprosy, a steady rise of HIV infections in some parts of the country, the persistence of unacceptable levels of mortality due to tuberculosis (TB), and the imperative to achieve goals related to maternal and childhood mortality, there is an increasing vulnerability to cross-border infections such as SARS (severe acute respiratory syndrome), H5N1, H1N1, Ebola, MERS (Middle East respiratory syndrome), and Zika that the world witnessed within the short span of a decade, calling for an unprecedented level of vigilance. Besides these threats, there are other equally important problems of antimicrobial resistance due to irrational use of antibiotics and a quality of care that is varied, questionable, and unregulated, both in public and private hospitals. High-cost corporate hospitals, too, are no exception to this assertion. Yet India's determined progress provides some scope for optimism. The last chapter of the book spells out the critical issues that India needs to pay heed to, for carving out a possible way forward.

Clearly then, resolving India's health crisis would require according high priority to health, addressing the issue of a weak and confused governance, and ensuring systems that foster strong leadership at all levels—political, administrative, and technical. The Indian state has to ensure that people's health and well-being become the raison d'être of development and health spending an investment and not be among the first few sectors that face 'expenditure' cuts for balancing fiscal deficits. Not doing so will be clearly going against what the Constitution of the country intended.

Notwithstanding the increasing political instability and a fragmented polity that explains the inconsistent style of governance, a frustrating lack of direction, a reluctance to adopt long-term perspectives required for building systems, and a proclivity towards pandering to irresponsible populism to ensure political legitimacy, the health and welfare of the people should be given due importance. It is clearly not a choice.

Health is a vast and multidimensional sector that cannot be exhaustively dealt with in a single book. I argue for a more focused and better informed leadership that values research and evidence in formulating policies and determining priorities. The Indian state has to deliver on its commitments to make universal access to safe tap water, sanitation, nutrition, and basic healthcare its primary obligation. The focus on our health policies should be grounded in the ideology of human welfare and to achieve the three basic goals of health systems—equity, efficiency, and quality. Appropriate funding profoundly impacts the health and well-being of our society and needs to be provided as a central justification for growth and development. We need to rethink our current mindset of how development needs to be defined and question its very purpose. We need to ensure that investments in public goods do not become victims of partisan politics.

Notes and References

1. A welfare state is a concept of government in which the state plays a key role in the protection and promotion of the economic and social well-being of its citizens.
2. Sabina Alkire, James Foster, Suman Seth, Mariana Emma Santos, Jose Manuel Roche, and Paola Ballon, 'Chapter 1', in *Multidimensional Poverty Measurement and Analysis* (Oxford: Oxford University Press, 2015), pp. 1–25.

3. Jeffrey D. Sachs, *Macroeconomics and Health: Investing in Health for Economic Development* (Geneva: WHO, 2001).
4. Timothy Evans, Margaret Whitehead, Finn Diderichsen, Abbas Bhuiya, and Meg Wirth, *Challenging Inequities in Health: From Ethics to Action* (New York: Oxford University Press, 2001).
5. Evans et al., *Challenging Inequities in Health*.
6. The 'citizen's perspective' of public policy that I got after my retirement profoundly impacted my thinking and, upon reflection, made me realize the limitations of our own understanding of the complexities of the environment in which we work.
7. China also has structures of governance consisting of the central committee and the politburo. But being a single-party state, decision-making and implementation are faster. In other words, China is not trammelled with the noise of democracy and elections. All it needs is for the highest decision-making authority to be convinced of the course.
8. Sir William Beveridge, *Social Insurance and Allied Services* (London: HMSO, 1942).
9. This is an important issue and explains why attempts to privatize the NHS in the UK face strong resistance—all citizens have a stake in it and refer to it as 'our' NHS. This is not the case in India where the better-off sections do not have any stake in the public systems since they have built their own alternatives.

Acknowledgements

When I retired in December 2010, some of my friends encouraged me to tell the National AIDS Control Organisation (NACO) story from an insider's perspective. Not only had my time at NACO been a moment of personal growth but, more importantly, it was also one of the few success stories in the annals of the health ministry. I undertook the challenge because I felt it would give me an opportunity to include the stories of several people who have dedicated their lives to the cause of fighting HIV/AIDS. Their names and work would neither be remembered nor acknowledged by our system. This would at least be my personal tribute to them. While we salute our armed forces, especially those killed in combat, we should also spare a thought for those who prevent people from falling sick and thereby save lives.

In 2012, I was invited by the Harvard School of Public Health (HSPH) as a leadership fellow to offer a credit course on leadership in India's health system. It was then that I looked at the evolution of the country's health system and was struck by the remarkable absence of political, administrative, or technical leadership in the health sector. That tremendous learning experience set me on this path of writing about India's health system.

I started writing this book in 2013 but it moved along in fits and starts due to my other engagements and frequent interruptions. There were several moments of despair when I threw up my hands and was ready to quit. The fact that the book exists at all is, therefore, largely due to the support of my friends Geetanjali Singh and Sunil Nandraj who did not let me give up. They patiently went through numerous revisions and drafts.

I have many to thank for their encouragement, for going through the drafts for accuracy, for providing suggestions, and for just being there for me. I am indebted to each of them: Ajay Reddy, Akhila Sivadas, Angela, Arnab Mukherji, Chitra and Gopi Gopalakrishnan, Dhruv, Dr Aman, Dr Bachani, Dr Govind Rao, Dr Raghavendra Rao, Dr Ramesh, Dr Rewari, Dr Shaukat, Dr Shobini, Dr Suresh Mohammad, Dr T.L.N. Prasad, Dr Venkatesh, Dr Vimlesh Purohit, Injeti Srinivas, Dr Jacob John, Dr Jana, K. Sudhakar, Dr K.R. Antony, Kavita Singh, Keshav Desiraju, Manjiri Bhawalkar, Manoj Gopalakrishnan, Manoj Jhalani, Mayank Agarwal, Meena Seshu, Michael Landesman, N. Devadasan, Nina Rao, Pranay Lal, Professor Venkataraman, Rajani Ved, Rajiv Ahuja, Rakesh Sarwal, Ravi Narayan, Sanghamitra Iyengar, Santosh Kraleti, Sankthivel Selvaraj, Shankar Prinja, Shiv Kumar, Shyam Ashtekar, Sindhu Khullar, Sundaraman, Surinder Singh, Sushena, Swarup Sarkar, T. Sundararaman, Tarun Seem, Thelma Narayan, Urvashi Butalia, Usha Tankha, Vidya Ganesh, Winnie Yip, and Yujwal Raj.

I would also like to thank officials in the Ministry of Health & Family Welfare (MOHFW) and NACO.

Finally, but most importantly, I thank Laxmi, a leader of the transgender community, for suggesting the title of the book. I cannot but agree to the title proposed as, sadly, from the viewpoint of the deprived and discriminated population groups living at the margins, India's health system just does not care for them.

Acronyms

ACA	Additional Central Assistance
AEP	Adolescence Education Programme
AIIMS	All India Institute of Medical Sciences
AIIHPH	All India Institute of Hygiene and Public Health
AMG	ASHA Mentoring Group
ANC	Antenatal Care
ANM	Auxiliary Nurse Midwife
APAC	AIDS Prevention and Control
ART	Antiretroviral Treatment
ASCI	Administrative Staff College of India
ASHA	Accredited Social Health Activist
AWW	Anganwadi worker
BCC	Behaviour Change Communication
BMA	British Medical Association
BMGF	Bill & Melinda Gates Foundation
BPO	Block Programme Officer
BSC	Blood Storage Centre
CAG	Comptroller and Auditor General
CAHP	Coordinating Agency for Health Planning
CBI	Central Bureau of Investigation
CBO	Community-based Organization
CCC	Community Care Centre
CCHFW	Central Council for Health and Family Welfare
CDC	Centers for Disease Control and Prevention
CEHAT	Centre for Enquiry into Health and Allied Themes
CGHS	Central Government Health Scheme
CHAI	Catholic Health Association of India

CHW	Community Health Worker	
CII	Confederation of Indian Industry	
CMH	Commission on Macroeconomics and Health	
CMO	Chief Medical Officer	
CND	Commission for Narcotics Drugs	
CoE	Centre of Excellence	
CPI(M)	Communist Party of India (Marxist)	
CSS	Centrally Sponsored Schemes	
CUP	Condom Use by Prostitutes	
DAPCU	District AIDS Prevention and Control Unit	
DBS	Dried Blood Spot	
DFID	Department for International Development	
DG	Director General	
DGHS	Directorate General of Health Services	
DIC	Drop-in Centre	
DMK	Dravida Munnetra Kazhagam	
DMO	District Medical Officer	
DPO	District Programme Officer	
EAG	Empowered Action Group	
EFC	Expenditure Finance Committee	
EQAS	External Quality Assurance Scheme	
FSSAI	Food Safety and Standards Authority of India	
GOI	Government of India	
GDP	Gross Domestic Product	
HBNC	Home-based Neonatal Care	
HDI	Human Development Index	
HEW	Health Extension Worker	
HFM	Health & Family Welfare Minister	
HIV/AIDS	Human Immunodeficiency Virus/Acquired Immune Deficiency Syndrome	
HLEG	High Level Expert Group	
HLL	Hindustan Latex Limited	
HLFPPT	Hindustan Latex Family Planning Promotion Trust	
HMIS	Health Management Information System	
HRG	High Risk Group	
HSS	HIV Sentinel Surveillance	
IAP	Indian Academy of Pediatrics	
IBBA	Integrated Behavioural and Biological Assessment	

ICC	Indian Chamber of Commerce
ICDS	Integrated Child Development Scheme
ICMR	Indian Council for Medical Research
ICTC	Integrated Counselling and Testing Centre
IDU	Injecting Drug User
IEC	Information, Education and Communication
IHO	Indian Health Organisation
IIHMR	Indian Institute of Health Management Research
IIPS	Indian Institute of Population Sciences
IMNCI	Integrated Management of Neonatal and Childhood Illnesses
IMR	Infant Mortality Rate
IPR	Intellectual Property Rights
IPHS	Indian Public Health Standards
IMF	International Monetary Fund
IRMA	Institute of Rural Management Anand
ISO	International Organization for Standardization
JIPMER	Jawaharlal Institute of Postgraduate Medical Education and Research
JSA	Jan Swasthya Abhiyan
JSR	Jan Swasthya Rakshak
KHPT	Karnataka Health Promotion Trust
LAC	Link ART Centre
M&E	Monitoring & Evaluation
MCI	Medical Council of India
MDG	Millennium Development Goals
MFC	Medico Friend Circle
MIS	Monitoring Information System
MMR	Maternal Mortality Rate
MNP	Minimum Needs Programme
MNREGS	Mahatma Gandhi National Rural Employment Guarantee Scheme
MOHFW	Ministry of Health & Family Welfare
MPI	Multidimensional Poverty Index
MS	Mahila Samakhya
MSG	Mission Steering Group
MSJE	Ministry of Social Justice and Empowerment
MSM	Men Having Sex with Men

NABH	National Accreditation Board for Hospitals and Healthcare Providers
NABL	National Accreditation Board for Testing and Calibration Laboratories
NAC	National Advisory Council
NACO	National AIDS Control Organisation
NARI	National AIDS Research Institute
NBTC	National Blood Transfusion Council
NCB	Narcotics Control Board
NCHRH	National Commission for Human Resources for Health
NCMH	National Commission on Macroeconomics and Health
NCMP	National Common Minimum Programme
NEET	National Entrance Examination Test
NFHS	National Family Health Survey
NGO	Non-government Organization
NHM	National Health Mission
NHS	National Health Scheme
NHSRC	National Health Systems Resource Centre
NICD	National Institute of Communicable Diseases
NICED	National Institute of Communicable and Enteric Diseases
NIE	National Institute of Epidemiology
NIHFW	National Institute of Health and Family Welfare
NIMS	National Institute of Medical Statistics
NPCC	National Programme Coordination Committee
NRHM	National Rural Health Mission
NRL	National Reference Laboratory
NSEP	Needle Syringe Exchange Programme
NSSO	National Sample Survey Office
NTWG	National Technical Working Group
OI	Opportunistic Infections
OST	Oral Substitution Therapy
PAR	Participatory Appraisal Report
PCR	Polymerase Chain Reaction
PE	Peer Educator
PEPFAR	President's Emergency Plan for AIDS Relief

PD	Project Director
PFI	Population Foundation of India
P4P	Performance for Payments
PGI	Postgraduate Institute of Medical Education and Research
PHC	Primary Health Centre
PHFI	Public Health Foundation of India
PIL	Public Interest Litigation
PIP	Programme Implementation Plan
PLWHA	People Living with HIV/AIDS
PMK	Pattali Makkal Katchi
PMU	Project Management Unit
PPP	Public–Private Partnership
PPTCT	Prevention of Parent to Child Transmission
PRI	Panchayati Raj Institution
PSA	Participatory Site Assessment
PSH	Partners of Sexual Health
PSI	Population Services International
PVOH	Private Voluntary Organizations for Health
PWC	PricewaterhouseCoopers
RAS	Rajiv Aarogyasri Scheme
RCH	Reproductive and Child Health
RKS	Rogi Kalyan Samiti
RoP	Record of Proceedings
RRE	Red Ribbon Express
RSBY	Rashtriya Swasthya Bima Yojana
RTI	Right to Information
RTW	Right to Work
SACS	State AIDS Control Society
SAEP	School AIDS Education Programme
SDG	Sustainable Development Goals
SHIP	Sexual Health Intervention Project
SHSRC	State Health Systems Resource Centre
SIAAP	South India AIDS Action Programme
SIHFW	State Institute of Health & Family Welfare
SLP	State Level Partner
SMA	State Medical Association
SMO	Social Marketing Organization

SOP	Standard Operating Procedures	
SRL	State Reference Laboratory	
STD	Sexually Transmitted Disease	
STI	Sexually Transmitted Infection	
TANSACS	Tamil Nadu State AIDS Control Society	
TI	Targeted Intervention	
TRG	Technical Resource Group	
TISS	Tata Institute of Social Sciences	
TSG	Technical Support Group	
TSU	Technical Support Unit	
U5MR	Under-five Mortality Rate	
UC	Utilization Certificate	
UHC	Universal Health Coverage	
UNODC	United Nations Office on Drugs and Crime	
UHIS	Universal Health Insurance Scheme	
UHM	Urban Health Mission	
UPA	United Progressive Alliance	
UPSC	Union Public Service Commission	
USAID	United States Agency for International Development	
UNICEF	United Nations International Children's Emergency Fund	
VAMP	Veshya Anyay Mukti Parishad	
VCTC	Voluntary Counselling and Testing Centre	
VHAI	Voluntary Health Association of India	
VHG	Village Health Guide	
VHSC	Village Health Sanitation Committee	
VHSNC	Village Health Sanitation and Nutrition Committee	
VYAPAM/ MPPEB	Vyavsayik Pariksha Mandal/Madhya Pradesh Professional Examination Board	
WCD	Women & Child Development	
WHO	World Health Organization	

PART I
India's Health System: Challenges and Constraints

The notion of what defines a health system has been evolving over time and has been variously conceptualized and defined by different scholars. While in India we still tend to largely view and measure health systems in terms of inputs and ratio of doctors, nurses, or beds to population, most countries also view it in terms of the financial resources mobilized and allocated, the organization of service delivery, flow and utilization of funds, and risk-sharing among different stakeholders. In its *World Health Report* of 2000, the WHO[1] defined the purpose of a health system as one that must achieve improvement in the health of the population it serves, respond to people's expectations, and provide financial protection against the costs of ill health by measuring them through the functioning of certain actions and policies of the government, namely stewardship, resource creation, service provision, and financing.

Broadly agreeing with the aforementioned, William C. Hsiao and his colleagues[2] from the Harvard School of Public Health (HSPH) sought to expand the understanding of what a health system is all about. Conceptualizing the health system as 'a set of relationships in which the structural components (means) and their interactions are associated and connected to the goals the system desires to achieve (ends)', they argued that such an understanding helps comprehend why a 'particular system yields a given outcome, what features of that system contributed the most to producing the outcome, or how one could restructure the system to achieve a preferable outcome'.[3]

Elaborating further, they theorized the health system at two levels: macro and micro. The macro focuses on the 'total size, shape, and functioning of the "elephant", that is, the health sector', while the micro 'explores behaviour and dynamics of individual firms and households'.[4] They argued that the interaction between these two levels can be understood through an analysis of the relationships among 'at least a dozen markets [that] compose the health sector' and the five control knobs that together impact health outcomes on the aggregate as briefly summarized ahead.

a) Financing, which consists of at least four principal instruments: financing methods (tax-based social or private insurance; out-of-pocket expenses that then determine the amount of funds available for healthcare; who controls the resources; and who bears the financial burden), allocation of funds (service delivery, medical and nursing education, capital and revenue expenses determining access to health services, and impact on health status), rationing (by making care unaffordable or by having poorly skilled or insufficient number of providers impacting equity and risk protection), and institutional arrangements for financing (competition; centralized or decentralized; to be financed through taxes, user fees, or insurance—commercial or social). These institutional arrangements then determine the extent to which the system is equitable and fair and its ability to reduce the market distortions of moral hazard and adverse selection.

b) Organization of service delivery that has four characteristics:

　i) Public monopoly versus competition, where monopolies over time can work more to protect the interests of their employees than delivering welfare, or where competition can entail large transaction costs and require a set of skills and competencies that governments often lack.

　ii) Decentralization of health planning or service delivery, which is often considered a good option to ensure that benefits reach the intended. However, in the absence of adequate mechanisms to ensure priority focus on the lagging regions that may not have the same level of fiscal space as the better-off regions or have a higher burden of disease and people in need, decentralization can result in decreasing both equity and financial-risk protection. Besides, though 'theorists suggest that public power, responsibility, and accountability should be delegated to the lowest level, local governments often lack sufficient capacity and human resources to manage the public health services'.[5]

iii) Vertical integration, which implies integrating the three different levels of service delivery—primary, secondary, and tertiary care services—as a continuum with patient flows regulated through a system of referrals (as is the case in the UK). However, in some countries such as the USA or India, the health system is organized in a fragmented manner that makes it more costly and inefficient. For example, in the USA, due to the low attention paid to preventing disease and focusing more on treatment, about 5 per cent of the patients consumed almost 49 per cent[6] of the total health expenditures (2002) and that, too, with uncertain outcomes. Such a situation is avoidable if there is a strong primary care that focuses on prevention and if hospital treatment is based on a system of referrals since prevention is cheaper than treatment.

iv) Ownership: public, private for profit, and not-for-profit. Ownership patterns impact the kind of care provided, type of patients seen, nature of diseases treated, and the extent of denial of care on grounds of affordability in environments that do not have any forms of financial-risk protection.

c) A payment system constitutes the incentive system that 'act[s] like a gravitational force, pull[s] individuals and organizations in a certain direction without coercion'[7] where the mode (a fixed budget, fee-for-service reimbursement, or case-based payment) and amount of payment (fee-for-service, capitation, or salary) impact the behaviour of different actors—patients and providers (health professionals, pharmaceuticals, institutional providers)—and help determine the distribution of risk and apportionment of rewards, affecting the cost, efficiency, and quality of care provided. International evidence suggests that on account of market failures, such as asymmetry of information, the providers often assume monopolistic tendencies notwithstanding the model of competition that may be in place, making government intervention inevitable.

d) Regulations that are enforced by the government through legislative enactments or administrative orders and guidelines to impose certain boundaries within which the professions have to function or manufacture and sale of pharmaceutical products and medical devices have to be organized. These instruments are to ensure patient safety; enhance the health goals of equity, efficiency, and quality; and correct market distortions.

e) Persuasion, where governments and private companies can influence people's beliefs, lifestyles, expectations, preferences, and behaviours through the power of advertising, campaigns, and dissemination of information. Persuasion also affects the supply side, justifying governments to regulate and organize medical education as service providers profoundly impact the availability, efficiency, and quality of healthcare through the medical ethics and beliefs they uphold.

Overall, Hsiao and others assert that national health systems are a product of their own historical traditions; cultural, political, and social contexts; and value systems. Thus, for example, while the European systems are rooted in egalitarian traditions and social solidarity, the US system is based on libertarian traditions that have constrained the country from achieving an equitable and fair health system despite being able to afford one. Viewed from these lenses, India's health system seems to be a confused one—articulated on egalitarian ideals but practised along libertarian principles. Again in India, public debate on health issues is typically not contextualized and often displays tendencies towards borrowing other countries' (UK, USA, Thailand, or Mexico) experiences to model our own.

Notwithstanding the above, a health system, in the ultimate analysis, is determined by certain structural components that provide a set of trade-offs and options to achieve multiple objectives within fiscal constraints. In a developing low-resource country, such trade-offs could range between inter-sectoral—like the exclusive focus on promoting industrial growth and infrastructure or neglecting social investment required to promote human capabilities through focus on education and health—and intra-sectoral, like primary care or focusing more on hospital treatment. Public policy, then, is required to not view these choices, preferences, and trade-offs in binary terms but provide a balance between competing demands. Such a balance is essential as economic growth is critical to affording universal healthcare. Likewise, primary care and hospital treatment are but two wheels of the health system.

The preferred choices and policy options are thus determined by political compulsions and the value system of our leaders, calling for the need to analyse health policies not in an abstract way but in terms of political economy. Such as analysis provides the framework to understand the 'different forms of power and the networks through which they flow, including the production of knowledge and the creation of legitimacy. Political economy analysis can help with understanding and changing the structure and allocation of power, for instance, through assessments of governance, accountability, participation, and voice.'[8] This, then, widens the debate. Not achieving improved health is not a question of a lazy government or insensitive doctors but a reflection of the relational power balances between the political and economic forces at play, competing priorities, implementational capacities of public institutions, the extent and strength of the prevailing structural inequalities and the effectiveness of public policies in addressing them, and so on.

Based on the previously discussed understanding and fully aware of the complexities involved, Part I of the book seeks to provide a broad understanding of the contexts that determined the evolution of public policy on health and the health system as a consequence, followed by the two determining pillars of health systems—financing and governance. While under financing, predominantly more of public finance and the impact of payment systems have been covered, under governance, regulation and persuasion have been included as part of the challenges confronting India's health sector. It is argued that a low funding of 1 per cent of the GDP on health has adversely impacted India's ability to achieve its goals of improved health status, financial-risk protection and health security, equity, efficiency, quality, and public satisfaction. Combined with poor governance, India's health system dangerously seems to be in a laissez-faire position, where 'because of market failures, such as asymmetry of information and imperfect agency relationship, a monopolistic, high-cost, provider-driven health services market will emerge. It's imperative for policymakers to understand the consequences of their action and non-action.'[9] Such an understanding continues to elude Indian policymakers.

Notes and References

1. According to this report, a health system includes all the activities whose primary purpose is to promote, restore, or maintain health. In summary, health systems have a responsibility to not just improve people's health but also protect them against the financial cost of illness and treat them with dignity.
2. His other colleagues were professors Michael Reich, Marc Roberts, and Peter Berman—all from HSPH, Harvard.
3. William C. Hsiao, 'What Is a Health System? Why Should We Care', Working Paper Series (Boston: Department of Health Policy and Management, HSPH, 2003).
4. Hsiao, 'What Is a Health System?'.
5. Hsiao, 'What Is a Health System?'.
6. M.W. Stanton, 2006, 'The High Concentration of U.S. Health Care Expenditures', *Research in Action*, 19, available at http://archive.ahrq.gov/research/findings/factsheets/costs/expriach/index.html (accessed on 15 September 2016).
7. Hsiao, 'What Is a Health System?'.
8. 'Report from Bellagio: Advancing Political Economy of Global Health to Understand and Influence the Drivers of Universal Health Coverage', 2015, *Health Systems & Reform*, 1(1): 20–1, available at http://dx.doi.org/10.4161/23288604.2014.991221 (accessed on 15 September 2016).
9. Hsiao, 'What Is a Health System?'

CHAPTER ONE

Evolution of India's Health System

The Inheritance

India had a tradition of understanding health in a holistic manner. Its comprehension of disease and its causation is in many ways superior to the allopathic system of medicine where treatment is largely symptomatic. Such traditional systems continue to be valid in the face of huge competition from modern pharmaceutical companies. We still have bonesetters who can outclass trained orthopaedics in some procedures, while practitioners of traditional systems of medicine—yoga and Ayurveda—are known to cure or provide relief for many ailments. With the onset of modernism in the seventeenth and eighteenth centuries and our enthusiastic embrace of it, much of this traditional wisdom got swept away. The first to brush it aside were the Portuguese who introduced the modern (allopathic) medical system in India.

Years later the British imposed modern medicine upon a reluctant people who trusted the traditional practices followed by 'vaids', 'hakims', and specialists or midwives—healers who lived amidst them in villages and towns. In viewing traditional medicine as irrational and referring to its practitioners as 'quacks', the British sought to assert their 'superiority', influence, and dominance. They argued on the basis of empirical science and observed data.

Health was not a priority for the British, who by the mid-eighteenth century were ruling large swathes of India's territory. During the period from 1889 to 1894, they barely spent 0.15 per cent of their revenues on health compared to the 4 per cent spent on education.[1] Unacceptably high death rates of over 69 per 1,000 and the debilitating impact of malaria, cholera, typhoid, and venereal diseases on the troops did, however, stir them into intervening in the area of public health. They also established hospitals in military cantonments and large civil stations that were manned by qualified doctors and nurses as privileged 'enclaves' to exclusively serve their needs.

Between 1863 and 1869, sanitary commissioners were appointed in the three provinces of Madras, Bombay, and Calcutta to implement public health measures establishing the linkage between environmental sanitation and disease. Improvements in the quality of water, public sanitation, and better housing helped to reduce mortality among soldiers and brought down morbidity due to waterborne diseases like cholera and typhoid from 40 per 1,000 in 1879–80 to about 10 per 1,000 by 1890–1900, while inoculation against smallpox, introduced around that time, reduced mortality from 200,000 to 20,000.

Preventive health measures were accompanied by a spate of enactments: the 1889 Village Sanitation Act empowered villages to levy a tax to mobilize resources for sanitation works, the various Contagious Diseases Acts between 1864 and 1869 regulated prostitution for reducing the prevalence of venereal diseases among soldiers that was as high as 52.5 per 1,000, the Epidemics Control Act in 1897 was enacted to control plague, and so on. The vigorous implementation of these acts, most particularly the one related to plague that empowered sanitary officials to enter houses, detain, segregate, and quarantine those suspected of having the disease, burning down villages rendering over 100,000 people homeless in the process, created huge resentment among local populations since they feared separation from their families, compromising their ritual purity, and hurting their family pride. Local bodies refused to raise revenues through taxation for sanitation and sewerage disposal works and instead accorded a higher priority to the 'cosmetics' of road watering and street lighting. Enforced in the spirit of authoritarian utilitarianism,[2] people responded to these activities with hatred for a foreign power that they perceived to be intruding into their cultural spaces, private beliefs, and imposing social ostracism.

In 1914, the post of sanitary commissioner was merged with the post of director general (DG) of the Indian Medical Service, thereby reducing the importance of public health. In 1933, the MCI was established and in 1940, the post of DG medical services was renamed as DG health services and the post of public health commissioner abolished. These two institutions continue to exist unreformed even today.

In 1943, a committee under Joseph Bhore was constituted to examine the state of health in India and to submit a blueprint for action. In 1946, this committee submitted its three-volume *Health Survey and Development Report*. The Bhore Committee made certain important recommendations, based on principles that must guide a health system: being close to the people, provision of care regardless of the ability to pay, and the active promotion of positive health through community engagement and linking ill health to environmental hygiene. It envisioned an ambitious architecture consisting of one bed for every 550 people and one doctor for every 4,600 people to be provided in every district that was to be the unit of implementation.

The conference of provincial ministers held in October 1946[3] endorsed the major recommendations of the Bhore Committee but diluted the proposed coverage norms. Instead, it resolved to make plans for establishing a health centre for every 40,000 people, 30 beds for every five centres, 200 beds in every district, and unanimously resolved to recognize, integrate, and support traditional medical practice; provide safe water to 50 per cent of the population in the next 20 years and 100 per cent in 35 years; and ensure adequate sewerage in towns having a population of 50,000 within 10 years.

The conference also accepted the recommendation to merge the two departments of medical services and public health. This meant amalgamating medical treatment for acute care for sick patients along with public health that essentially deals with population or community health such as infectious diseases. Both Madras and Bombay presidencies dissented to this—Madras felt that the coordination between medical and public health was already good and, therefore, saw no reason for the merger. Tamil Nadu's (Madras) high performance across all public health indicators is largely attributed to this fortuitous decision.

The financial implications of the aforementioned decisions called for a fivefold increase in per capita outlays—from Rs 1.4 to Rs 5.9 with a recurring expenditure of Rs 2.8 per capita for the first five years. With the implementation of the resolutions being contingent on support from the central government, the conference ended with a resolution 'for each state to do what it can given its finances'.[4] In 1946, India was spending 4 per cent of its expenditure budget on health against 20 per cent by the UK and 13 per cent by the US. Resources were to be mobilized by loans and taxes. 'If the rate of expenditure now incurred by the provincial governments [is] taken as an appropriate guide ... to determine financial limits ... any attempt to build a satisfactory system of health services would be fore-doomed.'[5]

India inherited a substantial disease burden: a crude death rate of 22.4 per 1,000 with 50 per cent of these deaths among children under five, infant mortality of 165 per 1,000 live births, maternal mortality of 2,000 per 100,000 live births, and life expectancy among men being 26.9. There were few doctors (1 for 6,500), nurses (1 for 40,000), and midwives (1 for 60,000) and barely 0.24 beds for every 1,000 people against a requirement of 10.

Reducing the disease burden required strong implementation of public health measures. But before leaving India, the British abolished the public health infrastructure consisting of the Public Health Commissionerate and the Indian Medical Service that provided the cadre of trained doctors and the licentiates who numbered at 29,870 as compared to a mere 17,654 trained allopathic doctors.[6] Instead, what was left behind was a co-opted elite consisting of the Western-educated, upwardly mobile middle classes, which believed that traditional medicine was quackery and allopathy a symbol of modern scientific temper. India's health structure was thus built upon a system of medicine that was contrary to the present-day realities and the levels of development prevailing in the country at that time.

Clearly, the seeds for the conditions that exist today were sown then—a neglected and weak public health policy of a diffident state, dominance of a Western-oriented medical system, fiscal conservatism with low priority and funding for health, an asymmetry that made states fiscally dependent on the centre for discharging their constitutional obligations, a huge burden of infectious diseases, and an ideal of ensuring health for all that was soon forgotten.

However, to be fair, the prevailing circumstances were daunting. India had won its independence in 1947 at a price: it was badly wounded with the world's most massive human migration occurring on its western borders, a famine in its eastern states that cost three million lives, a hinterland steeped in acute poverty, illiteracy, and deprivation, and no resources available. It was a fledgling democracy struggling to give itself an identity and expression—an anthem, a flag, a constitution. The mood in India was one of cautious optimism and hesitation that sought to underplay the tensions and anxieties that were a consequence of the stitching up of a highly fragmented and diverse social polity. It was a mood very different to that of a confident imperial Britain that had won World War II through its military might and a sound system of governance, leadership, and innovation. Understanding this background is important for, in our discourse, we often tend to wonder why India failed when the UK succeeded in launching its National Health Scheme in 1947. The environment, challenges, and capabilities could not have been more dissimilar. Over the years, with meagre resources in hand, India sought to build the foundations of a health system.

Initial Years after Independence

Relegating health to the Directive Principles of the Constitution, the focus in the initial years was on growth. With the country juggling between the urgency to spur economic development, to ensure food self-sufficiency, and to protect the country's unity from internal and external dissensions, its health policy focused on the immediate challenges—reducing the toll of infectious diseases, particularly deaths and morbidity on account of malaria that affected over three-quarters of its population, and ensuring maternal and child health. The National Malaria Control Programme was launched in 1953 with the help of the Technical Cooperation Mission of the USA and technical advice of the World Health Organization (WHO). With support from UNICEF, the WHO, and the Rockefeller Foundation, the BCG vaccination programme was launched to tackle TB alongside the vaccination programme for eradicating smallpox—TB and smallpox together were the cause of many deaths and took epidemic proportions in the country.

India was helped with expertise from various international agencies to build capacity to cope with the situation. Over the years, such help resulted in a tendency towards adopting a techno-managerial approach to disease control rather than undertaking the more difficult but sustainable policy of tackling the causative factors and linking disease with the social conditions that produce it—an understanding that continues to elude us to this day. Besides, dependence on external help also meant a reduced ability to reflect on what is best for us in our context.

The more damaging impact of this early approach, however, was seen in the neglect in building the foundation of the health system in accordance with the recommendations of the Bhore Committee. A decade later, in 1961, barely 2,600 primary healthcare units were established with less than half the human resources as envisaged by Bhore.[7] Meagre resources were spent on constructing AIIMS and other hospitals in urban areas. But then, even this investment was essential since India had barely any human resources and a demand for medical services that could not be ignored. Yet the thinking that rural areas can do with a few public health and disease control interventions while urban areas would need medical care took root at this time, resulting in the fragmented approach to the building of the health system.

Around the mid-1970s, the efforts to contain the high burden of infectious diseases began to show results. By 1976, malaria was contained at two million cases, down from the 75 million in 1947, and smallpox was eradicated.

As India settled down, populations and incomes grew, and so did the demand for health services and people's expectations. Demand outpaced supply resulting in the establishment of public and private hospitals in cities with large towns bursting at the seams with patients. Many of the patients were from the rural hinterland where people had limited access to medical care. Quality fell. Instead of addressing this growing demand, public policy shifted its attention to population control through expanding access to contraceptives.

Thus, during these first three decades of India's planned development, the health system was being shaped by three broad approaches. First, there was the dominant policy focus on controlling infectious diseases and family planning. The programmatic needs of these priorities then influenced the organization of primary health. Second, the focus was on teaching hospitals to produce the required human resources. Third, due to limited resources and weak prioritization, investments required for building a sound foundation of primary care were patchy and grossly inadequate.

Rather than basing the development of the health system on principles or a vision, the tendency was to appoint expert committees with specialists and clinicians to deliberate upon issues that were largely of public health significance. These expert committees constituted from time to time, such as the Mudaliar Committee (1959), the Chadha Committee (1963), the Mukherjee Committee (1965), the Kartar Singh Committee (1972), the Shrivastava Committee (1975), and so on (about 25 committees over the last seven decades), provided patchy solutions—such as tinkering with the front-line workers and tackling one problem at a time rather than taking a holistic view of the system, making recommendations such as adopting a target approach to sterilizations or disbanding malaria workers and refashioning them as multipurpose workers—that created a new set of problems. It was around this time that nutrition, water, and sanitation were also separated from the health department with nutrition being attached to the Department of Women and Child Development and water and sanitation to the Department of Rural Development.

The inadequate attention accorded to the provisioning of medical treatment and hospital care led to the mushrooming of a range of stand-alone diagnostic clinics, nursing homes, and hospitals in the private sector, particularly in urban and semi-urban areas, catering to different socio-economic strata of society. In this din of swanky hospitals, modern technology, shifting aspirations backed by the willingness to pay, the concept of a family doctor and the neighbourhood clinic that Bhore had envisioned was lost.

Alma-Ata Declaration (1978)

The insensitive implementation of family planning during the Emergency in 1976 and the resultant loss of the Congress's political power in 1977, followed closely by the Alma-Ata Declaration in 1978 where all countries committed themselves to providing universal access to comprehensive primary care brought a shift in thinking. In the meanwhile, there was also a churning with the emergence of civil society as a stakeholder in India's health landscape. The Jamkhed experiment launched by Arole and other NGOs under the banner of the Voluntary Health Association provided an alternative narrative. Opposing the medicalized approach of government policy, they reiterated social medicine and community participation through community health workers (CHWs). All such developments and the recommendations of the Shrivastava Committee Report of 1975 resulted in the introduction of the village health worker (VHW) scheme. Under this scheme, every village was to have a VHW who was to provide healthcare services to the community for a small monthly honorarium of Rs 50 and a medical kit. However, this scheme floundered due to the lack of training, supervision, and logistic support.

In 1983, the first National Health Policy (NHP) was released. Critical of the curative-oriented Western model of healthcare, the NHP of 1983 emphasized the need for a preventive, promotive, and rehabilitative primary healthcare approach, based on the foundation of community participation. It also called for an integrated approach as opposed to the verticalization of disease control and advocated the participation of the private sector in providing medical services and reducing the burden on government finances. Notwithstanding this articulation, the NHP did not lead to any fundamental changes in the policy or architecture of the health system: the budgets for health continued to be low and the approach to adopting selective healthcare delivery remained the same.

At another level, tectonic shifts were taking place on the global stage. By late 1970s and early 1980s, socialism was beginning to lose its influence to market forces. The concept of a welfare state that had emerged at the end of World War II in post-war Britain was being replaced and redefined by the state as a facilitator and financier of private enterprise. Post-war prosperity gave rise to new thinking: solidarity gave way to individualism and state to markets. In the 1960s, economists in the US began to argue that health was as much a marketable commodity as any other, making way for markets in the health sector. Led by Ronald Reagan in the US and Margaret Thatcher in the UK, this ideological shift began to impact thinking in India. The implications of a deteriorating economic environment and the shift towards the liberalization of economy held implications for the health sector that few understood.

Impact of Economic Liberalization in the 1990s

The ideology of liberalism that India sought to embrace post-1991 had three characteristics that questioned the state's ability to provide an alternative mode of service delivery:[8] the marginalization of the state, according primacy to markets, and ceding space to NGOs. Liberalism helped spike growth rates but not without widening the gap between the rich and the poor. Absolute poverty did not decline. Nor did the deprivation that poverty brings, in terms of denial of access to basic necessities. Nehru's brand of socialism had indeed become passé.

Political ideologies impact the nature of the health system more significantly and profoundly than is normally acknowledged or understood. Under the 'socialist' phase, the government was the dominant player in setting and implementing the policy agenda. The government funded, owned, and provided healthcare services to the people as a part of its responsibility. Costs were low as generic drug production was encouraged, personnel were salaried, and there was no pressure to generate revenues. The private sector that existed alongside was invisible and fragmented, treating sickness on a fee-for-service basis. As per a study, in 1963–4 private sector accounted for 61 per cent of the doctors—of whom only 11.4 per cent were working in a private hospital establishment—21.5 per cent of beds, and 16 per cent of hospitals.[9] The liberalization process of the 1980s and 1990s[10] changed the paradigm and the fundamental premises: over the following decades service became a commodity, hospitals became lucrative commercial enterprises, medical education became investment destinations, and patients became clients.

The shift from the family doctor to a professionally managed health machine was inevitable. In the face of technological innovation in medical devices, discovery of new drugs, rapid changes in disease profile towards non-communicable diseases that required better diagnostic tools, more sophisticated laboratory facilities, and institutionalized treatment, healthcare became specialist-dependent, organizationally structured, and resource-intensive. Facing a high fiscal deficit, the government had no option but to rely on the market to bring in the required investment to establish hospitals that could meet the demands of a rapidly growing, aspirational middle class. By 1990, private players accounted for 58 per cent of hospitals and 29 per cent of beds.[11] With budgets less than Rs 20 billion (Rs 17.43 billion during 1990–1),[12] the government struggled to build the primary healthcare infrastructure in rural areas as the principal strategic tool to achieve the global goal of Health for All by 2000.

However, even for that modest goal budgets did not keep pace with the commitments made in the plan documents that continued to reflect the gap between ambition in the text and the actual amounts provided by the Planning Commission (now NITI Aayog). Health under the Minimum Needs Programme of the central government proved to be inadequate, forcing people to resort to quacks or private facilities in accordance with their ability to pay, thereby fostering the entrepreneurial spirit of the private sector. It was no accident that Apollo, the first corporate hospital in India, established in 1984, was greeted with curiosity and measured relief by the rising middle classes since it brought in a new definition of quality with its corporate management and modern diagnostics. From then on, the growth of the private sector has been unstoppable: starting with tertiary hospitals, it seamlessly expanded to secondary care, medical and nursing education, and diagnostic centres and laboratories. By 2004, the private sector accounted for three-quarters of outpatient treatment, 60 per cent of inpatients, and three-quarters of the specialists and technology.[13]

By the mid-1990s, the economic collapse, the International Monetary Fund's (IMF) conditionalities to cut back on public expenditures to contain the fiscal deficit, and the ideological thrust towards the private sector impelled the government to introduce a two-pronged approach: the first was a further reduction of what was an already low government budget, and the second was to promote the private sector through fiscal incentives. During the period from 1974–5 to 1990–91, government health spending on medical care and public health, as a proportion to the total government expenditure, declined in real terms from 3.2 per cent to 2.7 per cent. Worse, the reduced spending had a higher proportion of salaries that increased from 39.93 per cent to 58.97 per cent and a corresponding decline in capital expenditures from 4.37 per cent to 2.58 per cent. In terms of GDP, public spending increased from 0.98 per cent in 1975 to 1.36 per cent in 1986, only to fall to 1.28 per cent by 1991[14]—this contracted even further to 0.9 per cent by 2000, resulting in the marginalization of the state as the primary player in health service delivery.

Entering the New Millennium

The lack of resources during the 1990s resulted in India abandoning the vision of Health for All as agreed to at Alma-Ata in September 1978. In fact, the fiscal crisis and the need for foreign exchange made the health ministry turn to the World Bank for funds for its important though limited set of national programmes. In 1993, the World Bank entered the stage espousing three important principles of engagement in developing countries: a) the concept of an essential health service package as opposed to the grand vision of comprehensive primary care articulated at Alma-Ata, b) confining the role of government to implementing selective disease control programmes justified on the principles of Disability-Adjusted Life Years (DALYs—a concept no one understood), and c) allowing markets to provide hospital and medical care with government engagement on the basis of public–private partnerships (PPPs).

Hitherto, the World Bank had provided loans only for the family planning programmes. In 1993, India received its first World Bank loan for HIV/AIDS control that was followed by funding for other national disease control programmes: blindness, TB, malaria, and leprosy. It was the push of the health secretaries of the day (both R. Srinivasan and Rajiv Misra) that got the World Bank to reconsider its lending policy and consider inclusion of strengthening the public health infrastructure, providing scope for the much-needed capital investment for block-level and district-level hospitals. Accordingly, under the Health Sector Reform (HSR), several states availed loans. Like all bureaucracies, the World Bank, too, had problems of coordination where the HSR teams barely talked to the teams working on, say, the Reproductive and Child Health Programme. Thus, though such strengthening of infrastructure capacity was undertaken during the decade after 1995 in states like Andhra Pradesh, Karnataka, West Bengal, Uttar Pradesh, and Rajasthan, institutional deliveries and hospital care for the poor did not follow until much after 2005 when the National Rural Health Mission (NRHM) was launched.

The wide portfolio of lending helped the World Bank expand its influence on policy. However, this growth in the World Bank's presence in the Indian health sector was similar to its expanding global presence, though not necessarily with equity-enhancing outcomes. Commenting on the rise of the World Bank's presence in the global health sector, Evans stated that '[e]quity entailing universal access to basic care [has been] replaced by [the] so-called Health Sector Reform under pressure from World Bank and IMF. HSR was perceived by them as priority selling of privatization and decentralization.'[15]

The aforementioned observation was insightful since in India too, under the projects for public health programmes, the World Bank also pushed the private-sector agenda, introducing the concept of PPPs. Justified on the grounds of improving organizational efficiencies, the concepts of 'outsourcing' and contracting services such as sanitation, laundry, diet, and the delivery of allied services took root, gradually expanding to co-opt NGOs and private-sector care providers as partners. User fees, based on a large number of 'willingness-to-pay' studies, was promoted as a means of mobilizing resources for the cash-strapped hospitals struggling to meet their very modest recurring costs. This argument did not impress many who commented: 'User fees are a mere mirage, for no one who can afford anything uses a government hospital; bribes ("transaction costs" as the World Bank calls them) notwithstanding, they are the only source of surgical and even minimally advanced medical care for the poor.'[16]

Initially, PPPs implied engaging NGOs for implementing government schemes. The practice of engaging NGOs had started imperceptibly in the late 1980s with the innocuous private voluntary organizations (PVOs) for health grant from the United States Agency for International Development (USAID) that enabled partnering with NGOs for family-planning programmes. The entry of the World Bank resulted in a more aggressive promotion of all national programmes for control of diseases—TB, blindness, HIV/AIDS, leprosy, and so on. Under a PPP, the government would contract NGOs to implement the schemes for which it would remunerate them. The attempt to create a parallel system of delivery through NGOs became clear with the consistent and illogical refusal to support and recognize societies formed by self-help groups.[17] Instead, funding of NGOs under the World Bank projects entailed complicated and complex processes of tendering, contracting, and auditing—all in the name of transparency and reducing corruption. The processes were often far beyond the capacity of the local NGOs, creating space for the emergence of international NGOs and the culture of highly paid consultants.

The establishment of the Insurance Regulatory Development Authority (IRDA) in 2000 stimulated the insurance markets in India and facilitated the entry of private companies in a big way. The IRDA sought to expand insurance in the health sector as well, by attempting to engage the health ministry to define clinical standards and treatment protocols, electronic patient records, codification of disease groups, and so on. In 2003, the Department of Financial Services, Ministry of Finance, with scant consultation with the health ministry, launched the Universal Health Insurance Scheme with a premium of Re 1 per day. Those insured under this scheme were provided with health services in accredited hospitals for an assured sum. Implemented by the four public-sector insurance companies, this scheme was a non-starter with most field staff buying up the premium in order to meet the targets.

In 2002, India came up with the second NHP. Prepared in-house by the health ministry, it broadly reiterated the tenor and recommendations of the first NHP. It called for a combination of policies such as decentralizing the delivery of services and focusing on building the primary healthcare infrastructure so as to expand access to services and enhance equity. It advocated for public investment to be increased to 2 per cent of the GDP with the central share hiked from the current 17 per cent to 25 per cent and that of states to 8 per cent of their revenue expenditure. The policy also indicated a set of programmatic targets to be achieved by 2010. Its significance lay in providing the broad framework and foundation upon which the NCMH (National Commission on Macroeconomics and Health) report as well as the design and approach for the NRHM programme were built.

By 2004, it was clear that the World Bank–IMF inspired policy had failed. Free services to a select list of interventions was an inadequate response to the unfolding social crisis with people either denying themselves timely care or getting into intergenerational indebtedness due to their inability to pay. The NSSO's household survey (60th round)[18] showed that 20 per cent people did not seek treatment even when they needed to, on account of financial reasons. The World Bank studies estimated that 3–6 per cent of the population sold their assets or borrowed at high rates of interest to pay their medical bills and that 40 per cent of those hospitalized were indebted.[19] Analysing data for 1999, Charu Garg and Anup Karan[20] showed that 3.24 per cent of the population or 32.45 million people were being pushed below the poverty line every year because of medical expenses. Of this, five states—Uttar Pradesh (10 million), Bihar (4.6 million), Maharashtra (3 million), Madhya Pradesh (2.7 million), and West Bengal (2.4 million) together accounted for 22.7 million people and, more importantly, 90 per cent of them were from rural households. This corroborated the impression that several farmer suicides were among the elderly who were unable to meet the cost of medicines and treatment for their chronic diseases. An analysis of the borrowings by self-help groups showed that almost 25 per cent of their borrowings were for health.[21] It was clear that the strategy of starving the public health sector of funds resulted in the collapse of the slender social security nets the poor had, particularly in rural areas, forcing them to go to private clinics for every blood test or treatment of fevers. The government's initiative towards launching universal health insurance policies also backfired as the markets failed to fill the vacuum created by the breakdown of the public health delivery system.

Gearing up a Response: 2005

By 2005, India was a sick country with huge morbidity and mortality and a dysfunctional health system. States where the poorest lived were also the sickest. Thus, Uttar Pradesh with nearly a third of its population below the poverty line had over 440 maternal deaths per 100,000 live births, while the risk of maternal mortality was at 1.90 per cent as compared to 0.20 per cent in Kerala that had a maternal mortality rate (MMR) of 96 per 100,000 live births.

India was responsible for over a third of global mortality on account of infectious diseases, even as hard-to-treat communicable and expensive-to-manage non-communicable and chronic diseases were re-emerging. Shamed on the global stage for its failure to eradicate polio or staying in denial over what was being perceived internationally an explosive HIV/AIDS scenario with 5.2 million HIV-infected people and their numbers growing rapidly, India quickly retracted its steps and launched the NRHM in April 2005.

During the period 1990–2005, the influence of the World Bank, the WHO, and donor agencies on policy formulation was strong, though the share of their funding was less than 2 per cent of the total health spending.[22] Complex health problems were simplified into single-line technical solutions—DOTS for TB, immunization for infant mortality, early diagnosis and distribution of chloroquine tablets for malaria, and cataract surgeries for blindness. Such deductive approaches invited strong reactions from another section of the civil society, largely of leftist persuasion.[23] The Voluntary Health Association of India (VHAI) brought out the report of the Independent Commission on Health in India— the first comprehensive assessment of India's health system. Earlier the Indian Council of Social Science Research (ICSSR) and the Indian Council of Medical Research (ICMR) had also brought out the volume *People's Health in People's Hands* (1994) advocating the need to steer public policy back on track and away from the policies being advocated by the donors and the World Bank in the name of spending efficiencies. Both reports argued that health policies were resorting to technological solutions while ignoring the social dimensions of disease causation and neglecting the importance of social determinants. In 2000, 18 civil society networks coalesced into the Jan Swasthya Abhiyan (JSA) as a pressure group to bring reason back in public policy, that had reduced public health principles to technological fixes and privatization. The JSA later gained a significant presence under the UPA I and they were deeply involved during the initial years in designing the NRHM.

The NRHM, launched in April 2005, was a programme designed and crafted in-house without donor influence. It was based on the two broad principles of decentralization and community engagement through the CHW and other community-based initiatives. States were provided with flexibility in planning and prioritizing their investment decisions. The main objective of the NRHM was to revitalize the rural primary healthcare system (see Chapter 5). Yet it was only a partial response to the crisis.

In confining the NRHM's focus to revitalizing primary care consisting of a few essential services, the issues related to addressing rural impoverishment on account of medical expenses were left unaddressed. Though one of the objectives of the NRHM was to address the issue of financial-risk protection, the health ministry, instead of seizing the opportunity, deflected this task to the Department of Financial Services that handled insurance. Attention now shifted to using insurance as a means of providing financial-risk protection against medical expenses to the poor and those working in the unorganized sector.

In a scenario where people were unable to afford high medical expenses while the hospitals had unfilled beds and unutilized technology,[24] Karnataka launched the Yeshasvini Health Insurance Scheme for farmers in 2005. Yeshasvini was an innovation pioneered by Devi Shetty and A. Ramaswamy who was the then secretary of the state's Department of Cooperatives. Under this scheme, a trust was constituted wherein farmers' contributions were deducted from their share capital. More than 200 hospitals were empanelled to provide over 900 surgeries at fixed rates that were arrived at through a process of negotiation. This model triggered interest in other states.

Building on the Yeshasvini experience, Andhra Pradesh brought further innovation in 2007 under the Rajiv Aarogyasri, which also provided cashless treatment for high-end surgeries with an assured sum of Rs 0.2 million per family and covered 85 per cent of the population under a more liberally constructed definition of the poverty line. The premium was paid by the state government on behalf of the beneficiaries to the government-owned trust with the scheme being administered in the initial years by a private insurance company. This was the beginning of the trend for government-sponsored insurance schemes where the state bore all the risk and under the guise of PPP, public resources were used to strengthen the private sector.

With this model of provisioning and financing of healthcare being opposed by the civil society that was actively engaged with the health ministry, the International Labour Organization (ILO) and the World Bank shifted their gaze to the Ministry of Labour. Since some time, the ILO had been advocating that countries enhance social security for their labour working in the informal sector.

More than 93 per cent of India's workers were engaged in the unorganized sector. Thus, under Schedule I of the Unorganised Workers' Social Security Act (2008) of the Ministry of Labour, the Rashtriya Swasthya Bima Yojana (RSBY)[25] was launched in early 2008, with the aim of extending access to quality care and reducing out-of-pocket and catastrophic health expenditures being incurred by families below the poverty line and other vulnerable groups. It was a modest health insurance scheme aimed at covering 70 million families below the poverty line by the end of 2012. This represented those in occupations ranging from construction, mining, railways, to street vendors, ragpickers, domestic workers, taxi drivers, and so on. Under this scheme, every target family was eligible for an assured sum of Rs 30,000 on a floater basis to access services in accredited hospitals. By the end of 2012, 13 states had brought in variations of such tax-funded insurance schemes providing cashless treatment to their citizens, predominantly for surgeries in 'empanelled' hospitals.

These developments entailed profound changes. Fragmented as they may seem, they contributed to the further strengthening of the private sector that was also in a crisis of sorts for want of an effective market and the slow growth of voluntary, commercial insurance. Thus, during the years 2007–14, India witnessed the strange playing out of a zero-sum game. On the one hand, the government, by deliberate policy, injected into the private sector over Rs 200 billion per year (public as well as private out-of-pocket expenditure that was tax-exempted) as premium for health insurance, thus helping it expand and consolidate its market presence in the secondary and tertiary care markets; on the other hand, it invested an equal amount of money under the NRHM for strengthening the public sector delivery system, largely in the primary healthcare segment. Such a dual policy further widened disparities between the public and private sectors while leaving unaddressed the problems of the two lowest income quintiles that desperately needed good-quality, comprehensive primary care services and not just risk protection for surgeries and hospitalization. This issue became more nuanced because the NRHM rapidly sank to promoting institutional deliveries as a proxy for primary care.

Strengthening primary care through such initiatives with limited secondary care in the public sector, while at the same time strengthening the private sector in secondary and tertiary care markets through insurance, reflected the government's confused and ambivalent thinking. While states initiated the RSBY and the tax-based tertiary insurance schemes in active collaboration with the private sector, they did not strengthen primary healthcare, promote prevention, and establish a referral system. Nor was there adequate investment in expanding the services and quality of public sector hospitals to enlarge access to affordable or free care. In other words, the government was not taking advantage of the supply-side finance. Treating insurance only as a demand-side intervention for empowering patients to make choices in accessing care gave rise to spending distortions. Money was available to conduct a heart surgery, a cochlear implant, or a C-section but not for essential medicines and basic diagnostics, preventive education, rehabilitative care, home nursing for the elderly, school health and adolescent care, or for addressing the direct causal factors of communicable and non-communicable diseases, or treatment of injuries, fevers, snake bites—conditions that were critically important for the poor.

The midterm review of the NRHM in 2010 clearly highlighted the achievements and gaps that had yet to be addressed. It argued that architectural corrections required time and money. The states, particularly the laggard ones, were not only increasing their absorption capacity by incurring higher spending of the resources assigned to them by the central government but also increased their own allocations. All evidence favoured a sharpening of focus and staying the course on the NRHM and expanding the scheme to the urban areas. But the Planning Commission had other ideas. By abandoning the NRHM, in a manner of speaking, it adopted the rhetoric of universal health coverage (UHC) to justify a further jettisoning of the public sector and speeding up the co-option of the private sector along the lines under implementation in Andhra Pradesh. The failure of the Planning Commission in pushing through its agenda exposed the fissures within the ruling party—one group wanting to co-opt the private sector, while another wanting to focus on strengthening the public sector to be the principle provider of essential care.[26]

The Twelfth Plan (2012–17)

Though civil society had been advocating UHC for over two decades, this issue gained traction and entered India's policy dialogue only through the Public Health Foundation of India (PHFI), an initiative of the McKinsey consulting company.[27] The PHFI,[28] a partnership between the government and the private sector, was established in 2006 to set up four to six public health schools and train about 10,000 public health professionals—a gap that the government could not fill owing to the lack of resources and inflexible processes related to the recruitment of human resources. Over time, the PHFI emerged more as a think tank and became a one-stop solution for all donor- and foreign-funded research, including the multinational pharmaceutical companies in the country.

Contracted to come up with a plan to advocate UHC, the PHFI was provided with handsome grants from the Rockefeller Foundation and had the political backing of the deputy chairperson of the Planning Commission. A High Level Expert Group (HLEG) was constituted. UHC, as defined by this group, was—to put it simply—all care (preventive, promotive, and curative) to all citizens on a cashless basis to be financed fully by taxes.[29] With a near absence of any analysis of the fiscal implications of this recommendation and the declining economic growth at 4.6 per cent in 2012 making prioritization inevitable, there was apprehension that rather than fulfilling its ethical obligation of addressing the basic needs of all citizens, the government may divert the already scanty resources and attention in favour of expensive diagnostic-based hospital treatment that had the backing of the corporate sector. At the heart of the issue was the large majority of Indians who still lacked access to safe water (44 per cent of the population has access to tap water and 47 per cent to toilets),[30] sanitation, nutrition, and were dying due to lack of access to cheap medicine for treatable conditions—TB, malaria, kala-azar (black fever), diarrhoea, respiratory infections—and to maternal and child care; this is in addition to morbidities and mortality due to non-communicable diseases that were by and large preventable in primary-care settings.

Despite the publicity advocating the aspirational goal of UHC, the health ministry was unimpressed and instead demanded that the Planning Commission fulfil the simpler assurances of providing universal access to free reproductive and child health services and treatment against minor ailments and infectious diseases. This objection was timely as fiscal pressures have entailed sharp reductions in the budgetary allocations for the NRHM, renamed as the National Health Mission. During the first two years of the Twelfth Five Year Plan a mere amount of Rs 349.78 billion was released for the NRHM against the total commitment of Rs 1.9 trillion for five years.[31]

In 2005, the Fourteenth Finance Commission submitted its report, adding a new twist to this already unhappy tale. As per the Constitution, it is the responsibility of the states to deliver health services. But they have not been able to do so for want of resources. To help states overcome their fiscal incapacities, the central government provides financial resources under programmes called Centrally Sponsored Schemes (CSS) that have often been resisted by states as an 'encroachment' on their turf. To correct this vertical asymmetry, the Fourteenth Finance Commission increased the proportional share of the states under unconditional grants from 32 per cent to 42 per cent of the total amounts devolved to the states, thereby reducing the central government's space for making discretionary grants under the CSS mechanism.[32] While the rationale for this strategic shift was to provide states with more fiscal space and flexibility to set their own priorities and spending preferences, the central government reacted by slashing budgets for several social-sector schemes that impact health—primary education, water supply, nutrition—and reduced the proportion of central share from 75 per cent to 60 per cent, burdening the states further. Though maintaining status quo in health, it slashed by 30 per cent the budget for HIV/AIDS and reduced the allocations for the NRHM in real and absolute terms—programmes that deal with the most marginalized sections of Indian society. Not unexpectedly, there is widespread concern about what the future holds.

Such concern is understandable. Governments have consistently accorded a low priority to health. Whether the growth rate is 3 per cent or 9 per cent,[33] negligible attention has been paid to those elements that constitute the basic building blocks of human development. Seventy years after Independence, India continues to have high levels of childhood mortality on account of contaminated water and poor sanitation—350 times more than the US and 7 times more than China—while we still chase the desired growth rate of 10 per cent that continues to elude us.

India's health system defies a uniform definition and is the outcome of strategies that seem to be working at cross purposes: a partially functioning primary care system, heavily overstretched public hospitals competing in the same space with well-funded private hospitals, varied insurance schemes with no single coordinating authority, and a remarkable absence of a sound regulatory environment to control the wild growth of the private sector. In addition, there is rampant corruption and low capacity to supervise, measure, and monitor health gains.

Profiteering from Healthcare?

The burgeoning private sector estimated at USD 230 billion (or Rs 15 trillion by 2020 and growing at 15 per cent per year) dominates every aspect of health policy formulation and implementation. Promoters of the corporate sector mobilize resources by sale of their own assets or borrowings from financial institutions such as banks, equity firms, venture capitalists, and share markets. In their pursuit of profits, they exploit the vulnerability of patients and auction medical seats to the highest bidders. It is this increasing trend towards the 'financialization'[34] of the health sector that is disturbing. The commitment, then, is not to the health outcomes of patients but to declaring dividends and safeguarding shareholders' interests.

The world over, a growing body of opinion considers such profiteering from the sick as unethical. In countries such as Germany, systems to insulate the doctor–patient relationship from being influenced by financial considerations were furthered 'by the political culture that emphasized the moral importance' of this issue. Even in the US, doctors initially resented the insurance companies who factored monetary considerations in clinical judgements.[35] This body of opinion, based largely on the European school of thought as well that of the UK and Canada, saw the commercialization of healthcare as a degradation of a humane service and was seen as unacceptable and a violation of the spirit of solidarity that must be the core governing principle of any civilized government. Such views advocate health to be a human right that governments must be obliged to provide free of cost, laying down the philosophical underpinning of the global movement for UHC.[36]

In India's health history, the emergence of privatization of the health sector appears to have been accepted without much contest. Unlike in the UK where the medical community, including the British Medical Association (BMA) and the general population, protested[37] against the ingenious manner in which Tony Blair sought to privatize the National Health Scheme (NHS), there have been no such protests in India.[38] There was no explicit outrage when medical education was being privatized in India, except for one incident in 1984 in Mumbai. In 1983, junior doctors in Maharashtra protested against the government proposal to permit private medical colleges to charge capitation fees on grounds that it favoured the rich and was unfair. 'The strike brought the healthcare system to a crawl and drew huge public support. Political leaders, student organisations, prominent citizens, trade unions, and senior doctors—including those from the IMA [Indian Medical Association]—marched in solidarity on the streets of Mumbai. When the government agreed to reassess the proposal we ended our strike.'[39]

In 2000 or so, the JSA—an NGO propagating health as a human right—issued a pamphlet on the growing commercialization of the health sector. Even as late as in 2016 when the circular of the MCI, issued in February, permitted promoters to take 300-bed district hospitals on a long-term lease of 33 or 99 years for establishing medical colleges, there has been only a deafening silence from the academics, civil society, or bureaucracy. The circular has serious implications since as a consequence, the trend that started in 2006 with the leasing out of the Bhuj district hospital to the Adani group in Gujarat will undoubtedly grow further. The latest example is the Chittoor district hospital in Andhra Pradesh being handed over to the Apollo group—initially on a five-year lease that was later extended to 33 years. The fiscal implications can be substantial in the absence of a policy for making commensurate investments to strengthen the hospitals below the district level for providing secondary care and instead handing over public hospitals to private corporates for providing tertiary care. Besides, in the short term it also implies denial of free care to the poor, largely due to the government's inability to enforce the conditions.

The 'non-visibility' of the alternative narrative of civil society seems to be largely due to the initial 'adversarial' positions it adopted against the government by refusing to engage with it and, thereby, reserving the right to critique its policies. The first time that civil society was actively engaged by the central government and provided a leadership role was in family planning programmes. Another instance of the central government's engagement with civil society was in late 1999—with a small WHO grant—under the programme to promote women's health that was to go beyond reproductive and child health, covering issues like self-worth, nutrition, exercise, HIV/AIDS, herbal medicine, and so on.⁴⁰ Civil society organizations were asked to develop learning materials, train facilitators, and prepare modules that were then vetted by the technical arm of the ministry.⁴¹ Subsequently, such interactions strengthened and matured under the NRHM. The Medico Friend Circle and others have provided a platform, yet dialogue and interaction continue to be weak and fragmented.

There can only be two plausible explanations for such a situation: firstly, socialist India never ever provided the resources for building a humane and caring health system in the way the war-torn UK did and India has no alternative models to compare with. The Left-ruled states, namely West Bengal and Kerala, failed to establish models demonstrating the benefits of public provisioning. In 2012, 53.8 per cent of women in West Bengal delivered babies in public hospitals, 19.8 per cent women in private hospitals, and 24.1 per cent delivered at home.⁴² Likewise, in both the states only a third of the primary health centres (PHCs) provided 24×7 services and an average of 20 per cent community health centres (CHCs) had the services of specialists. What is more worrying is the near-stagnant public health spending in Kerala. In 2011–12, Kerala's per capita public expenditure in real prices was Rs 282 as compared to Rs 287 in 2004–5, with nearly 50 to 70 per cent of it going into primary care, leaving the high-cost secondary and tertiary care to be purchased by individuals from the private sector. Given its high burden of non-communicable diseases, such spending explains why Kerala has high out-of-pocket expenditures, a situation that is addressed by providing Rs 100,000 over and above what is provided under the RSBY.

Secondly, the public and private sectors have coexisted in a seamless manner from the village quack to government doctors who run private nursing homes or pursue private practice in private hospitals. In other words, there was no professional organization that objected to, or resisted, the government's flirtations with the private sector. Perhaps the administrative and technical bureaucracies at the central and state levels could have provided evidence-based advice and focused more on analysing data, assessing implications, and providing options with the risks and benefits clearly laid out for enabling an informed decision.

Academic institutions, too, were not funded or incentivized to undertake high-quality operational research providing credible data on the nature and character of the private sector, comparing it to the public sector in terms of outcomes or unnecessary or exploitative behaviour to guide policy. Such research would have undoubtedly disabused the notion paramount among key policymakers that PPPs will 'help in cost reduction, improving efficiency, filling in the gaps, participatory planning, sharing of resources, quality assurance, ambulatory care, and in bringing about equity'.[43] Good research does prevent public policy from causing unintended harm.

Too overwhelmed with the urgency of implementing disease control programmes, the bureaucracies at the national and state levels failed to build the institutional capacities required to cope with the distortions that health markets entail. Asymmetrical information endows providers with power and authority over the patients who have incomplete information about what ails them. Providers often take advantage of such moments of vulnerability by ordering a battery of tests, unnecessary surgeries, or prescribing high-cost medicines, thus contributing to price inflation. What is, therefore, required are a set of strong regulations to reduce discretion in fixing prices, treatment protocols, computerization of medical records and monitoring for deviations, supervising for quality through patient-satisfaction surveys, and instituting grievance redressal mechanisms and a revamp of the existing systems of judicial redressal to make them less cumbersome and more accountable.

The current reality shows low public spending and 70 per cent of technology imported with no laws to regulate their location, utilization, or maintenance. In fact there are no regulations, accountability, and transparency regarding the functioning of private hospitals and diagnostic centres per se, though they provide a major share of care. Apart from illiteracy and absence of grievance redressal systems, information campaigns on unhealthy habits or behaviour have been severely compromised for want of funding and attention. India's strength was and continues to be, in part, its human resources—the country produces some of the finest doctors and nurses and has excellent training capabilities and systems. But this strength, too, is now witnessing a serious dent on account of multiple factors such as inadequate teachers, low salaries, more attractive alternative professions, the brazen commodification of medical and nursing education, and the migration of well-trained medical and non-medical professionals to foreign shores.

Narrow Options

The biggest challenge India faces today is solving this riddle called public–private mix in health care. The public–private mix model calls for restructuring the health system on five pillars:[44] first, of strong governance that clearly lays down regulatory frameworks for the assignment of roles between public–private/centre–state to avoid duplication and inefficiencies, minimize market failures, and protect the poor and vulnerable from the abuse of power. Second, financial systems that incentivize efficiencies in resource use and minimize wastage. The third is payment systems that regulate the behaviour of providers towards enhancing well-being rather than profiteering from sickness. Human resources in sufficient quantity, equal availability, and relevant to the needs of the times form the fourth pillar and the fifth pillar is transparency and information dissemination to empower individuals towards good health and technology that can save lives without impoverishing them in the process.

In short, a public–private partnership approach to health would require reworking these five pillars within an accountability framework, laying down clear functional boundaries between the centre and state, between public and private engagement, and public and private goods. Under the new thrust towards cooperative federalism, boundaries will need to be redrawn but in a manner that does not result in the centre abdicating its responsibility, but instead taking a higher responsibility in ensuring the achievement of national goals. In fact, under cooperative federalism the onus is more on the centre to ensure that a measure of equalization is brought in through resource transfers to those states that have the disease burden but not the fiscal capacity to address them.

States would need to show a vision and display a greater sense of innovation and renewed energy to rebuild the battered and broken public health system, revamping it in accordance with peoples' needs and the current epidemiological status, using the power of technology to overcome barriers. The centre and states have to work together to focus single-mindedly upon universalizing access to public goods and comprehensive primary care, abandoning the patchy approach consisting of a few essential services, and evaluating the impact of public policy on the poorest and most deprived. These ideas have been elaborated in Chapter 6.

The challenge will be to steer institutional reforms towards injecting new capabilities and competencies. While carefully sequencing strategies, there is a need to think diagonally[45] across horizontal and vertical spaces, prioritizing the immediate from the important. What is required in order to allow a plurality of views to be heard is to institutionalize systems that are consultative, open, and discursive, while the need of the hour is to establish regulatory systems and strong governance.

Making Healthcare a Human Right

Health is not a human right. The government has no legally enforceable accountability to its citizens to ensure access to, or denial of, health services. Taking the cue from the rights-based approach of the UPA II that had enacted laws making primary education and 100-days' employment a fundamental right, social activists keenly advocated making healthcare a justiciable right. This did not get any traction on account of the complexities and costs involved. At the policy level, there was always the apprehension that enacting a law making health a right in the absence of adequate funds and a fragmented, dysfunctional health system would only generate substantial litigation that the government would not be able to cope with.

Overcoming these obstacles, then, would undoubtedly require a strong leadership. What India has are formal structures of authority. Martin Linsky[46] argues that there is a distinction between leadership and authority, as there is between want and need. Most political leaders and senior managements stay within the scope of authority that is defined by law, accepted by the system of superiors and subordinates, and focuses on addressing wants. But leadership, Linsky argues, is all about taking risks to innovate, exceeding the scope by 'dancing on the edge of scope of authority', relentlessly pushing the envelope for change, not getting deterred by resistance, and moving beyond the status quo to address needs.

The Indian health sector can get out of its present quagmire only when we begin to accord equal value to all lives—irrespective of social or economic status and sexual orientation—and when the mindset of our policymakers shifts to defining development not in terms of GDP but as per the value scale of every citizen having equal opportunity to live life to the optimum. It is imperative that morality determines politics and economics. In the absence of that, the health sector will continue to suffer under a system that does not hold itself accountable to the people it is expected to serve. For more than the bricks and mortar, at the core of the health system are the values that drive it.

Notes and References

1. Mark Harrison, *Public Health in British India: Anglo-Indian Preventive Medicine, 1859–1914* (Cambridge: Cambridge University Press, 1994).
2. 'Those who know anything of the program of sanitary reform in England are aware that sanitation was to a great extent forced on the people … democratic governments have not waited until the people have risen en masse and howled for reform' (H.A.D. Phillips quoted in Harrison, *Public Health in British India*).
3. Minutes of the meeting available with the National Archives of India, New Delhi.
4. This attitude seems to find resonance today with the 2015 budget slashing central assistance to states in many social sectors.
5. *Indian Medical Journal* on Bhore Committee, March 1946, available at the National Archives of India, New Delhi.
6. As per the report of the Bhore Committee, 1946. The estimate is for 1941–2.
7. Mudaliar Committee Report, 1961, GOI.
8. For a more incisive discussion, see Aradhana Sharma, 2006, 'Crossbreeding Institutions, Breeding Struggle: Women's Employment, Neoliberal Governmentality, and State (Re)Formation in India', Division II Faculty Publications, Paper 40, available at http://wesscholar.wesleyan.edu/div2facpubs/40 (accessed in June 2016).
9. Sunil Nandraj, 1994, 'Beyond the Law and the Lord: Quality of Private Health Care', *Economic & Political Weekly*, 29(27): 1680–5. The Mudaliar Committee estimated the existence of 12,000 hospitals, 185,000 beds, and 88,000 doctors in 1960.

10. Many call this shift as neo-liberalism, a term I hesitate to use, since neo-liberalism is defined as an approach to economics and social studies in which control of economic factors is shifted from the public sector to the private sector. Drawing upon principles of neoclassical economics, neoliberalism suggests that governments reduce deficit spending, limit subsidies, reform tax law to broaden the tax base, remove fixed exchange rates, open up markets to trade by limiting protectionism, privatize state-run businesses, allow private property and back deregulation. (Definition from http://www.investopedia.com/terms/n/neoliberalism.asp.) We are trending towards that but still not quite there.
11. Sunil Nandraj, 2012, 'Unregulated and Unaccountable: Private Health Providers', *Economic & Political Weekly*, 42(4): 12–17.
12. Planning Commission, Sixth Plan (1980–5).
13. As per the Commission for Macroeconomics and Health, 2005.
14. K.N. Reddy and V. Selvaraju, *Health Care Expenditures by Government in India: 1974–5 to 1990–1* (New Delhi: NIPFP, 1994).
15. Evans et al., *Challenging Inequities in Health*.
16. Thomas George, 1994, 'Distorted Perspective on Health Care', *Economic & Political Weekly*, 29(30).
17. It was around this time that the Indian government sought to alleviate poverty though community-based self-help groups that were essentially aimed at saving and taking bank loans for economic activities. In Andhra Pradesh, self-help groups evolved from the anti-alcohol movement into vibrant conduits to self-empowerment and were an excellent means of advancing social agendas to the community such as educating every girl child, promoting savings, afforestation, and so on. Though self-help groups were constituted under the Societies Registration Act (1860), the World Bank never agreed to use them for the delivery of health services. It was much later that the World Bank gave the government of Andhra Pradesh loans to 'strengthen' (or weaken?) the movement.
18. The NSSO undertook this survey during January–June 2004.
19. David Peters, A. Yazbeck, R. Sharma et al., *Better Health Systems for India's Poor: Findings, Analysis, and Options* (Washington, DC: World Bank, 2002).
20. Charu C. Garg and Anup K. Karan, 'Catastrophic and Poverty Impact of Out-of-Pocket Payment for Health Care in India: A State-Level Analysis', Working Paper No. 23 (Institute for Human Development, 2004).
21. The Velugu Project, Government of Andhra Pradesh, interview with senior officials in 2013.

22. As per the National Health Accounts, 2004–5, Ministry of Health, GOI.
23. Imrana Qadeer, 'Universal Healthcare and Social Responsibility of the Private Sector', in *India Infrastructure Report, 2013–14* (Telangana: Orient Blackswan, 2010).
24. As Devi Shetty said at that time: 'I have the technology to save lives, but people are unable to pay even the minimum amounts to cover base costs.' He had offered to do a heart bypass at half the cost incurred in other private hospitals.
25. The RSBY provided an assured sum of Rs 30,000 for a family of five. The premium was shared by the central and state governments on a 75:25 ratio. The implementation was carried out by private insurance companies.
26. See Chapter 5 of this book for a more detailed analysis of this issue.
27. Barry Bloom, the then director of the HSPH, broached the idea of this initiative to Rajat Gupta, the then head of McKinsey.
28. Chaired by a corporate honcho, the PHFI was set up with a corpus of Rs 0.65 billion from the Indian government, Rs 0.65 billion from the Bill & Melinda Gates Foundation (BMGF), and about Rs 0.4 billion of contribution promised by other corporate leaders.
29. The HLEG report (2011) submitted to the Planning Commission of India thus defined UHC:
    Ensuring equitable access for all Indian citizens, resident in any part of the country, regardless of income level, social status, gender, caste or religion, to affordable, accountable, appropriate health services of assured quality (promotive, preventive, curative and rehabilitative) as well as public health services addressing the wider determinants of health delivered to individuals and populations, with the government being the guarantor and enabler, although not necessarily the only provider, of health and related services.
30. For example, as per the 2011 census 3 per cent and 18 per cent of the rural Bihar has access to tap water and sanitation respectively.
31. As per the data released by the NRHM Division, Ministry of Health, GOI, October 2015.
32. See Chapter 2 for a detailed explanation on this.
33. In the first few decades after Independence, India's growth rate hovered around 2–3 per cent. In 2009–10, it touched a high of 10.3 per cent only to slip to 5.1 per cent by 2012 (World Bank). In 2015, the growth rate was estimated to be around 7 per cent and the growth rate indicated for 2016 is around 7.6 per cent.
34. Financialization is the process by which financial institutions, markets, etc., increase in size and influence. (Definition from http://

www.oxforddictionaries.com/definition/english/financialization, accessed on 21 November 2015.)
35. See Paul Starr, *The Social Transformation of American Medicine* (New York: Basic Books, 1982).
36. It implies a comprehensive access to all services—preventive and curative.
37. Thousands of people marched in protest against the plan to reform the NHS and the BMA frontally attacked government policies to privatize through media, public speeches, and so on. See John Lister, *The NHS after 60: For Patients or Profits?* (London: Middlesex University Press, 2008).
38. Julian Tudor Hart, *The Political Economy of Health Care: A Clinical Perspective* (Bristol: Policy Press, University of Bristol, 2010); Colin Leys and Stewart Player, *The Plot against the NHS* (London: Merlin Press, 2011).
39. Sanjay Nagral, 2016, 'Symptoms Documented, But What about the Disease?: Medical Council of India under Parliament Scrutiny', *Economic & Political Weekly*, 51(14).
40. This information was gathered through a personal discussion with Thelma Narayan of SOCHARA, Bangalore, 2016.
41. Kameshwari Jandhyala, 2001, 'Women's Health Training Programme: An Assessment of the Programme in Karnataka' (unpublished).
42. As per the District Level Household Survey IV, Indian Institute of Population Sciences (IIPS), Mumbai, GOI.
43. Qadeer, 'Universal Healthcare and Social Responsibility'.
44. Harvard University defines health systems as consisting of five pillars: financing, payment systems, organization, regulations, and persuasion.
45. Julio Frenk, Octavio Gómez-Dantés, and Felicia M. Knaul argue that health policymaking cannot be linear. It needs to look diagonally at other sectors that cause disease and impact health outcomes. Julio Frenk, Octavio Gómez-Dantés, and Felicia M. Knaul, 'The Health Systems Agenda: Prospects for the Diagonal Approach', in Garrett W. Brown, Gavin Yamey, and Sarah Wamala (eds), *The Handbook of Global Health Policy* (Chichester: Wiley-Blackwell, 2014).
46. Professor Martin Linsky, Harvard University, class notes, 2013.

CHAPTER TWO

Health Financing

*D*espite India graduating to a lower-middle-income country and accounting for one-fifth of the global disease burden, its public spending on health continues to hover around 1 per cent of its GDP. Low public spending has resulted in lowered risk protection with households bearing the brunt of medical expenses. The high cost of healthcare has resulted in an estimated 32 million people being pushed into poverty. Of them 22 million are the rural poor.[1] Worse, a fifth of the ill in both rural and urban areas deny themselves treatment.[2] A more recent estimate suggests that every year 3.5 per cent of India's population becomes impoverished and 5 per cent faces catastrophic expenditures due to medical bills. Formal insurance schemes are meagre, accounting for not more than 7.6 per cent of the current health expenditures. India is, therefore, a nation struggling to meet its two objectives—improving the health status of its people and reducing impoverishment of households due to the high cost of healthcare.

Health financing in India is largely private. Public spending accounts for only 28.6 per cent of the total health expenditures (states and central government combined [NHA 2013–14]). Households incur about 67.74 per cent (including premium for health insurance), which translates to about 5.73 per cent of household incomes.[3] Since medicines, diagnostics, and ambulatory care are estimated to constitute 70 per cent of this payment, it is estimated that if all outpatient treatment could be provided for free, then only 0.5 per cent people will sink into poverty due to health expenditures.[4]

Inpatient treatment and hospitalization are estimated to account for about 32 per cent of out-of-pocket expenses. Expenditures that account for more than 40 per cent of non-food spending or 10 per cent of household expenses are considered as catastrophic. An estimated 13.68 per cent of Indian households face this situation, incurring these expenditures out of their savings or borrowing in informal markets that have interest rates ranging from 24 to 60 per cent,[5] thrusting many into intergenerational poverty.[6]

Due to the extensive market failures, irrespective of the ideological persuasion of the political system—social solidarity or individual choice—government intervention seems inevitable in order to ensure equity and social stability. Accordingly, in Europe, the UK, and Canada, every citizen is entitled to free healthcare paid out of tax revenues. But then, health spending in these countries also accounts for 9 to 12 per cent of the GDP and about a third of the revenue budgets. In other middle-income countries such as Turkey, Thailand, Brazil, and China, tax-based financing accounts for about three-quarters of the total health spending.

In according primacy to choice and market competition, the US, on the other hand, has limited public intervention that is extended to the elderly and the poor. Though US dominantly has a privatized health system with mandatory health insurance for all employees in the organized sector, public spending in the country accounts for nearly half of the estimated 18.5 per cent of the GDP spent on health. In the absence of universalism, close to 30 million people have no access to medical care—a situation that the new Affordable Care Act (2010), popularly known as Obamacare, is seeking to redress.

In this context, the current system of health financing in India is considered to be both regressive and inequitable. It is an open, unregulated marketspace where individuals pay in accordance with their financial capacity and providers charge in accordance with their choice. Irrespective of the political party in power or the level of economic growth, government allocations for health have been stagnant.

Given a federal polity, raising public spending for health in India has been a challenge. States need to almost treble their spending from the current level of 2.47 per cent to 8 per cent, which is a problematic issue due to restricted fiscal capacities and competing demands. Besides, three-quarters of disease burden is concentrated in about nine states that also account for an equal number of the poor. The per capita income ratio between them and the better-off states is 1:5, making it impossible for any central government to bridge the divide. In other words, those that need to spend do not have the fiscal space. The problem is further compounded with 93 per cent of people working in the informal sector and over 40 per cent having no assets or steady incomes. This seriously limits the scope to mobilize resources by expanding the tax base or copayments and user fees.

To find a solution to this conundrum, an understanding of public financing of health, particularly of the central government's allocation and spending priorities, is critical for two reasons: a) to assess the allocative and technical efficiencies in the little money that governments spend, and b) to assess the processes put in place for ensuring efficiencies in spending. It is believed that deep reforms are required in resetting priorities at the macro level as well as the sector level in order to mobilize additional resources and get better value for money.

This chapter explores a few assertions. First, it argues that the chronic underfunding of health is not accidental but the result of a development model adopted in the early years of India's independence and the mindset of economists who shape the agenda, earmark priorities, and determine spending.

Second, interstate disparities in health status are the result of vertical and horizontal asymmetries embedded in the constitutional division of power and responsibilities, where the states are made responsible for ensuring welfare while the centre has the resources.

Third, the institutional mechanisms created by the Constitution and an executive order—Finance Commission (FC) and the then Planning Commission—have failed to bridge the vertical imbalance in terms of functions and finances between the union and the states as well as the horizontal imbalance in terms of offsetting the interstate fiscal disabilities and bringing in a measure of equalization through the process of resource transfers.

Fourth, apart from the centralization of decision-making and funding, the central government acts more like an auditor. Systems and procedures are geared more towards delaying the release of funds, while budgeting cycles and the arbitrary manner of imposing cuts or withholding approved budgets lead to uncertainty—severely eroding the credibility and sustainability of the public health delivery system.

Fifth, the fragmented and disconnected manner of introducing health insurance and other demand-side interventions have strengthened an already unregulated and aggressive private sector and undermined the public sector, creating supply-side distortions. Besides, these interventions have only partially succeeded in reducing out-of-pocket expenditures and enhancing equity.

Historical Context

Both education and health are of foundational importance for building human capability as Amartya Sen never tires of reminding us. But this requires a model of development to which these concerns are central. To understand why this is not the case in India, it is important to look at the historical context and shifts in the political understanding of growth and development, the institutional arrangements for resource sharing between the centre and the states, and the states' inability to meet the demand for services, resulting in the gradual shift towards utilizing other fiscal instruments such as insurance and the private sector to provide services.

Model of Development

The Nehruvian model of development sought to leapfrog into modernity by harnessing science, technology, and natural resources through a centralized system of planned development. The development philosophy rested on two premises—that growth would over time benefit all and increased incomes would automatically translate to accessing good nutrition, health, and education. While the low base of private capital led to stimulating industrial growth through the public sector, the focus on achieving food self-sufficiency and reducing dependence on imports meant public investments in river-water projects and agriculture. With over 50 per cent of the population below the poverty line and the fledgling nation state facing famines, increasing food production through better farming methods and irrigation were legitimate priorities during the initial two decades of India's independence.

The model did not provide for central control over natural resources like river waters and electricity generation, the two important levers of development, which meant that states had to take on resource-intensive projects such as power plants and irrigation dams, restricting the fiscal space for social sector expenditures. Thus, for example, Andhra Pradesh invested over half of its resources during the first three decades after Independence on irrigation works and became the rice bowl of the country without any compensation from the centre. With the centre and states focusing on economic growth measured in terms of GDP, India's planning process clearly failed to prioritize the everyday aspirations of the common people wanting income and employment but also health, education, and a home with tap water and a functional toilet.

India's story of a planned development was, however, in real contrast to China's that also had a large population, immense poverty, and a colonial past. Both could not have been more dissimilar in the manner in which they tackled health problems that were common to them at a comparable economic level. While India in the early years of Independence focused on a narrow public health agenda of containing malaria and promoting family planning and medical education, China located barefoot doctors within the communities and launched multiple campaigns to change individual behaviour towards consumption of boiled water, public hygiene, sanitation, and cleanliness. In terms of population health, while China witnessed a remarkable decline in waterborne diseases and increased life expectancy, India even now is struggling with a high burden of diseases such as diarrhoea, frequent epidemics of waterborne and airborne diseases, and an under-five mortality rate that is seven times higher than that of China.

Clearly then, it is not true that postcolonial compulsions led to making choices between economic development and social development as every finance secretary made me believe in the initial years of my career. Non-availability of resources for health has more to do with the mindset and political priorities envisioning economic growth in binary terms, where spending on health or education is seen as an expenditure (of lower priority) and providing subsidies to private industry as an investment. Besides, the growing tendency towards populism as a means of asserting the legitimacy of the ruling power has meant frittering away scarce resources on extending financial subsidies to those already better off and also more vocal.

Over time, resource allocations have been guided more by political pragmatism than national welfare. Addressing basic needs and rights, whether pertaining to healthcare or other elementary goods, are increasingly perceived as acts of patronage seeking electoral returns instead of entitlements that the political system should be duty-bound to deliver. Since investment in health and well-being, particularly averting disease, does not have the same dramatic electoral impact as distributing cycles or food coupons, it continues to have a low priority in terms of resource allocation.

Resource planning and allocation from among competing demands need to be understood within this larger framework of political priorities such as providing gas subsidies and the macro-economic structure of public finance—extent of past liabilities and future commitments, level of taxation, and proportion of public expenditures as a ratio to GDP—and the institutional capacity of the public health financing system to absorb the increased inflow of resources.

Resource Mobilization

Government spending on health in India, whether by the centre or states, is largely based on tax and non-tax revenues. In the past few years, the nature of spending tax funds has diversified from spending on health facilities and programmes to procuring private care through insurance. But such a shift has not implied any additionality in resources by way of, say, copayments or enhancing the overall budgetary allocations.

With a view to raising the states' fiscal capacity to discharge their constitutional responsibilities, the central government devolves a proportion of the resources—following the principle of cooperative federalism—through the institutional mechanisms of the FC and the former Planning Commission (now directly by the finance ministry).

Institutional Mechanisms for Resource-sharing

Schedule VII of Article 246 of the Constitution provides the legal basis for the division of functions between the centre and the states. In the health sector, the centre has wide concurrent powers on medical education, medical profession, mental health, food adulteration, drugs, population control and family planning, social security and social insurance, maternity care, prevention of infectious diseases, and vital statistics including registration of births and deaths (concurrent list). The states are responsible for public health and sanitation, and hospitals and dispensaries (state list). Such a division created an asymmetry since the resources required by states for service delivery outstripped availability over time, making them dependent upon the centre for resources to meet their various obligations.

Besides earmarking responsibilities, the Constitution also delineated the resource base of the central and state domains separately and also those resources that are to be mobilized by the centre but shared with the states. The political question, then, was how, and based on what norms and principles, would these shareable resources be distributed among the states and utilized. To determine this issue, the Constitution provided for an FC to recommend the devolution of central taxes to states every five years, while the utilization of central funds was to be determined by the Planning Commission that was established by an executive order in 1950. The idea behind constituting this body was to have a think tank of experts who would analyse data, carry out evaluations, and suggest blueprints for development in the form of five-year plans. Such a state-guided approach, it was believed, would help to achieve growth with equity and in a balanced manner.

With the institution of the Planning Commission, an artificial accounting construct of Plan and Non-Plan expenditure was created. Plan came to represent expenditures incurred during the five-year-plan period and Non-Plan reflected the commitments on revenue expenditures. So the construction of a hospital would be a Plan activity while its maintenance in the following plan period would be Non-Plan. This construct was then divided with the FC looking into the Non-Plan component of expenditures and the Planning Commission handling the larger pie of Plan funds. With this the political control over the issue of resource sharing with states was made absolute. This artificial distinction has been removed starting this fiscal in 2016.

Thus, central transfers to states consisted of the transfers awarded by the FC and those allocated by the Planning Commission. Together these central transfers were to reduce interstate disparities and enable greater equalization. Instead, what we see over the years is a widening of disparities. It is generally believed that transfers through the two commissions failed to reduce interstate disparities as these were 'too insufficient to offset fiscal disabilities', with the Planning Commission's Gadgil formula and the Central Sector Scheme mechanisms 'having a weak equalization impact'.[7]

Since both these bodies set the tone for spending priorities and were an important source of revenue, an understanding of their mandate and why they failed to focus on health and education would be in order.

Finance Commission

Articles 275 and 280(1)(b) provide for making grants to states for a general or specific purpose. Article 270 provides for sharing of union taxes. Finance commissions can give both general and specific purpose grants. However, while grants can be conditional, the devolution of taxes and grants given to meet the post-devolution revenue gaps are unconditional. Through the years, the grant-in-aid component of the FC award grew from 7.72 per cent during the Seventh FC to 18.87 per cent in the Twelfth FC—an increase from Rs 16.09 billion to Rs 1.42 trillion. In all these years, a minimal amount of Rs 108 billion has so far been allocated to health. Combined with the states' lack of preference for investing in health and the low priority accorded to it under the grant-in-aid mechanism, the FC has been a virtual non-player in the health sector despite health being central to all human development.

Such 'neglect' of health by the successive FCs was a consequence of the general understanding that resource transfers should enable states to 'allocate among the competing purposes according to their best judgment'.[8] It was also believed that growth would automatically translate to well-being, as an individual, being rational, will consume and behave in a manner that will be conducive to good health. The fact that these assumptions had no basis in reality was never considered in any depth.

The principles of examination were set out by the First FC which, among others, stated that '[g]rant in aid [was given] to help equalize standards of basic social services in the different states by bringing up the levels of such services in the poorer states', and taking account of 'special needs or obligations of national concern' or 'grants ... to further any beneficent service of primary importance'. This provided the FCs with scope to earmark funds for subjects that were predominantly governed by the state under the grants-in-aid mechanism.

All through the years, the FCs, particularly the Fifth, Sixth, Seventh, and Ninth FCs, expressed their concerns and despaired at the 'need for equalization' and the widening disparities between states as well as the necessity to narrow them—for which they saw Article 275 as the main instrument. The Sixth FC laid down three principles for grant-in-aid: fill fiscal gaps, narrow disparities in the availability of various administrative and social services between the developed and less developed states, and take into account the 'spending burdens cast on a state because of its peculiar circumstances or matter of national importance ...'[9] In terms of ideas, the Seventh FC was the first to discuss the concept of equalization while determining that the role of transfers is to:

> narrow, as far as possible, disparities in the availability of various administrative and social services between the developed and less developed states, the object being that every citizen, irrespective of the state boundaries within which he lives, is provided with certain basic national minimum standards of such services. While the long-term objective may be to provide to each citizen the services at the levels obtaining in the most advanced states, due regard should be had to the feasibility of upgrading these standards in the shorter term.[10]

While such articulation and principles would be eminently suitable for providing resources for health that qualified on all counts for serious consideration, none did.

The health sector had to wait until the Twelfth FC that sought to develop a normative framework for resource allocation to assure that 'total funds match total needs' in a two-step approach that consisted of the following: a) all states to spend a certain proportion of their total revenue expenditure on health and education, and b) identifying those falling short and providing a cover of 30 per cent of the distance to reach the group average. Based on this norm, seven states were provided Rs 58.87 billion for health (4 per cent) out of a total grant of Rs 1.42 trillion. But these transfers turned out to be ineffective as the 'conditionalities were too complicated'. The grants were also treated in isolation and not contextualized in accordance with the current policy. Further, it was also assumed that state spending as a share of total expenditure reflected preference. Consequently, the grant was not linked to 'lower resource availability and different income elasticity of demand for health expenditures'.[11]

The Thirteenth FC took a different view. Allocating Rs 50 billion (out of the 1.7 trillion awarded, which comes to 2.9 per cent), the Thirteenth FC made its releases to states conditional to the improvement in infant mortality rates (IMR), taking the Sample Registration System (SRS) data of 2009 as the baseline. In operational terms, this was difficult to implement resulting in the better-off states availing the first tranche of funds as compared to those most in need. Out of Rs 15 billion released in the first instalment,[12] six states and high achievers together got almost Rs 10 billion.

Being small, these transfers were of marginal value and not worth the elaborate procedure laid down to access them. In the absence of a shared vision driving the process of resource transfers, 'the fiscal allocations have been ad hoc and the utilization more in the nature of gap filling, failing to offset the fiscal disabilities of the poorer states leaving them with large unmet expenditure needs'.[13]

The report of the Fourteenth FC is different from the earlier FC reports on four grounds: a) it removed the artificial construct of Plan and Non-Plan while taking a holistic view of the available resources, b) it enhanced the unconditional component of central devolutions from 32 per cent to 42 per cent of the divisible pool,[14] c) it removed all discretionary grants other than what was required for meeting post-devolution revenue gaps, disaster relief, and local bodies, and d) it sought to bring in a measure of fairness by providing revenue grants to overcome the fiscal disability imposed by debt and liabilities. The report, however, exhorted states to meet their basic obligations of providing public goods such as drinking water but made no specific reference to either health or education or even the concept of the multidimensional nature of poverty and want. It based itself on the premise that it is up to the elected governments at all levels of governance to make choices regarding spending preferences.

With the 'reduction' of fiscal space for discretionary spending by the centre, the 2015 budget drastically cut down allocations to the social sector, justified on the ground that the FC had allocated more resources to the states to discharge their constitutional obligations. This was, however, not true since the devolution recommended by the FC was within 63–5 per cent of divisible resources. The change lay in the states having the discretion to spend their resources than being determined by the centre. In other words, the central government continues to have adequate fiscal resources to transfer to states for programmes of national importance, if it so wishes.

Besides, in addition to the sharp cuts in budget allocations, the central government has also reduced its share of the centrally assisted schemes from 75 per cent to 60 per cent. This revision is in accordance with the recommendation of the expert committee under the chairmanship of Shivraj Chauhan, the chief minister of Madhya Pradesh. Also, the committee did not list out any sector for prioritization, thereby leaving the discretion upon the states to choose which sector to prioritize.[15] In such a situation, Andhra Pradesh can choose to invest on industrial corridors and a capital, while Telangana may choose to focus on building temples, a new secretariat, an assembly building, or a water grid. No state may consider health or education to be of any importance.

In the short term, therefore, it is likely that health and the social sector may face a handicap. In the face of the low priority that states have accorded to critical sectors such as health and education, and given the absence of any 'national goals' driving prioritization, it seems worrying that future allocations to health will now depend upon the extent of support that the state governments choose to accord to this sector.

Overall, the FCs failed to define equalization and basic services in the context of public goods and merit goods that must be the first charge on development funds and the first obligation of the state to fulfil. This could have been enforced through conditionalities and guidelines for states pushing them to prioritize spending on building up health infrastructure; laying down water grids for tap water in all houses, sewerage lines, drainage, and waste disposal systems; and dissuading states from focusing on subsidies for private goods that only benefit the middle classes. Had the successive FCs interpreted their directional role in this manner, the disease burden would have been half of what it is today and the overall productivity levels higher impacting economic growth.[16] If indeed India wants to reap the demographic dividend, investment in human capital is imperative and the country can ill afford to court a disaster instead of a dividend in the future.

Planning Commission (1950–2015)

The Planning Commission provided the divisible resources to states as loans and grants under three broad heads: central sector projects, additional central assistance (ACA), and the CSS. The resource devolution of central assistance was as per the Gadgil formula. An analysis of the CSS shows that since the Ninth Five Year Plan, the proportion of CSS to Gross Budgetary Support (GBS) grew from 31.3 per cent to 41.59 per cent, that is, from Rs 990.02 billion to Rs 6,605.06 billion. During the last three plan periods, the elasticity of per capita CSS and central sector transfers with respect to per capita GDP has been 2.5 per cent, showing that for every 1 per cent increase in the per capita income, central transfers have been 2.5 per cent. While this has been a 'progressive' step, the focus on health and social determinants has been relatively small.[17]

Since health outcomes are multifactorial necessitating horizontal approaches across sectors and administrative boundaries, the Planning Commission with its convening power was considered the right forum to ensure a coordinated policy framework where health action is suitably enhanced by an equal amount of resources and attention being paid to its other determinants. During the Eleventh Plan, of the total amount of Rs 6,987.01 billion released for 15 flagship schemes, health (NRHM, 9.34 per cent), drinking water (5.69 per cent), sanitation (0.94 per cent), and nutrition (Integrated Child Development Services Scheme [ICDS], 5.58 per cent) accounted for Rs 1,505.79 billion (21.59 per cent). Since most grants are subject to sharing with the states (ranging from 15 per cent to 50 per cent), it has been argued that such schemes create distortions in states' ability to set their own priorities. Maharashtra, for example, was required to earmark 10 per cent of its revenue budget to avail of the CSS grants.[18]

During the initial years, powerful state chief ministers resisted the centre's attempts to encroach into state domains. Equitable sharing of resources was always a bone of contention and was the main issue of discussion in all National Development Council (NDC)[19] meetings. For political exigencies, the states actually surrendered their powers of taxation resulting in the gradual shrinking of their fiscal space to meet people's growing aspirations for a better quality of life. To address this gap, the states would accept grants and financial assistance from the centre for whatever programmes and on whatever conditions offered.

Political dimensions apart, a more consistent criticism against the CSS, however, has been that it essentially encroaches upon and violates the constitutional principles of sharing responsibilities, often resulting in duplication and immense distortions, such as the central government providing the transport charges of a community health worker while the states struggle to meet the high costs of medical education.

Centrally sponsored schemes are conceived, formulated, and designed by the central ministries and the states are merely expected to provide their share of funds as required and implement them. While central grants to states, particularly those that are cash-strapped, have helped to keep focus on primary care and disease control, in the absence of making grants conditional to those states that provide clear strategies for addressing systemic deficiencies, allocation of greater funds has not, in several instances, helped achieve the desired outcomes.

Instead, centrally sponsored schemes create several systemic problems. For example, there is no certainty or predictability regarding the release of funds. Though the financial outlay for the five-year period is finalized and physical targets indicated, every year the issues are revisited and much time lost in the uncertainty of what quantum of funds would be available for the following year, or worse, reducing fund availability in the middle of the year. This happens because there is no real correlation between the funds allocated and the targets fixed that keep moving from year to year and plan to plan. In fact, ministries spend nearly two months of peak 'implementation' time drawing up the annual proposals only to be allocated an incremental amount to keep up with the inflation.

Furthermore, though grant allocations to states are to be made according to their needs, the ultimate releases depend on fulfilling the conditionalities, including the submission of utilization certificates (UCs). With the most needy states underutilizing their allocations due to several systemic reasons, funds allocated to them are redistributed to the states that fulfil the conditions and have better utilization capacity. In such a scenario where there is no provision for multi-year utilization or a system of non-lapsable funds meant for the underperforming states, and no relationship between the original allocation and ultimate releases, disparities have only widened though gross allocations of central assistance may have increased.

The situation has now dramatically changed with the abolition of the Planning Commission and the establishment of the NITI Aayog with effect from 1 January 2015. But such winding up should be replaced by better instruments of planning since we need an agency with the capacity to frame policy options based on evidence and insulated from political compulsions. Over time, hopefully a culture of formulating policies based on data analysis to ensure better quality of decision-making will develop. As of now, it is yet to be seen how this body will function and how it will seek to harmonize the varied demands, reduce interstate disparities by improving fiscal disabilities, and what priority it will accord to the social sector, namely health and social determinants. For now, health is a low priority for NITI Aayog and there is no clarity regarding the future.

Public Spending on Health

As has been already noted, India's public spending on health has been persistently low—within the narrow band of 0.8 per cent to 1.1 per cent of the GDP. In 1986–7, the total public revenue expenditure was at its peak: 20 per cent of the GDP with a capital expenditure of 7 per cent. To finance the increasing revenue expenditures, states resorted to borrowings that meant more money being committed to interest payments and consequently, a debt trap compelling a structural adjustment loan from the IMF that came with stiff conditions of expenditure compression. By 1996–7, revenue expenditures came down to 14 per cent and capital expenditures plummeted to 2.39 per cent by 2000–1. Most revenue expenditures went into sustaining the salary increases as a result of the Fifth Pay Commission that wrecked the economy of the states as well.

During the years 1995–2002, there was only a marginal increase in aggregate health spending from 0.88 per cent of the GDP to 0.9 per cent—that, too, on account of pay revisions—which declined to 0.83 per cent in 2001–2.[20] During this decade, state spending was estimated to be 0.46 per cent of the GDP. During 2004–5, the highest public spending in per capita terms among larger states was by Maharashtra at Rs 348 while the lowest was by Bihar at Rs 124. Per capita health expenditures increased by 1.95 per cent to every 1 per cent increase in per capita incomes, indicating a health expenditure growth of 18 per cent per annum in nominal terms and 11 per cent in real terms.[21]

The Eleventh Plan (2007–12) trebled the central government allocations for health. During this period, India spent about 4.1 per cent of its GDP on health.[22] Of this, the total public spending (states and centre) was 27 per cent, up from 17 per cent in 2002, the rest being spent by households, with marginal amounts by private sector or external aid.

The central government's own share of financing of health sector expenditures (its own spending and grants to states for the health sector) increased from Rs 15.2 billion in 1990–1 to Rs 97.86 billion in 2013–14 that includes expenses incurred by central and state governments, local bodies, and on social insurance (NHA). During this period, the relative share of the centre, in public financing of the entire health sector, increased from 20.3 per cent to 28.3 per cent.[23] The central government increased health spending 2.5 times over the amounts incurred during the Tenth Plan, while the states together spent only 2.14 times more, together accounting to 1.15 per cent of the GDP.[24] In terms of per capita expenditures incurred by central and state governments in nominal terms, this amount translates to Rs 593 and Rs 786 (NHA 2014) if all expenses are taken into account, against Rs 304 in 2004 (NCMH) with wide variations across states.

Such centralization of financing is evident from the centre's increasing role in the planning and designing of policy and the increased dependence of the states on the centre. Such dependence aggravated the interstate differentials due to unequal resource capacities—an inequality that federal transfers clearly failed to mitigate.

Interstate Variations in Spending[25]

Health spending by states in proportion to the total revenue spending was 7.02 per cent in 1984–5 that steadily declined to 5.7 per cent and 3.4 per cent in 1995–6 and 2003–4 respectively, increasing to 4.4 per cent in 2011 and falling to 3.78 in 2014. None of the states achieved the original 7 per cent even though these were years of economic prosperity. Among the larger states, except for Kerala, Goa, and Rajasthan that spent more than 5 per cent as a ratio of aggregate expenditure,[26] the rest of the states averaged between 3 per cent and 4 per cent. The lowest spending was by Haryana (3.4 per cent), Odisha, and Madhya Pradesh at about 3.5 per cent. In other words, despite a substantial increase in central funding, state spending continued to be in the range of 3–5 per cent with 4.4 per cent as the national average,[27] up from 3.4 per cent in 2003–4. These ratios have been consistent over the decade from 2000–12. This is of vital importance as the overall public spending of 3 per cent of the GDP is dependent upon the ability of the states to treble their spending to a minimum of 8 per cent of the total revenue spending.

Impact of IMF Conditionalities

Fiscal deficit management in India is nearly always done by expenditure cuts and not by raising additional resources. Needless to say, the worst-hit under such a strategy are the social sector and capital expenditures. The already poorly designed and badly implemented public health policy suffered a further setback with the harsh conditionalities the IMF imposed on the government to reduce its fiscal deficit.[28] The social sector and health in particular were easy targets for such cuts. Reduced budgets resulted in the shutting down of training schools, vacant positions with no new appointments, no recurring expenditures for drugs and consumables, and a near-complete suspension of all capital expenditures—buildings, equipment, or vehicles. The programmes that the health departments at the central and state levels implemented during the period 1990–2004 were those for which World Bank loans were available, namely infectious disease control programmes, family planning, and child immunization. States like Andhra Pradesh, Karnataka, West Bengal, Tamil Nadu, and Uttar Pradesh obtained World Bank loans for the construction of district and sub-district-level hospitals.

Selective primary care was an inadequate response to the rapidly changing epidemiology, lifestyles, an ageing population, and an increasingly assertive middle class triggering demand for medical and acute care, surgeries, latest diagnostics, branded drugs, and clean hospitals backed by a willingness to pay.

The void created by the virtual withdrawal of the state was met by the private sector—by default. Since the late 1980s, within a span of 20 years, the private sector accounted for 60 per cent of inpatient treatment and 80 per cent of all outpatient treatment.[29] In 2004–5, the average private per capita spending was four times that of public spending at Rs 959 against Rs 242. In the absence of insurance policies, an aggressive, unregulated, and rapidly proliferating private sector became the only option for many. However, the increasing costs of care—growing at the rate of 15–20 per cent per year—and the unpredictable, lumpy nature of health expenditure began to put pressure on the middle classes while impoverishing the poor who were clearly outpriced.

Low Capital Spending

Capital expenditures in the health sector have been low. The share of capital expenditure in the total health expenditure was just about 13.7 per cent in 2012–13 and the share of the central government's capital expenditure in the total expenditure was just about 1.2 per cent. In fact, throughout the period, capital expenditure remained low, marginally increasing from 8.4 per cent in 1990–1 to 12 per cent in 2000–1 and finally to 13.7 per cent in 2012–13, then falling to 7 per cent in 2013–14 (NHA).

India's ability to expand universal access to primary healthcare is seriously hampered by the persistent gaps in infrastructure required to deliver a basket of services. There is still a normative gap of 3,469 CHCs for a population of 0.1 million, 5,887 PHCs for every 30,000 people, and 27,430 sub-centres for every 5,000 people. Seventy per cent of the gap is in the poorly performing states that also have the disease burden. Besides, the existing facilities are not equipped properly and have inadequate infrastructure with 10 per cent of the PHCs and 35 per cent of the sub-centres housed in thatched huts or single rooms. Worse, almost 174 districts in seven major states have thousands of sub-centres located more than 3 km away from the village, seriously impacting access.

In 2012, the Ministry of Health & Family Welfare (MOHFW) issued the revised Indian Public Health Standards (IPHS) detailing the services, equipment, building area, human resources, and drugs that ought to be available at each of these facilities. A costing exercise to implement the IPHS undertaken by the MOHFW showed that a nonrecurring amount of Rs 1.11 trillion[30] and a recurring amount of Rs 482.21 billion per year would be required for establishing new facilities and strengthening the existing ones to the IPHS.[31] Of this, Rs 923.13 billion of capital investment and a recurring amount of Rs 379.34 billion per year is required only for rural areas. Seventy per cent of this money is required in the northern states that have low fiscal capacity. Against this huge capital investment gap in primary care, a measly Rs 60 billion or so might have been spent during the Eleventh Plan period.

The IPHS norms are idealistic, very costly, and quite clearly unaffordable for most states to achieve in the short and medium terms. They should be reviewed in terms of need and functional relevance. Three factors compel such a reassessment: (a) substantial development in road and transport communications, (b) technological advances, and (c) choice of providers. Mapping of all facilities could help rationalize infrastructure needs and develop strategies to ensure equitable access to health services in a more economically sustainable manner.

Apart from funds from the centre, states also have their own spending. During the period starting from 1996, several states like Andhra Pradesh, Karnataka, Tamil Nadu, Odisha, West Bengal, Rajasthan, Maharashtra, and Uttar Pradesh availed World Bank loans for the construction of district and sub-district hospitals. The main problem has been the maintenance of these assets since Non-Plan expenditures are the first to get slashed in times of financial stringency. Likewise, starting from 2010, the central government has also been heavily investing in establishing institutions similar to AIIMS, providing assistance to states for upgrading their medical colleges and setting up nursing schools, and upgrading its own hospitals and colleges.

Not investing and limiting public expenditures required for infrastructure—physical buildings and equipment—is self-defeating as the backward states are lagging behind precisely because they have no infrastructure. Low capital investment has made the public health system dysfunctional. At a time when there is huge technical innovation and shift in epidemiology towards diseases that need better diagnostic support and inpatient care, inadequate investment in health infrastructure is forcing people to opt for expensive private care at the cost of spending on food or education, entailing intergenerational consequences. For many countries infrastructure is such a critical determinant that Thailand put a moratorium on any spending in urban areas during the five-year period from 1995 to 2000 until the infrastructure in rural areas was strengthened. This enabled Thailand to launch the UHC policy in 2002.

Impact of Central Transfers through NRHM, 2005–12

In 2005, the central government launched the NRHM with a threefold increase in budgets to contain the crisis that had engulfed the health sector and revitalize the ailing primary healthcare system in rural India. The NRHM was a financing mechanism based on three core financial principles: a) flexibility in funding to enable states address their needs with a 0.3 per cent increased weightage to the 18 low-performing, high-focus states; b) enhancing the central share in proportion to the total public health spending by increased grants-in-aid to the states; and c) devolution of funds and decentralization of priority-setting and planning to the implementing agencies.

During the Eleventh Plan period, an estimated Rs 596.36 billion[32] (the centre and state share combined) was incurred under the NRHM.

Releases under the NRHM were made under three pools: the NRHM pool, the reproductive child health (RCH) pool, and funds for disease control programmes. Though the intention behind structuring the NRHM funds into pools was to allow greater flexibility, each pool has defined spending heads and inter-transfers are restricted and need prior approval of the central government. Likewise, due to the weak absorption capacity of the high-focus states, the more organized and better-off states such as Maharashtra and Tamil Nadu disproportionately utilized the NRHM funds. Thus, against 1.3 times of resources allocated to the 18 high-focus states, only 0.8 times was utilized during the period 2007–12. Within states, too, the better-off districts tended to utilize more funds widening the disparities further. In a study conducted in Karnataka, the differentials in per capita expenditures were wide as seen in Bangalore Rural that spent Rs 84.67, the highest, compared to Rs 44.5 in Davangere, the lowest. Such studies indicate that the central funds were inadequate for scaling up the absorption capacity of the poorer districts.[33]

The NHP of 2002 identified three financial goals to be achieved by 2010: a) increase in public health expenditure from the existing 0.9 per cent to 2.0 per cent of the GDP, b) increase in share of central grants to at least 25 per cent of the total health spending, and c) increase in state sector health spending from 5.5 per cent to 7 per cent of the budget by 2005 and further increase to 8 per cent by 2010.

Since achieving Goal 1 is dependent on a threefold increase in the state sector spending in proportion to the total public spending, the central government imposed two other conditions for the release of central grants: a) to provide 15 per cent share of the amount being released for the NRHM (that has now risen to 40 per cent), and b) to increase health allocations to 10 per cent of the total revenue expenditures. The purpose of these goals was to ensure that the central transfers were not being substituted by states diverting equal amounts to other aspects of healthcare not funded by the NRHM as argued by Rao and Choudhury[34] in their paper where they found that there was a 'substitution effect' with the tendency of states to resort to shifting expenditures to central grants.

By the end of the Eleventh Plan period, health spending against Goal 1 was 1.04 per cent of the GDP as in 2012;[35] Goal 2 was achieved on an all-India basis with wide interstate disparities, where critical states like Uttar Pradesh had a central spending of about 15 per cent; and under Goal 3 data shows that the central transfers did not stimulate an appreciable increase in health spending by states that continued to average between 3 per cent to 5 per cent, having increased by 1 percentage point to pre-NRHM levels. Finally, expenditure patterns show that NRHM funding to high-focus states was not 1.3 times relative to others but instead continued to be given to those that had the capacity to spend.

To understand why these goals were not achieved, the manner of utilization of the funds released, the quality of spending, and the expenditures incurred by 19 states[36] representing 90 per cent of the country's population during the two years 2007–8 and 2011–12 (baseline and end line of the Eleventh Plan) were analysed. In addition to the issues raised earlier, two more questions were studied:

a. Whether the relative proportions of spending under primary, secondary, and tertiary care were being maintained, particularly with the Twelfth Plan target asking states to spend 70 per cent of their health budgets on primary care.
b. Whether there is an optimality or effectiveness of spending assured by having a balanced mix of the various critical components impacting outcomes—salaries, drugs, equipment, infrastructure, and so on.

Analysis of 19 Major States[37]

Data obtained from the states' Demand for Grants, expenditure statements of the NRHM, State AIDS control organizations, and the allocations made under the Central Sector Schemes for non-communicable diseases as well as the RSBY (that was then with the Ministry of Labour) were analysed under four categories: a) by assessing the total expenditure incurred by the health department as a whole and as indicated in the revenue/capital accounts—Plan/Non-Plan; b) by assessing the distributional preferences in the allocation of budgets between primary, secondary, and tertiary care, for which programme data was also collected to triangulate it with the budget outlays; c) by assessing the allocative efficiencies and quality of spending on primary care in terms of the balance in inputs among the various components required for an outcome; and d) by assessing the share of central and state governments. The state spending patterns for the two years were then collated to understand the financial flows related to absorption of funds.[38] The findings of the budgetary data of 19 states have been discussed further.

Central Transfers: Substitution or Supplementation

As a proportion of the GDP, public health spending increased only marginally from 0.9 per cent to 1.1 per cent during the Eleventh Plan period. Of importance is the increase in central funding in proportion to the total public spending from 17 per cent during 2001–2 to 24 per cent[39] in 2012, reducing to that extent the burden on the states.

However, such increases were uneven across states. While among the high-focus states, Chhattisgarh and Bihar accounted for over 39 per cent and 33 per cent respectively of their spending to central grants, the proportions for West Bengal, Uttarakhand, and Uttar Pradesh were about 18 per cent. Among the large states, Andhra Pradesh had the lowest proportion of central funding at 16 per cent while relatively better-off states such as Maharashtra and Karnataka accounted for 31 per cent and 28 per cent respectively, showing that states with greater implementation capacity made better use of the

NRHM and other central sector funds. All states increased in gross terms (current prices) the allocation for health and, barring Andhra Pradesh, most provided their share of 15 per cent of the NRHM matching funds. In fact, it is interesting to note that Bihar increased its own resources earmarked for health by 12 percentage points—from 33 per cent in 2008–9 to 45 per cent in 2011–12—reducing its dependence on the centre and Madhya Pradesh did the same by 7 percentage points. During this period, states maintained a 74 per cent share of the total government spending on health.

Table 2.1 gives a comparison of the average per capita public spending on health incurred in 19 major states during 2004–5 and 2011–12. During this seven-year period, per capita spending increased from an average of Rs 230 to Rs 312 (at 2004–5 prices), indicating a steady rate of over 11 per cent growth per year. The spending on primary care was Rs 244 per capita in real prices. In current prices, the total health spending was Rs 537 and Rs 390 per capita on primary care. There was doubling of expenditures in states such as Gujarat, Madhya Pradesh, and Karnataka and an impressive spending in the new states of Chhattisgarh, Uttaranchal, and Jharkhand. While it is clear that all states have increased their spending, an outlier is Kerala where public health spending in real terms was stagnant at Rs 287, lesser than in 2004–5. Considering that Kerala is facing a huge non-communicable disease burden, public health spending should have gone up to provide the necessary risk protection. It clearly appears that the state withdrawal from the health sector has been significant in recent years (See Table 2.1).[40]

Analysed in real terms, the gap between the highest and lowest states appears to have narrowed only marginally by 0.4 times, given the significant push under the NRHM. For example, in 2004–5 (prior to the NRHM) the highest spenders were Maharashtra, Punjab, and Kerala at Rs 348, Rs 326, and Rs 319 per capita respectively, 2.5 times more than Bihar that had the lowest spending at Rs 124 per capita. In 2011–12, Bihar continued to be the lowest spender at Rs 182 per capita (at 2004–5 prices) against the highest spending by Tamil Nadu at Rs 475 that was 2.6 times more.

TABLE 2.1 Interstate Comparison of Average Per Capita Spending in 19 Major States: 2004–5 and 2011–12 (in 2004–5 Prices)

State	Total population in crores as per census 2011	Per capita health expenditure 2004–5	Per capita health expenditure 2011–12 in 2004–5 prices
Odisha	4.10	179	238
West Bengal	9.10	205	297
Goa	0.15	798	1,790
Gujarat	6.00	187	439
Maharashtra	11.20	348	397
Bihar	10.30	124	183
Chhattisgarh	2.50		364
Haryana	2.50	189	353
Himachal Pradesh	0.68	486	970
Jharkhand	3.20		307
Madhya Pradesh	7.20	164	328
Punjab	2.70	326	438
Rajasthan	6.80	198	304
Uttar Pradesh	19.90	150	224
Uttarakhand	1.00		528
Andhra Pradesh	8.40	216	408
Karnataka	6.10	231	469
Kerala	3.30	319	282
Tamil Nadu	7.20	248	475
Average for 19 States	**112.33**	**230** (All India 304)	**465** (All India 312)

Source: Column 1: Census 2011, Column 2: NCMH, Column 3: Expenditures incurred by 19 states under the state budget, the NRHM, the NACP, and the RSBY totalling Rs 60.4 billion.

Note: 1 crore equals to 10 million.

What this shows is that health inflation is eating into the increased resources with the same services needing higher spending. The higher spending in southern states such as Tamil Nadu and Karnataka at Rs 408 per capita as compared to Rs 310 by northern states is reflective of better utilization of health services and the epidemiological divide. Reduction in childhood mortality increases lifespans but also shifts spending from the young to the old, on diseases that are more expensive to treat. Overall, since the percentage of the rate of growth in public spending is lower than health prices, there is an increasing share of spending on health in the total household expenditures with about 40 per cent of the non-food component being incurred on medical treatment.[41]

Overall, stacking one variable of central funds transferred to the states as CSS against the other variable of state health budgets does not appear to provide evidence of state governments substituting central funds with their own (except Andhra Pradesh). Instead, evidence suggests increased health spending in gross terms though not in proportion to the total government spending or gross state domestic product (GSDP).

Allocative Efficiencies and Quality of Spending

There are two aspects that determine allocative efficiencies: distribution of resources among different levels of care and the amounts allocated to different activities at a particular level. The first is also dependent on the epidemiological status of a people and the nature of demand. For example, while India spends most of its money on primary and secondary care, in the US 90 per cent of the total spending is consumed by just 1 per cent of the patients. Tertiary care guzzles far more resources and therefore, if not carefully monitored, can crowd out other levels that are in equal need of resources.

Second, in the health sector it is not enough to merely spend but it should be ensured that the spending is balanced out among the various components. A doctor in a facility without drugs or equipment will be only partially productive. Besides, in times of financial stringency it is the salary component that is safeguarded and budgets for drugs or maintenance often slashed. Very often, during the last quarter of the financial year, the Ministry of Finance imposed a unilateral 10 per cent cut[42] as a means of containing the fiscal deficit, which is often compensated by not paying for the drugs procured resulting in delay of supplies or cutting down of drugs supply. Such measures have often resulted in increasing drug resistance as patients have either been denied the life-saving drugs or been provided only half the dosage.

In the Twelfth Plan document, the Planning Commission has called for earmarking 70 per cent of the health budget for primary

TABLE 2.2 Allocative Efficiencies in Spending in 19 Major States during 2007–8 and 2011–12 (Rs Crores)

Region and State	Primary Care		Secondary Care		Tertiary Care & Medical Education		Others		Total	% against All States
	Exp	%	Exp	%	Exp	%	Exp	%	Exp	
EAST INDIA										
Odisha										
2007–8	269	36%	71	9%	153	20%	257	34%	750	3%
2011–12	727	44%	143	9%	305	19%	468	28%	1,643	3%
West Bengal										
2007–8	666	40%	798	48%	176	10%	37	2%	1,677	7%
2011–12	1,827	44%	1,713	42%	562	14%	10	0%	4,112	7%
Sub Total										
2007–8	935	39%	869	36%	329	14%	294	12%	2,427	10%
2011–12	2,554	44%	1,856	32%	867	15%	478	8%	5,755	10%
WEST INDIA										
Goa										
2007–8	NA	NA	NA	NA	NA	NA	NA	NA	NA	NA
2011–12	160	39%	137	33%	99	24%	19	5%	415	1%
Gujarat										
2007–8	922	57%	185	11%	434	27%	76	5%	1,617	7%
2011–12	2,115	54%	470	12%	1,189	31%	124	3%	3,898	7%
Maharashtra										
2007–8	NA	NA	NA	NA	NA	NA	NA	NA	NA	NA
2011–12	3,883	66%	243	4%	1,059	18%	707	12%	5,892	11%

(Cont'd)

TABLE 2.2 (Cont'd)

Region and State	Primary Care		Secondary Care		Tertiary Care & Medical Education		Others		Total	% against All States
	Exp	%	Exp	%	Exp	%	Exp	%	Exp	
Sub Total										
2007–8	922	57%	185	11%	434	27%	76	5%	1,617	3%
2011–12	6,158	60%	850	8%	2,347	23%	850	8%	10,205	18%
NORTH INDIA										
Bihar										
2008–9*	1,432	85%	42	3%	181	11%	20	1%	1,675	7%
2011–12	1,982	68%	202	7%	660	23%	77	3%	2,921	5%
Chhattisgarh										
2007–8	347	61%	59	10%	76	13%	90	16%	572	2%
2011–12	805	58%	105	8%	178	13%	311	22%	1,399	3%
Haryana										
2007–8	NA	NA	NA	NA	NA	NA	NA	NA	NA	NA
2011–12	958	65%	13	1%	288	20%	207	14%	1,466	3%
Himachal Pradesh										
2007–8	226	70%	89	28%	6	2%	0	0%	321	1%
2011–12	509	61%	154	19%	156	19%	10	1%	829	1%
Jharkhand										
2007–8	391	68%	66	12%	105	18%	11	2%	573	2%
2011–12	826	61%	135	10%	241	18%	163	12%	1,365	2%
Madhya Pradesh†										
2007–8	1,089	62%	173	10%	309	18%	191	11%	1,762	8%

2011–12	1,772	51%	445	13%	926	26%	358	10%	3,501	6%
Punjab										
2007–8	449	54%	150	18%	139	17%	101	12%	839	4%
2011–12	1,143	59%	312	16%	288	15%	198	10%	1,941	3%
Rajasthan										
2007–8	920	50%	103	6%	511	28%	324	17%	1,858	8%
2011–12	1,768	47%	361	10%	870	23%	754	20%	3,753	7%
Uttarakhand										
2007–8	215	59%	88	24%	42	12%	19	5%	364	2%
2011–12	558	62%	138	15%	143	16%	64	7%	903	2%
Uttar Pradesh										
2007–8	2,323	56%	827	20%	952	23%	49	1%	4,151	18%
2011–12	3,999	60%	1,190	18%	1,460	22%	49	1%	6,698	12%
Sub Total										
2007–8	7,392	61%	1,597	13%	2,321	19%	805	7%	12,115	52%
2011–12	14,320	58%	3,055	12%	5,210	21%	2,191	9%	24,776	44%
SOUTH INDIA										
Andhra Pradesh										
2007–8	1,509	53%	345	12%	677	24%	328	11%	2,859	12%
2011–12	2,521	46%	499	9%	2,118	38%	364	7%	5,502	10%
Karnataka										
2007–8	918	47%	354	18%	693	35%	7	0%	1,972	8%
2011–12	1,419	42%	615	18%	1,345	40%	5	0%	3,384	6%
Kerala										
2007–8	NA	NA	NA	NA	NA	NA	NA	NA	NA	NA

(*Cont'd*)

TABLE 2.2 (Cont'd)

Region and State	Primary Care Exp	%	Secondary Care Exp	%	Tertiary Care & Medical Education Exp	%	Others Exp	%	Total Exp	% against All States
2011–12	766	75%	145	14%	95	9%	13	1%	1,019	2%
Tamil Nadu										
2007–8	1,344	58%	103	4%	594	26%	262	11%	2,303	10%
2011–12	2,856	54%	188	4%	1,312	25%	906	17%	5,262	9%
Sub Total										
2007–8	3,771	53%	802	11%	1,964	28%	597	8%	7,134	31%
2011–12	7,562	50%	1,447	10%	4,870	32%	1,288	8%	15,167	27%
ALL STATES										
2007–8	13,020	56%	3,453	15%	5,048	22%	1,772	8%	23,293	100%
2011–12	30,594	55%	7,208	13%	13,294	24%	4,807	9%	55,903	100%

Source: All data submitted by states except for Goa, Punjab, and Maharashtra. The information on state budgets for Goa and Maharashtra is taken from the state budget books for 2011–12 and for central contributions to these states from GOI. The information for Punjab is taken from the state budget for 2011–12 available on the RBI website and central contribution to the state from GOI.

Note: 100 crores equal to 1 billion.

* Expenses for Bihar are for 2008–9 as those for 2007–8 are not available.

† Medical education expenses for 2007–8 and 2011–12 have been taken as differential to the total budget from that given on the RBI website.

care. Though the basis for such a target is not clear, it is nevertheless important that primary care is protected against other sectors, particularly when the health budget itself is not increased.

Though in percentage points some states reduced their budgets for primary care or kept it stagnant, in absolute terms the amounts increased across the states. Comparing two reference points—2007–8, the first year of the Eleventh Plan, and 2011–12, the end year—expenditure trends become easier to appreciate (See Table 2.2). Thus, while Tamil Nadu spent Rs 28.56 billion in 2011–12 on primary care, in percentage terms spending had reduced from 58 per cent in 2007–8 to 54 per cent in 2011–12. Likewise, Gujarat also increased its primary care spending from a low budget of Rs 9.22 billion in 2007–8 to Rs 21.15 billion in 2011–12, but in percentage terms there was a reduction from 57 per cent to 54 per cent of the total health spending.[43] Bihar and Chhattisgarh also indicated reductions from 85 per cent to 68 per cent and 61 per cent to 58 per cent respectively. However, given the huge gaps in primary care in these two states such reductions may not appear to be justified. Overall, the average for all states was 56 per cent in 2007 that came down by 3 percentage points in 2011–12.

The outlier is Andhra Pradesh where the budget for primary care dwindled by 7 percentage points from 53 per cent to 46 per cent during the period 2007–12 because the money got diverted to the state-sponsored insurance scheme called Rajiv Aarogyasri Scheme (RAS) under which patients got cover for high-cost surgeries that were being provided by corporate hospitals.

With improvement in service delivery and shifts in the epidemiological profile towards non-communicable diseases, the proportion of expenditures on primary care comes down. For example, in the UK it is only 30 per cent. If, therefore, 50 per cent is taken as the cut-off point, then both Odisha and Rajasthan have to spend more. While expenditure in Odisha went up from a low of 36 per cent in 2007–8 to 44 per cent by 2012, Rajasthan reduced spending for primary care from 50 per cent to 47 per cent, which is inadequate in view of the health status in both these states.

In analysing such expenditures there are three points to observe: a) these figures also include the devolutions from the central government under the NRHM and, therefore, the actual state effort will need to be read by subtracting the central government's funding; b) this data shows the steady increase in state capacity to absorb and utilize funds; and c) such increased spending on primary care has been at the cost of secondary care in some states, such as Tamil Nadu that spent only 4 per cent on district hospitals—perhaps because NRHM funds could also be incurred for improving district hospitals. The relatively high percentage of spending on secondary care, say, in states such as Uttar Pradesh or Uttarakhand, is also reflective of the need to respond from the supply side to the pressures triggered on the demand side under conditional transfer schemes such as the Janani Suraksha Yojana (JSY) that provides Rs 1,400 to a pregnant woman for delivering in a government facility. With the primary health centres in disarray, most deliveries take place in the poorly endowed district hospitals that have of late been improved with the introduction of wards, labour rooms, and operation theatres with the NRHM assistance.

Composition of Spending

Regarding the composition of spending, almost all states except for Odisha, West Bengal, Gujarat, and Punjab showed an increase in salaries (see Table 2.3). This increase could be on two counts: the impact of the Sixth Pay Commission and the NRHM funding support for appointing personnel on contractual terms. This then explains the dramatic increase in spending under this head in Uttar Pradesh where filling up long-pending vacancies resulted in an increase in expenditure from 39 per cent to 60 per cent. Likewise, Madhya Pradesh also increased spending from 38 per cent to 54 per cent, Rajasthan from 53 per cent to 63 per cent, and Bihar from 27 per cent to 37 per cent.

As a norm, salaries and wages should account for 50 per cent and drugs for 10 per cent of the total spending. It is pertinent to see how little Bihar, Punjab, Rajasthan, Jharkhand, Himachal Pradesh, Maharashtra, Gujarat, and Uttarakhand spent on drugs—all ranging from 1 per cent to 3 per cent—while southern states like Andhra Pradesh and Karnataka spent about 14 per cent. The data does not, however, help derive any pattern on drug spending that appears to be more of a state-level decision. Similarly, capital expenditure has also been minimal at 8 per cent. Most expenditure was incurred under 30 per cent of the NRHM pool budget earmarked for taking up refurbishing of facilities or construction of new ones. In fact, capital expenditures were equivalent to the amounts provided as grants to local bodies (6 per cent) and incentives to CHWs (7 per cent; demand-side interventions) that ought to have been twofold as after a point demand gets impacted by quality that is a supply-side function. Overall, spending appears to have been driven more by the schematic approach prescribed by the central government rather than the states' own needs. Yet given the huge demand and the meagre resources, states struggled to do their best.

An analysis of health financing under the NRHM and health spending in 19 major states shows clearly that alongside an increase in the quantum of funding, there is also a need to improve the policy design and quality of spending to ensure closer alignment with health outcomes. For example, if the desired outcome is to increase institutional deliveries in public hospitals to 75 per cent of the total deliveries in a state like Uttar Pradesh, then greater spending on increasing the bed strength and reducing the supply-side deficiencies should have been accorded an equal priority alongside demand-side interventions like the JSY—a situation dissimilar to that prevalent in Tamil Nadu or Kerala.

While central funds were used in addition to supplement states' own efforts, it would also be correct to assert that states continued to accord a low preference to health even when the resource pie had expanded, indicating that the mere enhancement of resource devolution without conditions has limited impact. In other words, the additional resources from the centre to improve primary care in rural areas perversely incentivized states to instead invest their own funds on buying health insurance (Andhra Pradesh, Chhattisgarh, and Karnataka) despite their primary health systems being weak. In Chapter 6, a table has been provided to show the list of services that should be available in primary care facilities. As can be seen, out of the 30 such activities, barely a dozen are being fully or partially provided due to the paucity of funds.

TABLE 2.3 Interstate Comparison of Spending by Component: 2007–8 and 2011–12 (Rs Crores)

State and Year	Salaries		Supplies and Drugs		Major Works		Equipment		Incentives		Maintenance and Minor Works		Grant-in-aid		Others		Total	% against All States
	Exp	%	Exp	%	Exp	%	Exp	%	Exp	%	Exp	%	Exp	%	Exp	%	Exp	%
EAST REGION																		
Odisha																		
2007–8	73	27%	54	20%	17	6%	2	1%	78	29%	2	1%	9	3%	34	13%	269	2%
2011–12	202	31%	93	14%	36	5%	14	2%	23	4%	2	0%	103	16%	183	28%	656	3%
West Bengal																		
2007–8	381	57%	41	6%	5	1%	5	1%	0	0%	4	1%	106	16%	124	19%	666	5%
2011–12	899	50%	83	5%	53	3%	30	2%	0	0%	12	1%	272	15%	436	24%	1,785	7%
Sub Total																		
2007–8	454	49%	95	10%	22	2%	7	1%	78	8%	6	1%	115	12%	158	17%	935	7%
2011–12	1,101	45%	176	7%	89	4%	44	2%	23	1%	14	1%	375	15%	619	25%	2,441	9%
WEST REGION																		
Goa																		
2007–8	NA	NA	NA	NA	NA	NA	NA	NA	NA	NA	NA	NA	NA	NA	NA	NA	NA	NA
2011–12	98	62%	14	9%	3	2%	3	2%	1	1%	1	1%	8	5%	30	19%	158	1%
Gujarat																		
2007–8	601	65%	54	6%	17	2%	1	0%	0	0%	6	1%	21	2%	222	24%	922	7%
2011–12	1,250	58%	107	5%	195	9%	11	1%	3	0%	17	1%	15	1%	564	26%	2,162	8%
Maharashtra																		
2007–8	NA	NA	NA	NA	NA	NA	NA	NA	NA	NA	NA	NA	NA	NA	NA	NA	NA	NA
2011–12	NA	NA	NA	NA	NA	NA	NA	NA	NA	NA	NA	NA	NA	NA	NA	NA	NA	NA

Sub Total																			
2007–8	601	65%	54	6%	17	2%	1	0%	0	0%	6	1%	21	2%	222	24%	922	7%
2011–12	1,348	58%	121	5%	198	9%	14	1%	4	0%	18	1%	23	1%	594	26%	2,320	9%
NORTH REGION																			
Bihar																			
2008–9*	382	27%	44	3%	52	4%	15	1%	5	0%	132	9%	0	0%	802	56%	1,432	11%
2011–12	630	31%	118	6%	267	13%	9	0%	22	1%	116	6%	0	0%	859	43%	2,021	8%
Chhattisgarh																			
2007–8	175	50%	42	12%	31	9%	11	3%	44	13%	4	1%	0	0%	40	12%	347	3%
2011–12	455	56%	38	5%	61	8%	21	3%	73	9%	8	1%	0	0%	157	19%	813	3%
Haryana																			
2007–8	NA	NA	NA	NA	NA	NA	NA	NA	NA	NA	NA	NA	NA	NA	NA	NA	NA	NA
2011–12	591	80%	24	3%	0	0%	10	1%	5	1%	0	0%	3	0%	107	14%	740	3%
Himachal Pradesh																			
2007–8	176	78%	8	4%	15	7%	1	0%	1	0%	0	0%	0	0%	25	11%	226	2%
2011–12	396	66%	6	1%	12	2%	0	0%	1	0%	3	0%	0	0%	185	31%	603	2%
Jharkhand																			
2007–8	164	42%	20	5%	139	36%	16	4%	15	4%	1	0%	0	0%	36	9%	391	3%
2011–12	449	53%	20	2%	136	16%	4	0%	84	10%	16	2%	1	0%	134	16%	844	3%
Madhya Pradesh																			
2007–8	409	38%	197	18%	50	5%	12	1%	249	23%	43	4%	0	0%	129	12%	1,089	8%
2011–12	944	51%	145	8%	164	9%	29	2%	291	16%	55	3%	1	0%	210	11%	1,839	7%
Punjab																			
2007–8	373	83%	3	1%	9	2%	0	0%	1	0%	2	0%	0	0%	61	14%	449	3%
2011–12	569	56%	15	1%	10	1%	25	2%	18	2%	0	0%	0	0%	376	37%	1,013	4%

(*Cont'd*)

TABLE 2.3 (Cont'd)

State and Year	Salaries		Supplies and Drugs		Major Works		Equipment		Incentives		Maintenance and Minor Works		Grant-in-aid		Others		Total	% against All States
	Exp	%	Exp	%	Exp	%	Exp	%	Exp	%	Exp	%	Exp	%	Exp	%	Exp	%
Rajasthan																		
2007–8	489	53%	24	3%	79	9%	1	0%	0	0%	13	1%	0	0%	314	34%	920	7%
2011–12	1,106	63%	58	3%	95	5%	22	1%	20	1%	12	1%	12	1%	443	25%	1,768	7%
Uttar Pradesh																		
2007–8	906	39%	106	5%	629	27%	5	0%	1	0%	78	3%	0	0%	598	26%	2,323	18%
2011–12	2,402	60%	166	4%	296	7%	2	0%	145	4%	45	1%	0	0%	952	24%	4,008	16%
Uttarakhand																		
2007–8	91	42%	7	3%	66	31%	2	1%	3	1%	8	4%	1	0%	37	17%	215	2%
2011–12	305	55%	10	2%	46	8%	5	1%	7	1%	8	1%	0	0%	176	32%	557	2%
Sub Total																		
2007–8	3,165	43%	451	6%	1,070	14%	63	1%	319	4%	281	4%	1	0%	2,042	28%	7,392	57%
2011–12	7,847	55%	600	4%	1,087	8%	127	1%	666	5%	263	2%	17	0%	3,599	25%	14,206	55%
SOUTH REGION																		
Andhra Pradesh																		
2007–8	845	56%	141	9%	28	2%	2	0%	117	8%	35	2%	66	4%	275	18%	1,509	12%
2011–12	1,634	65%	368	15%	65	3%	3	0%	105	4%	44	2%	63	2%	239	9%	2,521	10%
Karnataka																		
2007–8	463	50%	92	10%	27	3%	1	0%	100	11%	14	2%	36	4%	185	20%	918	7%
2011–12	907	64%	201	14%	36	3%	27	2%	50	4%	20	1%	46	3%	126	9%	1,413	5%

Kerala													
2007–8	NA NA	NA NA	NA NA	NA NA	NA NA	NA NA	NA NA	NA NA	NA NA	NA NA	NA NA	NA NA	NA NA
2011–12	NA NA	NA NA	NA NA	NA NA	NA NA	NA NA	NA NA	NA NA	NA NA	NA NA	NA NA	NA NA	NA NA
Tamil Nadu													
2007–8	597 44%	112 8%	16 1%	5 0%	30 2%	NA NA	47 3%	303 23%	NA NA	234 17%	NA NA	1,344 10%	
2011–12	1,301 46%	134 5%	86 3%	82 3%	39 1%	NA NA	55 2%	559 20%	NA NA	552 20%	NA NA	2,808 11%	
Sub Total													
2007–8	1,905 51%	345 9%	71 2%	8 0%	247 7%	NA NA	96 3%	405 11%	NA NA	694 18%	NA NA	3,771 29%	
2011–12	3,842 57%	703 10%	187 3%	112 2%	194 2%	NA NA	119 3%	668 10%	NA NA	917 14%	NA NA	6,742 26%	
All States													
2007–8	6,125 47%	945 7%	1,180 9%	79 1%	644 5%	389 3%	542 3%	3,116 4%				13,020 24%	100%
2011–12	14,138 55%	1,600 6%	1,561 6%	297 1%	887 3%	414 2%	1,083 4%	5,729 22%				25,709	100%

Source: For Goa and Maharashtra, information on state budgets is taken from the state budget books for 2011–12 and information on central contributions to state is taken from GOI. For Kerala and Punjab, information on state budgets for 2011–12 is taken from the RBI website and information on central contributions to state is taken from GOI. Such analysis for Kerala and Maharashtra is not available because the lump sum allocations made to the local bodies made it difficult to assess what the funds were spent upon. Overall, the analysis of state budgets showed the absence of any standardization of budget books in terms of subheads, language, and so on.

Notes: * Expenses are for 2008–9 as those for 2007–8 are not available.

Expenditures included under each of the detailed heads is given below:

a. *Salaries*: all salaries, contractual employee costs, and wages.

b. *Office expenses*: all costs related to office management and administration.

c. *Drugs and supplies*: all costs related to drugs, consumables, and supplies.

d. *Machinery and equipment*: all costs related to machines and equipment purchased, including vehicles other than maintenance.

(*Cont'd*)

TABLE 2.3 (Cont'd)

e. *Scholarships and stipends*: any cost provided to the staff or beneficiaries for pursuing academic studies.

f. *Major works*: all costs related to construction of new buildings.

g. *Maintenance and minor works*: all costs related to the maintenance of building, equipment, and vehicles and also minor works related to repair and refurbishment of the same.

h. *Grant-in-aid*: grant-in-aid provided to the other local government bodies (panchayats and zilla parishads).

i. *Compensation*: all costs incurred on ASHAs and other volunteers. This also includes incentives provided to clients for family planning, blood donation, and so on.

j. *Other works*: this covers any other costs including those of training, EMRI services, health camps, and so on.

Besides financial devolution, much of the quality of spending and outcomes is compromised on account of the archaic procedures and processes that govern financial releases and utilization at the central and state levels. As elaborated further ahead, until these structural issues are not comprehensively addressed, a mere increase in budgetary allocations will be inadequate.

Expenditure Management

Expenditure management involves a whole set of new issues: classification of funds, processes laid down for their release to implementing agencies, and auditing how funds are utilized. Government budgets at the central or state levels consist of two classifications: Plan and Non-Plan budgets; they include revenue and capital and the latter is nearly always under Plan. The central government collects its resources through a wide range of instruments: income tax, sales tax, excise, and custom duties. However, resource allocation and use make for a more complicated story. The structure of expenditures consists of interest liabilities, defence, administration, pensions, social and economic sectors, loans and advances, and others. Nearly 50 per cent of the central money just goes into paying interest liabilities and other commitments while another 30 per cent of central funds are for defence and subsidies for fertilizers, LPG cylinders, and the like. States tend to spend 30 per cent of their resources on economic sectors.

Resource Allocation and Utilization (First to Twelfth Plans)

The process of resource allocations among departments in the central government was a highly formal exercise.[44] With the abolition of the Planning Commission, the processes proposed for expenditure management are unclear. Up until 2015 when the NITI Aayog came into being, the process of fund allocation consisted of a sequence of states as under. At the start of every five-year plan period, the concerned ministries would constitute working groups consisting of subject experts. The Planning Commission in turn constituted a steering committee consisting of a wide range of experts, NGOs, activists, and academicians to reflect on the recommendations of the working groups. Inputs from these then fed into the sectoral plan that allocates resources scheme-wise, laying down priorities and indicating targets to be achieved at the end of the five-year period.

All sectoral plans had to be approved by the full Planning Commission chaired by the prime minister along with five other cabinet ministers and members of the Planning Commission. This is where the inter se priorities were determined and the political dimension of the exercise came into play. Informal discussions were held on the size of the plan and the thrust areas of the government. The plan would then be placed before the NDC that consisted of the chief ministers of all states. Once approved, the document would become the basis for making annual allocations to all departments and reviewing the progress of implementation.

Individual departments prepared their annual plans based on the funds allocated for the year. Every year the departments were told to prepare their plans as per need but invariably ended up with a ritualistic 10 per cent increase 'to absorb inflation'. Over the years, the annual plan formulation lost much of its importance. Despite the five-year allocation, the departments were never able to undertake advance planning to meet their actual requirements since every year the charade of vetting and 'fixing' the plan size would be played out, creating constant uncertainty.

Central budgets again have two components: funds to be spent centrally and those to be given as grants to states. The central components consist of procuring equipment and drugs to be supplied to the states and for the centre's own use, appointing personnel, and so on. For each of these sub-items, different committees are constituted and procedures laid down. For procurement, based on the bids received, the lowest tender is finalized by committees chaired by the Directorate General of Health Services (DGHS). If the tender is above a certain limit, the approval of the minister has to be obtained.

Issues related to the appointment of personnel are yet another time-consuming exercise. Any formal appointment has to be made by the Union Public Service Commission (UPSC) that takes close to three years for the recruitment process, by when most candidates (particularly the employable ones) take up other employment or leave the country. In fact, due to the recruitment policies, inflexibility in salary packages, and the inability to distinguish the really meritorious from the mediocre, the government does not attract the best talent. Moreover, the former prime minister Nehru himself was reported to have inspired the best to serve in premier institutes such as AIIMS and imbibed in them the value of public service and nation-building. Such recruitments are impossible now, bound as we are with procedures and quota considerations. Compounded with inordinate delays, government hospitals are the most affected with unfilled vacancies or persons of lesser experience being recruited. Besides, financial scrutiny for sanctioning posts is very tight and given after much haggling. Such tight controls on a sector dependent on human resources have been unproductive. And in order to cope with all these impediments in public employment, departments increasingly depend upon consultants appointed on an annual contract entailing trade-offs that urgently need attention.

Release of Funds

Release of funds to implementing agencies is a major challenge. At the beginning of the five-year plan period, every individual programme such as the NRHM, HIV/AIDS, mental health, and blindness control has to be approved by the Expenditure Finance Committee (EFC) chaired by the expenditure secretary. The EFC makes sure that the expenditure plans are in conformity with the funds allocated. A cabinet note is then prepared containing a detailed justification for the funds, the targets to be achieved, the strategies to be followed, and the funds required on an annual basis as well as comments, if any, of the related departments. This whole exercise can take anywhere between three months to a year or more. The process is the same for availing foreign grants for any of these programmes or any new scheme, and the same exercise has to be conducted before signing any agreement. New schemes invite greater scrutiny to ensure that financial implications for the future are within reasonable bounds. In fact, all new schemes require the explicit approval of the finance department, which again causes a lot of delay. For small schemes of less than Rs 0.5 billion, the secretary of the department is the approving authority as the chair of the Standing Finance Committee (SFC)—the representative of the finance department is also a member of this committee. Such delegation is of recent vintage and has helped speed up decision-making.

Despite all the elaborate approvals, the actual release of money to the concerned implementing authority is highly procedure-bound. As can be seen in Figure 2.1, every stage provides a scope for delay. It is because of this that field officers complain of budgets being received at the fag end of the year.

For every 'approved' item of expenditure, the file has to go with all the details of the scheme to the financial advisor (FA; who reports to the department secretary) as well as to the expenditure secretary in the finance department. At times, the FA can cause delays.

Any variation within an approved scheme requires financial approval contributing to further delays. In December, the revised estimates are fixed based on the actual expenditures incurred. But when there is a fiscal crisis, arbitrary cuts are imposed across the board on grounds of financial stringency, nullifying all the efforts made and approvals obtained to incur expenditures or place orders for supply of drugs or equipment.

If getting funds is one battle, spending them is another. The central government releases funds to the states and implementing agencies in four tranches at quarterly intervals. The first is released immediately after Parliament approves the budget. For releasing the second tranche in July, UCs of previous expenditures are insisted upon. Delay in the release of the second tranche is due to this insistence, often resulting in funds getting released only at the end of the year. Since rules require 'unspent funds' as on the last day of the financial year to be remitted to the treasury, much fudging is done to show utilization even when funds may have been

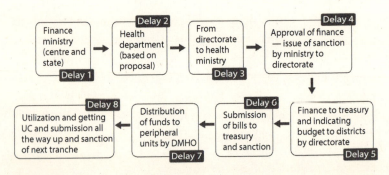

FIGURE 2.1 Financial Resource Flows
Source: Author.

received only on the last day. If that is not possible, much time is spent obtaining a revalidation from the finance department.

UCs are difficult to obtain, particularly from states or when the implementing agency is outside the government. Typically, social sector projects have small funds spread over several agencies and accounting heads. For example, if a professional organization is outsourced to undertake the procurement of drugs or equipment, a UC can be submitted only after the signed receipts from those to whom the goods have been delivered are submitted. These could run into hundreds if the consignees are below district levels. Likewise, the states also have to obtain UCs from all those units such as panchayats to whom small grants of Rs 10,000 are disbursed under the NRHM. The procedure is the same for NGOs. Such procedures affect implementation as neither the field agencies nor NGOs have the resilience to hold on for months.

For the second tranche of releases, the department has to also submit the audit statements for the releases made during the previous year. This is yet another problem. Thus, most of the time of the senior officials in the ministry is spent on managing the release of funds and chasing states and agencies for obtaining the UC and audit certificates. In the absence of such submissions, further releases are held up. Low releases or utilization in the month of December could then endanger the next year's outlay and so on, notwithstanding the allocations approved for the department for the five-year period.

Mostly, fiscal crisis is managed by imposing expenditure controls, not by improving resource mobilization. In health, this affects procedures such as the procurement of vital drugs. Non-supply of drugs to the field is often then managed by either administering half the dosage or giving drugs for a week instead of a month—at times leading to chances of drug resistance and poor patient management, and in the long run breaking the credibility of the public system.

In this complex process of releasing and utilizing funds, the attention paid to processes and UCs is disproportionately high, leaving little time for implementation and utilization. Reviews are focused on how much money has been spent, not on how many lives have been saved. Nobody, at any time, wonders how the programme is being implemented—whether drugs are reaching the facilities on time or funds are being released to the implementing agency; often this happens on the last day of the financial year. There is no effort to synchronize inputs that are critical for saving a life or to differentiate between critical programmes and the not-so-critical ones.

While the process of supplementary budgets provides flexibility for mid-course corrections, it also entails a state of continuous planning. Very often important activities as approved by Parliament are dropped halfway and the unimportant and less complicated ones get into the queue. In fact there is variation between budget estimates (BE), revenue estimates (RE) of December, and the actual FE that are available only in the following year or later. Besides, it is only at the FE stage that one knows what has actually been spent and on what. Until then, all releases are assumed as 'expenditures'. This is also a reason for the discrepancies between the 'expenditures' of the central government departments, which are releases, and the 'expenditures' of the state governments that are actual spends. The process of reconciliation can be quite problematic.

Weak Financial Oversight

Part of the problem mentioned in the preceding paragraphs is also due to the systemic deficiencies and lack of attention to financial oversight—the poor capacity to deal with financial matters both in the central ministry as well as in the states and districts. For example, in the absence of guidelines the financial administration of the NRHM was a virtual mess in 2009. The programme, handling an annual budget of Rs 200 billion, had one director—a relatively junior-level IAS officer in charge of finance and assisted by some consultants who were comparatively inexperienced in public finance. In contrast, NACO, with a budget of about Rs 12 billion, had a team of nearly 10 finance officers on deputation from government and three senior consultants with experience in public finance. In states the situation has been equally bad. For example, in Andhra Pradesh, prior to 2010, an accounts officer hired on a one-year contract managed the NRHM funds. Upon termination of his service, he took away the hard disk of the computer. As a result, today financial information for the earlier years is not available.

The replication of NACO's finance systems[45] was initiated in 2010 by bringing in a senior officer of the Indian Audit and Accounts Service (IAAS) as the director of finance. It is important that the finance department be made responsible for putting in place appropriate financing and audit systems, with accountability and oversight by third parties.

Allocation of resources, utilization in the manner prescribed, and accounting are all critical elements of expenditure management. But unfortunately, disproportionate attention is focused on accounting. Combined with the diffused accountability of the finance ministry in respect to achieving departmental goals, obtaining results is tough and most often the fault of non-implementation of a scheme or failure to achieve a target is entirely the responsibility of the department. As a result, nothing really ever gets done in the desired manner and speed, and if it does, the effort is monumental. The constant 'struggle' with the finance department wastes much time and energy, diverting from monitoring actual implementation. It can also be very frustrating as the attitude of finance is still colonial—treating every release as a favour and not a responsibility.

Until systems for public financing are reformed and timeliness ensured, there can be no improvement in the absorption or utilization of funds. It is time that the medium-term plans[46] are held as sacrosanct and releases made on a rolling basis. This is because the procedures for procurement of goods or services at the initial stages are time-intensive and require adherence to transparency necessitating public disclosures at every stage with the probability of a court stay at any time. Similarly, expenditures are at times lumpy when final payments for completion of a building or procurement of equipment or drugs are made. Therefore, a certain amount of automaticity should be ensured in the release of funds in keeping with the specific needs of a particular activity and the multiple levels and frequency of approvals should be reduced. Focus should instead shift on what has been achieved and how. Though efforts to address some of these issues by computerization have helped, they are inadequate. Computers cannot substitute the reforms required in expenditure management and audit processes. This is an issue of far-reaching importance and urgency, particularly as new actors are being made eligible for public funding.

Expenditure Management in States

The procedures for expenditure management are similar in the states too, only worse. The budget proposals from the directorates take half the year to reach the secretariat and get approvals from the finance department and actual releases from the district treasury take an equally long time, particularly in states that have a fiscal crisis. Grants received from the central government are diverted or their releases held up in the personal deposit (PD) account to show a better balance-of-payments position. There are instances when the finance department would approve the sanction orders and promptly call up the district treasury officer not to release the funds.

Even after the finance department's approval, there are delays in the release of orders to the directorate, requiring the directorate-level officers to lobby. The funds are released to the directorates that, in turn, release them to the districts. At the district level, another round of pleadings take place—this time with the district treasury officer who can reject the 'bill' for any reason, such as the bill number not written properly or the date not entered or the sanction not received by them from the finance department.

Formation of Societies

To circumvent these procedural delays, health societies were registered at the state and district levels. State health societies were constituted and funds released directly by the centre through account payee cheques, bypassing the state finance departments. This procedure ensured quicker utilization of funds, made the unspent funds non-lapsable, and provided flexibility in spending decisions. Subsequently, funds were released directly to the district health societies by e-transfer. There was a huge merit in this policy design. States' absorption trebled and since the funds were substantial, state governments also increased their health budgets.

Health societies provide a greater ease of operation. However, in the absence of rules and stringent oversight on a concurrent basis, the flexibility and autonomy provided to them could be misused. For this reason, as also the protests from states for bypassing them, in 2014 the finance ministry rescinded its earlier permissions to release funds directly to societies and brought back the 'treasury route'. It would have been more advisable if instead the long-winding procedures having the potential to delay at every stage had been rationalized and grant releases to states made conditional to putting in place rules and procedures and institutional capacities for financial and audit functions. Such systems and infrastructure are necessary to minimize the scope for siphoning off funds, misutilization and fraud, and systems of accountability.

Restoring the treasury route without resolving the basic reasons as to why social sectors looked at alternate mechanisms for financing in the first place has been a regressive step, taking the clock back. In placing discretion with an accounts clerk or a treasury officer without any accountability for the non-release of funds only encourage corrupt practices. Neither NGOs nor the government departments get funds in time and once again, in every state, funds are choked up and not reaching the implementation levels as in the pre-NRHM days. Once again the old problems of delayed release of funds, drug stock-outs, and suspension of implementation of activities have emerged.

The existing systems of resource-sharing are rigid and useful for accounting and auditing purposes but not amenable to development spending. Budgetary processes need to facilitate spending and measure efficiency in terms of process outcomes achieved and not just follow accounting principles.

Public–Private Partnerships

The concept of PPPs emerged in the 1990s. It has been defined as 'the combination of a public need with private capability and resources to create a market opportunity through which public need is met and profit is made'.[47] Multiple objectives drive PPPs. The term is misleading as it seeks to convey that there is an element of relational equality between the government and the private entity where each does something for the other to achieve a common good. In reality, it is simply the government procuring services or goods from private agencies.

PPPs in the context of health financing cost three times more than in government. When budgets are limited, diverting such funds to buy expensive care rather than the government building up its own capacity can be questionable. There are trade-offs that need to be carefully assessed on a case-to-case basis as a PPP for every intervention may not always be uniformly advantageous.

Besides, there are some prerequisites for realizing the full benefits of PPPs: availability of data and pricing information; the skill to negotiate to maximize gain and minimize risk; the ability to draft contracts that are enforceable and have adequate safeguards built in to penalize fraud and reduce risk; developed IT platforms to monitor against quality markers; and ensured institutional capacity to enforce contracts effectively so that the contractor does not cut corners, defraud, or provide poor quality. Such capacities are scarce at the district levels and below—levels where most PPPs are being rolled out.

Accordingly, including PPPs within the government financing systems would need reforms to enable making payments are as per the agreed schedules. Reneging on payments often undermine the system as the holding-out capacity of private agencies is time-sensitive. The absence of timely payment then often hurts the patients as the providers charge the patients or quote a higher price at the time of filing tenders to take care of such contingencies. In extreme cases they even stop provisioning of the service. The current system of running around finance departments and treasuries for approval of every bill will, therefore, not be workable.

In the absence of sound audit and accountability systems being institutionalized through the various levels of implementation, merely pushing PPPs can just become another way of 'privatizing profits and nationalizing losses' and a one-sided game with the private sector taking advantage of the loopholes most of the time and gaming the system. Overall, engaging with the private sector in the short run may be more expensive, but over time as knowledge is gained, and if institutional checks and balances are built in, efficiencies between both parties may kick in and even out.

Demand-side Financing

Insurance or demand-side financing works on the principle of cross-subsidization—mobilizing premiums from the healthy, young, and rich to spend on the poor, sick, and old. In India, social and private health insurance accounts for about 7.6 per cent of the total current health spending. The entry of health insurance was waiting to happen, given the chronically low levels of public spending trapped in a cycle of stagnation and the consequential emergence of a large network of private hospitals providing services on a fee-for-service basis. Since the cost of treating non-communicable diseases such as cancers or heart ailments is expensive, private expenditures have been very high. With a higher incidence of such expensive-to-treat non-communicable diseases, Kerala accounts for the highest per capita out-of-pocket expenditures of Rs 2,663, nearly 10 times more than public expenditure. In contrast, Bihar has a per capita private expenditure of Rs 420. The gap between states is a reflection of both demand and supply factors as well as the income elasticity of health expenditures. In his paper, Bhat[48] argues that private health expenditures as a percentage of per capita incomes increased from 2.7 during 1961–70 to 5.53 during 2001–2. During the decade 1991–2003, private health expenditures are reported to have grown at 10.88 per cent per annum in real terms while per capita incomes grew at 3.76 per cent per annum.

The government's response to this emerging crisis was initially indifferent and patchy, at times even incoherent and self-contradictory. Its response to addressing financial distress on account of medical care had a two-pronged approach: on the one hand, it invested in building health delivery infrastructure to provide free services and on the other, it launched the JSY in the 18 high-focus states. The JSY is a conditional cash-transfer scheme introduced in 2005 under which a cash incentive of Rs 1,400 is provided to women delivering in public hospitals.

In 2008, the Ministry of Labour launched the RSBY for all families of informal workers providing a risk protection of Rs 30,000 with the government paying the premium directly to the insurance company. On the other hand, the government allowed private commercial health insurance companies to set up shop and exempted insurance premium from tax. The emergence of insurance as a mode of demand-side financing was due to the convergence of several factors: demands for health services that were consequently pushing the already poor into greater impoverishment, pressure from private insurance companies to expand business, and the lobbying of private-sector corporate hospitals to increase utilization of their built-in capacity. Given this confluence of powerful interests, it was a matter of time before insurance against health risks began to gain traction, which it did with the establishment of the IRDA in 2000, giving rise to a new form of health financing in India.

By 2015, over 280 million people had some form of health security under four types of insurance programmes concurrently under implementation in India entailing a premium amount of about Rs 323 billion per annum (tax-based and out-of-pocket private):

(a) The Central Government Health Scheme (CGHS) under which all government employees drawing their salaries from the Consolidated Fund of India obtain total health cover for a nominal premium deducted at source from their salary bills.
(b) States having different schemes for their own employees in addition to their own tax-based insurance schemes aimed largely at those living below the poverty line.
(c) Implemented by the government of India (Ministry of Labour), the RSBY is a national health insurance scheme for those in the informal sector. At the same time, it also provides a health cover for the employees in the formal system.
(d) Private insurance where private individuals pay the premium for an assured sum.

In 2003, the Indian government launched a truncated universal health insurance scheme with a premium of Rs 365 on a 'one rupee a day' slogan. The scheme did not do well and was aborted. The first to scale a successful health insurance policy was Yeshasvini in Karnataka. Yeshasvini was an innovative scheme under which the Cooperative Department released the premium amount of Rs 20 per farmer member to a trust (chaired by the secretary of

TABLE 2.4a Government-sponsored Health Insurance Schemes

	RAS (Erstwhile Andhra Pradesh)	VAS (Karnataka)	CM Health Insurance (Tamil Nadu)	Yeshasvini (Karnataka)	RSBY (GOI)
Launched in	4/2007	2/2010	6/2009	2003	4/2008
Launching process	In a phased manner	In a phased manner	Big bang	Big bang	In a phased manner
Main population	State BPL (7 crore people)	State BPL (4.5 crore people). Recently included APL also (1.8 crore people)	State BPL + HHs with income < INR 72,000 pa + members of 26 welfare boards (3.6 crore people)	Members of cooperative society (0.3 crore people)	Central BPL. Other population groups, such as MGNREGS beneficiaries, construction workers, domestic workers, and so on (14.8 crore people)
Unit of enrolment	Family	Family	Family	Individual	Family
Enrolment process	Automatic	Automatic	Automatic	Active enrolment	Active enrolment
Premium collected from community	Free	Free for BPL; part payment for APL	Free	INR 210/individual/year	INR 30/family/year
Enrolment rate	100%	100%	100%	14% (30 lakh out of 2.2 crore—2014)	60%
Unit cost	INR 270/family	INR 200/family	INR 500/family	INR 350/individual	INR 400/family/year
Administrator of the scheme	Independent trust with > 150 staff members	Independent trust with TPA > 100 people	Dept. of Health	Independent trust	MOHFW

(Cont'd)

TABLE 2.4a (Cont'd)

	RAS (Erstwhile Andhra Pradesh)	VAS (Karnataka)	CM Health Insurance (Tamil Nadu)	Yeshasvini (Karnataka)	RSBY (GOI)
Role of the administrator	As detailed[1]	Idem + quality assurance provisions like death audits, grievance redressal mechanisms.	As detailed[2]	Idem	Formulating policies, developing packages and prices.
Insurer of the scheme	Erstwhile Govt. of Andhra Pradesh, now Dr. NTRVST★ in Andhra Pradesh and AHCT† in Telangana	Govt. of Karnataka	United India Insurance Company	Govt. of Karnataka	Insurance company
Benefit package	Secondary and tertiary care: 938 packages from 31 specialties	Tertiary care: 567 packages from 7 specialties	Secondary and tertiary care: 1,016 packages from 51 specialties	Secondary and tertiary care. Surgical procedures: 892 Excludes implants	Secondary care: 727 packages.
Upper limit for package	INR 200,000/family/year in AHCT in Telangana; INR 250,000/family/year in Dr. NTRVST in Andhra Pradesh	INR 150,000/family/year	INR 100,000/family/4 years	INR 200,000/individual/year	INR 30,000/family/year
Utilization rate	1.1/1,000/year	0.75/1,000/year	7.5[3]/1,000/year	NIL	18/1,000/year
Providers	Public = 97, Private = 352	Public = 24, Private = 120	Public = 56, Private = 636	Public = 29, Private = 421	Public = Nil, Private = > 3,000

	50 beds with infrastructure and HRH	50 beds with infrastructure and HRH	50 beds with infrastructure and HRH		10 beds
Eligibility criteria for empanelment					
Provider-payment mechanism	Case-based	Case-based	Case-based	Case-based	Case-based
Gatekeeping	Pre-authorization	Pre-authorization	Pre-authorization	Pre-authorization	Nil
Top five conditions	Oncology	Cardiac surgery	Orthopaedics	Gynaecology	Medical admissions
	Cardiac surgery	Oncology	Oncology	Ophthalmology	Cataract
	Poly trauma	Nephrology	Nephrology	Cardiac	Hysterectomy
	GU surgery	Neurology	ENT	General surgery	Delivery
	General surgery		Cardiac surgery		
OOP payments	Yes	NA	NA	Yes	Yes
Copayments	Nil	Yes for APL	Nil	Nil	Nil
Waiting time	Nil	Nil	Nil	Yes	Yes
Exclusion of conditions	Yes	Yes	Yes	Yes	Nil
Medical audits	Yes to some extent	Yes	Nil	Nil	Nil
Grievance redressal	Yes	Yes	Nil	Nil	Nil

[1] Formulating policies, IEC; managing contracts with hospitals; developing the packages and prices of the same; managing pre-authorization claims, reimbursements; and monitoring the scheme.

[2] Formulating policies, developing the packages and prices of the same, and monitoring the scheme.

[3] Preauths, not claims.

Notes: *Dr. NTR Vaidya Seva Trust.
†Aarogyasri Health Care Trust.

TABLE 2.4b
Other Health Insurance Schemes in the Country

State	Name of the Programme	Primary Care	Secondary Care	Tertiary Care	Maximum Benefit
Himachal Pradesh	Critical Care (RSBY Plus)	No	No	Yes	Rs 175,000
Meghalaya	Megha Health Insurance Scheme (MHIS)	Partial	Yes	Yes	Rs 160,000
Kerala	Comprehensive Health Insurance Scheme (RSBY-CHIS)	No	Yes	Yes	Rs 30,000 (RSBY) + Rs 70,000
Karnataka	Yeshasvini Cooperative Farmers Health Care Scheme	No	Yes	Yes	Rs 200,000
Chhattisgarh	Chief Minister Child Heart Protection Scheme	No	No	Yes	Rs 180,000
Chhattisgarh	Sanjeevani Kosh	No	No	Yes	Rs 300,000
Gujarat	Mukhyamantri Amrutam Yojana	No	Partly	Yes	Rs 200,000
Maharashtra	Rajiv Gandhi Jeevandayee Arogya Yojana	No	No	Yes	Rs 150,000

Source: NHA, September 2015.

cooperatives) on behalf of its members to pay for services against an assured sum of Rs 100,000 in accredited hospitals.[49] Meetings were organized with doctors, the benefit package designed, and rates fixed. Insurance was only for the members and solely for the purpose of surgeries. The response was positive and inspired many other variations in the country.

In 2007, Andhra Pradesh launched the RAS to provide risk protection against catastrophic expenditures that 'have the potential to wipe out life time savings of poor families'. The justification offered was that there was an effective demand for treatment of non-communicable and chronic diseases, low investment in public hospitals, and a burgeoning private sector that is unaffordable for most. Y. Rajasekhara Reddy, a doctor-turned-chief minister, is credited with the initiative and decision to establish the RAS.[50] Despite pressures from the ICICI to replicate their insurance scheme implemented in Assam,[51] the Yeshasvini model was adopted as a more feasible one in terms of design features.

Under this scheme, high-cost, low-volume procedures were to be covered for an assured sum of Rs 150,000 extendable to Rs 200,000 per person per year. Administered by a trust chaired by the chief minister, the package gradually expanded to 983 procedures covering tertiary and secondary care. The rates were fixed reportedly in consultation with some corporate hospitals and the CGHS and were uniformly applied in all hospitals whether they were located in Hyderabad or in districts or whether they had any accreditation or not.

In covering over 85 per cent of the population, the RAS was the first 'universal coverage' programme of sorts. The state government directly released the premium amount on behalf of all the 'below poverty line' citizens to the RAS trust. Keeping pace with the increased utilization, the premium nearly trebled from Rs 212 in 2007 to Rs 597 in 2013. In the initial years, 90 per cent of the payout went to private hospitals—in particular, the corporates based in Hyderabad. Reimbursement rates were also very generous. Stung by public criticism, efforts were made to expand coverage in government hospitals as well and government surgeons were incentivized with 30 per cent of the total value of the surgical procedures performed being paid to them as bonus. Many poor and not-so-poor benefited. The media was very enthusiastic about it and it was rumoured that this scheme influenced a 5 per cent swing in favour of the ruling party in the 2009 elections. Since what matters in politics is perception and the RAS generated an immediate feel-good reaction, it inspired half-a-dozen states to replicate it.

But there is a thin line between perception and reality. Several people have critiqued it as having provided a steady revenue stream strengthening the private corporate and medium-level hospitals without necessarily reducing health expenditures or improving health outcomes and benefits.[52]

While there are no systematic evaluations to assess the impact of the RAS, a recently conducted survey in Andhra Pradesh by Access International, covering 8,623 households, showed an overall reduction in out-of-pocket expenditure and increased hospitalization but a limited impact in reducing impoverishment or indebtedness among the two lowest quintile groups. For example, while per capita expenditures for inpatient treatment nearly trebled from Rs 391 in 2004 to Rs 1,083 (2012) for the poorest quintile, it was down to Rs 1,174 from Rs 1,819 for the fourth quintile group. Likewise, while the proportion of those incurring catastrophic expenditures more than doubled from 1.1 per cent to 2.8 per cent and 1.2 per cent to 3.4 per cent for the two lowest quintiles, the richer quintiles faced reductions. Such wide disparities are attributed to the concentration of half the accredited hospitals in seven districts (towns) that accounted for 48 per cent of the eligible hospitals and over 50 per cent of the claim reimbursement. Such gross deficiencies on the supply side made access difficult and unaffordable for those residing in backward districts, who are also likely to be poorer.

Secondly, 49 per cent of reimbursement was for cardiac, cancer, and kidney failure (38 per cent of patients or 0.5 per cent of the population), while the two bottom quintiles suffered impoverishment, premature mortality, and disability due to lower-respiratory infections, diarrhoeal diseases, TB, ischaemic heart diseases, and malaria—conditions eminently preventable and treatable with effective primary care. Besides, partaking of the RAS benefits implies forced hospitalization for outpatient care, increasing the risk of hospital-acquired infections and higher indirect expenditures that the poor cannot bear.

Thirdly, the primary healthcare system that the earlier Telugu Desam Party government accorded high priority to had all but collapsed, with the state consciously choosing to abandon primary care for universal coverage of a select set of tertiary and secondary care conditions. Among 19 major states, Andhra Pradesh incurred the lowest expenditure of central grants (NRHM and disease control programmes) in proportion to its total health spending during 2011—16 per cent against 31 per cent and 28 per cent by Maharashtra and Karnataka respectively. It was also the only state to slash its primary care budgets from 53 per cent to 46 per cent and allocate just 9 per cent for secondary care, down from 12 per cent during 2007–12. In comparison, the RAS was provided 23 per cent of the health budget for less than 1 per cent of the population (not necessarily poor) or 11.3 per cent of the total hospitalization.

The RAS is reportedly one of the better designed schemes in terms of the IT platforms it has established, enabling instant prior authorizations for surgeries and payments with minimum hassles for the patient. This is admirable but its important aspects such as pricing and quality are worrying. While the RAS has 150 people working in the head office, there are no chartered accountants or health economists. Prices are set by a committee of doctors in negotiation with the private sector—not necessarily based on unit-costing exercises or an understanding of input prices or standards of care to ensure value for money. Pricing is generous and costs are likely to escalate further, impinging on the fiscal space of the two new states of Telangana and Andhra Pradesh. The RAS reimbursement rates, say, for hysterectomy, laparoscopy, appendectomy, or coronary bypass, are higher when compared to the other schemes in the country. Further, package rates provide the scope for gaming the system. In the absence of standards to measure quality and regulations to control provider behaviour and fraud, perverse incentives are created, as reflected in unnecessary diagnostics, procedures, and surgeries.

Quality is understood in simplistic terms. The RAS teams inspect hospitals and list them. Only 18 of the hospitals have the slightly tougher National Accreditation Board for Hospitals and Healthcare Providers (NABH) accreditation. The more difficult but critical parameters such as readmission rates or hospital-acquired infection rates are not monitored and outcomes in terms of quality of life not measured.

Worse, the conflict of interest and the growing nexus between politics and the private sector with several instances of unreasonable price-fixing and empanelling undeserving hospitals have also created distortions that will be difficult to set right. It is not without reason that the chief minister chairs the trust, not a professional. Not unsurprisingly, the outgoing government enhanced the prices just before elections and the new government enhanced the package rates just after the elections. Thus, while primary care is weak, in the absence of regulations to control provider behaviour and the tendency to seek a specialist corporate-style hospital, the two states of Telangana and Andhra Pradesh are irrevocably on the high-cost path. They are riding a tiger they will find difficult to dismount.

The RSBY was yet another intervention that attracted attention for the wrong reasons. With an assured sum of Rs 30,000 for a family of five, the RSBY expanded at a breathtaking speed regardless of the quality of care being provided. States like Kerala that had a good public health infrastructure took full advantage of this scheme for providing financial-risk protection to its patients visiting the public hospitals while also providing a revenue stream for the cash-strapped facilities. However, the experience was poor in states with severe supply problems that resulted in low pre-qualifying criteria for empanelment at 10 beds. With such a condition, over 12,000 hospitals were empanelled by the end of 2014. A basic understanding of health economics is enough to know that 10 beds can never be economically viable for providing even a minimal quality of care. Here, too, it was the poor living in the backward regions who lost out. For example, Udaipur, a tribal district of Rajasthan, had just a hundred claims in 2012, while Haryana showed no interest in implementing it.

Due to the inclusion of all hospital services in the scheme, there was a substantial duplication of services. In other words, of the top-five conditions covered under the RSBY were deliveries and IOL cataract operations—services that the government had already budgeted to provide free-of-cost to the poor. This has only increased corruption as it is an open secret that most government doctors also own or work in private hospitals and, therefore, have serious conflicts of interest. C-sections and hysterectomies increased with no impact on outcomes. In other words, there was no concept of demarcating the government and private sector roles in a manner that could supplement, complement, and strengthen them. Instead, it was competition in non-level playing fields, arbitrated by a political system that colluded with the private sector to the disadvantage of the public sector. High prices were paid for low-quality products but since the payment delays were high, the well-performing hospitals opted out. It was a scheme that came to be known as 'for, by, and of the insurers'. The Ministry of Labour undertook a thorough evaluation in consultation with the states (See Table 2.4a). Before any action to rectify the issues could be taken, the scheme got transferred to the health ministry.

Without necessarily addressing design and incentive issues, the current government has increased the sum assured from Rs 30,000 to Rs 100,000. Combined with the fact that most corporate hospitals are facing a problem of underutilization of bed capacity, the provocation for trebling the assured amount seems driven by a desire to help the private sector as well as expand the scope of services to include those that go beyond secondary care.

Is Health Insurance the Way to Go?

With the current government increasing the FDI cap for insurance, the rapid financialization of the private medical industry and substantial interests in this form of financing taking deep roots is expected. The options to health insurance also seem to be getting restricted. Instead, what is being seriously considered is the adoption of the principles of insurance (distributing risk) but with premiums paid for, which is to be managed by the government by creating new institutional mechanisms like a government trust or authority, much like the RAS.

The NCMH report in 2005 suggested the establishment of a social health insurance corporation pooling in all the government-funded insurance programmes (CGHS, Employees State Insurance Scheme [ESIS], and UHS) to provide the necessary traction and also to avoid their fragmentation since consolidation would enhance market power. The NCMH model had a two-tiered level of services: a public-funded and administered primary care and a strong secondary care. While primary care was to be provided mainly by the public sector and a not-for-profit private sector, secondary care was to be provided by a network of hospitals competing with each other. Such a network approach was considered essential since private facilities and services at the sub-district levels are fragmented with substantial duplication. Most nursing homes, for example, provide treatment for minor ailments and reproductive care services. If a package can be guaranteed, then these facilities could enter into partnerships to ensure all the required services included in the package are made available. Here, too, it was envisioned that the government would address at least 50 per cent of the demand. Institutionally, the NCMH recommended the establishment of authorities at the district and state levels with technical capacity to negotiate and purchase services. At the central (apex) level, it was recommended that an institutional mechanism be established to act as a reinsurer, along the lines prevalent in Chile and the National Bank for Agriculture and Rural Development (NABARD) nearer home. It was also proposed that such a mechanism be named the Social Health Insurance Corporation.

The undue focus on primary care was largely justified on two grounds and one consideration. Since tertiary care addresses 1–2 per cent of hospitalization, a strong primary healthcare system could, on the one hand, avert disease by promoting healthy lifestyles and timely diagnosis, and on the other hand ensure that patients go to higher facilities only on referral. The consideration was containing costs and making it sustainable.

The HLEG suggested a similar set-up but also advocated for networks providing a single window—primary to tertiary care—argued on the principle of continuum of care and payment systems that incentivize prevention. This was along the lines of managed care in the US where hospitals and providers form networks and provide a one-window solution to all the health needs of an individual. Under this model there is one key provider who owns or, on franchise model, develops a network of providers to provide services to their clients as per a negotiated fee structure.

The managed care model attracted attention as, in order to contain costs, it encouraged preventive health and early diagnosis and exercised a tight control on provider fees. Yet experience and data shows that costs have not been contained and it was also felt that the very sick and high-risk patients were not treated or did not get any attention. In the Indian context, this model was considered inadvisable due to the apprehension that the corporate sector could use its financial muscle to strengthen its hold on primary, secondary, and tertiary sector, which could over time fragment the health care system into monopoly chains.

Another solution offered by the HLEG to contain costs was changing the form of payment from fee-for-service to capitated payment systems as is being done in Thailand. This is an important recommendation and had also been made by the NCMH, but only for mandatory services to be provided in primary-care settings. For capitation, it is essential to have clarity on the schedule of benefits and the cost of provisioning them. In Thailand, the capitation amount was based on historical spending at the district level and below as the government is the only provider.

In India, not only is the public sector a small partner but the pricing in the private sector is also extremely varied, making any such aggregation of prices impossible. Besides, neither the public nor the private sector provides the full complement of services that constitute primary care. This, then, needs to be defined and unit-costing of those services worked out to understand the full implications for the government before it commits to make capitation payments. However, the more immediate reasons for not considering capitation are that it is a management challenge and also needs a far greater outlay of resources besides information, data for monitoring, and enforcement capacity.

Interest in health insurance emerged once again with the new BJP government flagging the National Health Assurance Mission (NHAM) as one of its important policy initiatives. In 2015, the RSBY was transferred to the health ministry from the Ministry of Labour, which is bound to facilitate better coordination and some adherence to quality and standards of care. An expert group was constituted in July 2014 to submit a blueprint of how an NHAM can be implemented. This report laid bare the deficiencies in the current system and the patchy research and scanty evidence available, making it difficult to provide more precise implications for government finances. It highlighted the immediate need to establish a national health assurance authority; a trust to implement the financing of the NHAM; a benefit package that consists of a comprehensive set of primary healthcare to be provided by a restructured primary healthcare system in the public sector, including the charitable NGO sector where desirable; secondary care providing assured hospitalization for Rs 50,000 and outpatient treatment in public hospitals; and tertiary care limited to heart, paediatric surgeries, cancers, and emergency care with private participation to supplement government efforts. A 15-year time frame was indicated for its full realization as the barrier to the NHAM is not money but human resources and infrastructure. We estimated a requirement of over Rs 180 billion per annum with the premium for 60 per cent of the population being paid by the government. Several preparatory steps to be taken in a sequential manner were detailed. Given the extensive caveats and riders, it was clear that India was not ready to implement the plan as proposed and it is feared that the usual rough-and-ready approach may be taken that is bound to entail adverse consequences in future. The government continues to be in denial of the problems it needs to resolve and refuses to build in the capacity and resilience required for the long haul.

The reason for such pessimism stems from several apprehensions. First, India has not carried out its due diligence. Its refusal to regulate and its inability to enforce even the minimal regulations that exist is a kind of subsidy to the private sector to thrive in these imperfect markets. Pushing health insurance without laying down standards, pricing, quality parameters, monitoring systems, and supervisory controls and grievance redressal systems can only be suicidal in the long run. It is pertinent to note that the US, despite having a strong legal architecture covering some of these aspects, is unable to cope with the adverse consequences of commercial insurance in health on access and the cost of care.

Second, there are serious supply-side deficiencies that have to be addressed in the first instance. In more than half the country there are no facilities to provide even a limited benefit package of services in the public or the private sector. And if quality parameters are any consideration, applying even the minimal quality indicators can result in a majority of the hospitals losing their eligibility. So even to form the network model as is being proposed, there is an initial need to invest heavily in building up the required infrastructure. In the absence of such capital investment, it is the city-based middle classes that will benefit leaving the larger majority of the population with a 'notional coverage', since absence of access due to distance will be a major barrier. In the short and medium terms, health insurance in such a dysfunctional system will widen disparities and enhance inequity. It is precisely for this reason that most countries, namely the US, the UK, Thailand, and Brazil predicated universal insurance on capital investments in building up the delivery system.

Third, the manner in which health insurance has evolved as of now, primary care and all preventive health is being undermined, which in the long run will make the system unsustainable.

Fourth, health insurance in India is highly fragmented. Harmonization of at least the tax-based schemes could give greater leverage to governments to get better-quality services at lower costs.

Fifth, the payment system—whether tax-funded or private, out-of-pocket—is based on fee-for-service that is inherently inflationary. Therefore, several insurance schemes have come up with package rates, but then over time this, too, has not succeeded due to the large-scale gaming of the system.

Sixth, in providing a cap to the amounts that are reimbursable in cases like cancer—where the treatment pathways have a certain extent of uncertainty—can result in the treatment being left halfway if the patient is unable to afford the expenses beyond the insured amount. For this reason, it is believed that capping does not guarantee quality of the outcomes.

Seventh, in the existing tax-based insurance models the risk is totally borne by the government with nothing shouldered by either the provider or the user, creating scope for inefficiencies to creep in, thereby making it unsustainable in the long run, more so since there are no regulations, weak redressal systems, and corruption. Risk must be borne by all stakeholders to ensure no misuse or overuse. Free service has resulted in the overuse of services. It should not mean a non-payment where one does not share even a small portion of the premium or pay a part of the whole cost. Such behavioural characteristics are important issues that should be carefully studied and designed in such a manner that the policy is both sustainable as well as equitable.

Eighth, the current system that has a mix of payment systems—fee-for-service and third-party insurance—provides scope for increasing prices. It is for this reason that government should be the sole payer. In mixed systems hospital managers and providers have the choice to opt out if the rates being paid are not up to their expectations and resort to fee-for-service or provide substandard care to the 'insured' against those paying fee for service. Conversely, when the reimbursement rates are high, the tendency is to accord priority to those 'covered' under insurance at the risk of ignoring those not covered. In a single-payer system where the government is the sole monopoly purchaser, such a choice to opt out is not available, forcing greater compliance to both standards and prices.

Ninth, and most importantly, are the moral considerations as well as cost-effectiveness. The question starts with what defines the ethical obligation of the state. When funds are fungible, does it seem right to spend vast amounts treating a terminal case of cancer or conducting a bypass when large numbers of people are dying for want of a simple bed net that costs two US dollars? Which is more cost-effective: ensuring that a case of diarrhoea does not occur by promoting access to uncontaminated tap water and proper waste disposal and sewerage systems or providing cashless treatment to multiple episodes of diarrhoea? In rural Bihar, only about 2.3 per cent of the households have access to tap water, more than two-thirds of the population have no access to toilets, and over a third of the children are malnourished. Infectious diseases continue to take a toll on the lives of earning members in poor families with devastating impacts at the household level. Breakdown of family systems, agricultural stress resulting in migration and unplanned growth of slums, unemployment, and rising food prices are contributing to alcoholism, drug addictions, and chronic diseases such as diabetes and blood pressure, calling for strategies to prevent and manage stress. These multifactorial aspects of poverty and want need to be addressed in the first instance.

The principal issue, then, is not the question of insurance coverage but sequencing public investment focused on strengthening a comprehensive and wider definition of primary care on the one hand and supply-side deficiencies on the other by rapidly building public hospitals and incentivizing the not-for-profit[53] and non-commercial enterprises to supplement government efforts.

Basically, the bottom line is that tax-based spending in India should be increased substantially to make the system more affordable and equitable. As insurance schemes—private or tax-based—provide partial coverage against an assured sum and are based on fee-for-service systems of payment, India's financing system is considered to be regressive, iniquitous, and highly inflationary. Increased resources should be accompanied by a strategy of how, and on what to spend these additional resources.

India traverses different time spans and epidemiological profiles and thus cannot have one national design. Different strategies need to be applied as relevant to different areas. But in all this, it is essential that the Indian state continues to focus on public goods being made universally accessible in the first instance. That itself is a huge challenge that the state has to address without losing any time.

The Way Forward

There are clearly three concerns that typify India's current status: (a) improving the health standards of its people, (b) reducing disparities and promoting equity among states and social groups, and (c) increasing the fiscal space to achieve them. It is in this context that two definitions need to be recalled. One by Peter Heller who defined fiscal space as 'the availability of budgetary room that allows a government to provide resources for a given desired purpose without any prejudice to the sustainability of a government's financial position', and the second by the WHO that defined an equitable health system as providing 'access to key promotive, preventive, curative and rehabilitative health interventions for all at an affordable cost'.[54]

Increased Public Spending

For achieving the first two objectives of improving health and reducing disparities, government spending has to be increased appreciably. During the Twelfth Five Year Plan, barely 53 per cent of the Rs 2.68 trillion provision has been allocated, even while expanding the number of schemes to be implemented. Besides, central transfers should be based on having all states achieve a minimum level of well-being and quality of life. There is also a need to revamp the system of delivery of services and build the health system on the strong foundations of primary care. It is more cost-effective in the long run than a system that is treatment-oriented. In Chapter 6, these two ideas have been elaborated.

Strengthening the delivery system would require diverting 1 to 1.5 per cent of the GDP towards capital investment to build the required infrastructure. Another 1 per cent may be needed to provide free universal access to comprehensive primary care, secondary care, and a select set of tertiary conditions, namely heart, cancers, trauma, emergencies, and paediatric surgeries for 60 per cent of the population. If all care for all people is to be free, a doubling of resources would be needed. Since medical care alone does not make people healthy or productive, what is equally important is to invest in universal access to social determinants. This will need an upfront investment of at least 2 per cent of the GDP, mainly for the infrastructure related to public sanitation and waste disposal, tap water and nutrition, and housing.

Such increases should be accompanied by systemic reforms on issues related to expenditure management where the allocation of funds is seamless and not tyrannized by 'governatalism'. Flexibilities should be built in to address unpredictabilities and public health emergencies such as swine flu or H1N1 that come unannounced. Such predictability and uninterrupted flow of funds will be key issues in working with private hospitals on a legal agreement basis. In situations of fiscal stringency, priority is accorded to fulfilling legal contracts at the cost of the more critical activities related to infectious diseases. Emphasis should be placed on prioritization of interventions as well as on equity and quality.

Sourcing Funds: Increasing Fiscal Space

Despite the constant call for increasing health budgets, they remain stubbornly the same. This is due to the structure of public financing that gives little room for dramatic increases. India's tax-to-GDP ratio is low at 17.24 per cent (2012) as compared to the UK or Canada where it is over 30 per cent. Of this, 10.14 per cent is of the central government. Second, it follows that the central government's revenue expenditure-to-GDP ratio is about 15 per cent. Of this, only about 25 per cent is available for developmental expenditure, out of which 5 per cent is earmarked for health. Third, it should concern the health sector that two-thirds of the disease burden and infrastructure deficit is in states that have low per capita incomes. In 2011–12, Bihar and Uttar Pradesh had a per capita income of Rs 13,178 and Rs 18,249 respectively as compared to Gujarat and Haryana where it was four times more at Rs 57,508 and Rs 62,927 respectively.[55]

In such a scenario, increases for health and social determinants by three to four times would require a radical restructuring of the budget—reprioritizing its spending and raising resources by hiking revenue to GDP to at least 20 per cent. This would require a range of policies: reducing taxes foregone; expanding the tax base; improving collections by reducing corruption and tax evasion; levying surcharges on 'unhealthy' products such as liquor, tobacco, fast foods, and medical tourism[56] (the consumption for which is higher among the better-off sections); increasing wealth and property taxes; and perhaps also exploring copayment from the 40 per cent better-off sections of the population.

Managing Public Funds: Improving Systems and Accountability

One reason for the poor absorption of funds and utilization of budgets is explained previously. Structural reform in the manner of decentralization of funds to district levels and below is required. This, then, could imply having a rolling budget and releases made in two tranches with a review after the third tranche. Systems for a measure of automaticity and timeliness of releases could be incorporated so that the implementation of the activity does not suffer at any cost.

In the years to come, districts will emerge as the units of health action. Decentralization to the district level should be in tandem with the capacity to discharge responsibilities in a cost-conscious manner and in sync with the national goals. Constituting special financial authorities at the district level for purchasing services, procurement of goods, and making payments to service providers with trained professionals is required as against the present arrangement of clerks. In other words, the purchasing function needs to be separated from the administrative. Computerization of accounts and designing reporting formats as well as having supervisory teams to make random checks and inspections would be needed. The finance systems of releases, utilization, and auditing need to be restructured accordingly.

Payment Systems

The structure of incentives and mode of payment of service providers have a profound effect on the overall productivity levels. Should providers be paid a monthly salary or should they be paid based on their performance during that month? Fixed salaries are believed to be not motivating enough to do more than the minimum. Pay-for-performance, on the other hand, incentivizes providers to do more than necessary at times. India's experience is mixed. Salaries have been found to be dampening but then there are institutes like AIIMS where doctors as salaried employees are comparably productive. Under pay-for-performance, the volume of work is seen to be more but it does not necessarily guarantee quality of outcomes. The surgeon is paid for the surgery even if they botch it up and the patient does not survive.

The third is a mix of two. A base salary is paid and further topping is based on performance. It is similar to what the general practitioners in the UK follow with the difference that additional earnings are calibrated based not on the quantity of work but on the outcomes achieved. Payment systems influence provider behaviour and, thereby, outcomes. We need to experiment and model these different payment systems to see what works best in the Indian context.

Role of the Private Sector

Julian Hart[57] refers to the phenomenon of the 'inverse care law' that 'relentlessly subordinates human values to pursuit of profit' by providing more care and consultation time to those with the ability to pay and less to those who have a higher need. We see this in India where areas inhabited by the poor who suffer from diseases caused due to malnutrition or lack of safe water and hygiene and with a low paying capacity are the least preferred for investment, creating inequities and wide regional disparities in access.

Unlike other sectors, the health sector is characterized by extensive market failures. Distortions are created by barriers to entry (as only the accredited can provide services) or the asymmetry of information and the consequential inability of the patient to objectively evaluate medical advice that could well be tainted by commercial considerations. Misrepresentations and conflicts of interest dot the present-day landscape of the medical industry, heightening the acute vulnerability of patients to exploitation. Strong psychological predispositions of trust in a particular doctor or a provider's motives for personal gain neutralize competition or choice, controlling prices or the rational distribution of resources. Besides, public goods such as immunization or antenatal care services are neglected by markets on grounds of non-profitability, making public policy intervention an imperative and public spending a necessity.

But then, political and economic compulsions are such that the private sector cannot be wished away. There are several areas in which the private sector is more efficient and also cheaper. These strengths ought to be leveraged for public good. Public policy in India falls short in not defining these strengths and utilizing them with appropriate incentives.

In the geographically challenged areas where even the government finds it difficult to function (close to 200 districts), it needs to come up with financial packages to either establish government facilities or incentivize the not-for-profit sector and social enterprises to set up facilities and provide a market for them over the medium term. Whatever be the policy, supply deficiencies need to be addressed in the first instance before setting out for universal coverage.

Financing of health is at the centre of the health system and is a critical pillar on which it rests. Attention to its reform and restructuring is vital for achieving health system goals. It has been said that '[e]conomics is the study of choice. It does not tell us what to choose. It only helps us understand the consequences of our choices.'[58] If this is indeed true, then it is time that our economists, whose advice our political leaders depend upon, bring out clearly the economic consequences of neglecting health.

Notes and References

1. Charu C. Garg and Anup K. Karan, 'Health and Millennium Development Goal 1: Reducing Out-of-Pocket Expenditures to Reduce Income Poverty—Evidence from India', Working Paper 15 (New Delhi: Institute for Human Development, 2005).
2. As per the NSSO survey report (60th round).
3. Sakthivel Selvaraj and Anup K. Karan, 2012, 'Why Publicly-financed Health Insurance Schemes are Ineffective in Providing Financial Risk Protection', *Economic & Political Weekly*, 47(11).
4. Renu Shahrawat and Krishna D. Rao, 2011, 'Insured yet Vulnerable: Out-of-Pocket Payments and India's Poor', *Health Policy and Planning*, 27(12): 213–21, DOI:10.1093/heapol/czr029.
5. As per the NSSO survey (71st round), 2014.
6. Selvaraj and Karan, 'Why Publicly-financed Health Insurance Schemes are Ineffective'.
7. M. Govinda Rao, *Inter-State Equalization of Health Expenditures in Indian Union* (New Delhi: National Institute of Public Finance and Policy, 2008).
8. Otto Niemeyer's report quoted in B.P.R. Vithal and M.L. Sastry, *Fiscal Federalism in India* (New Delhi: Oxford University Press, 2001).
9. Ministry of Finance, *Report of the Sixth Finance Commission* (New Delhi: GOI, 1973).
10. Ministry of Finance, *Report of the Seventh Finance Commission* (New Delhi: GOI, 1978).
11. Rao, *Inter-State Equalization of Health Expenditures*.
12. As per the Ministry of Finance, GOI, 2010.
13. Vithal and Sastry, *Fiscal Federalism in India*, p. 148.

14. The divisible pool consists of the gross tax revenue collections of the centre excluding the revenue from cesses and surcharges and the cost of collecting taxes.
15. As per the NITI Aayog, GOI, 2015.
16. Reportedly, 12 per cent of absenteeism among industrial labour is on account of ill health.
17. Anita Rath, 2013, 'Growing Centralization of Social Sector Policies in India', Special Article, *Economic & Political Weekly,* 48(4).
18. Rath, 'Growing Centralization of Social Sector Policies in India'.
19. The NDC is chaired by the prime minister and all state chief ministers are its members.
20. *Report of the National Commission on Macroeconomics and Health* (New Delhi: MOHFW, GOI, 2005).
21. Ramesh Bhat and Nishant Jain, 2006. 'Analysis of Public and Private Healthcare Expenditures', *Economic and Political Weekly*, 41(1): 57–68.
22. Planning Commission, *Faster, More Inclusive and Sustainable Growth*, Twelfth Five Year Plan Report, Vol. II (New Delhi: SAGE, 2013).
23. *Indian Public Finance Statistics, 2013–14* (New Delhi: Department of Economic Affairs, Ministry of Finance, GOI, 2014).
24. Planning Commission, *Faster, More Inclusive and Sustainable Growth*.
25. Much of the analysis regarding interstate comparison detailed in this chapter was done by me for the Fourteenth FC, background paper through the Centre for Economic and Social Studies, 2013. See also National Health Systems Resource Centre, 2016, 'National Health Accounts Estimates for India (2013–14)', MOHFW, GOI.
26. RBI, 2016, Statement 27: Expenditure on Medical and Public Health and Family Welfare—as Ratio to Aggregate Expenditure.
27. RBI, Statement 42: Expenditure on Medical and Public Health and Family Welfare—as Ratio to Aggregate Expenditure.
28. 'The IMF merely conditioned reduction in the deficits. There was no condition that social sector spending should be reduced. The government chose to adopt an easy way because social sector spending did not have a political constituency.' Private communication with Govinda Rao in 2015.
29. As per the NSSO, Survey on Morbidity and Health Care (60th round), 2004–5.
30. All in current prices as of 2013.
31. The existing facilities are calculated at 50 per cent of the amount required for new facilities.

32. As per the Department of Health, MOHFW. The Planning Commission has estimated an expenditure of Rs 661.27 billion in the chapter on Health in the Twelfth Five Year Plan.
33. Gayatri K., 'District Level NRHM Funds Flow and Expenditures: Sub National Evidence from the State of Karnataka', Working Paper 278 (Institute for Social and Economic Change, 2012).
34. M. Govinda Rao and Mita Choudhury, 'Health Care Financing Reforms in India', Working Paper No. 2012–100 (New Delhi: NIPFP, 2012).
35. The RSBY, drinking water, sanitation, the ICDS, and mid-day meals together took the total spending to 1.94 per cent of the GDP. See Planning Commission, *Faster, More Inclusive and Sustainable Growth*.
36. Background Paper for 14th FC, CESS, 2013.
37. This analysis was undertaken for the Fourteenth FC.
38. It is a matter of grave concern that this was an enormously difficult task on account of the fragmentation of data between budget, society grants, and the like. The data sets of the central government and states do not match, though both claimed sourcing from audited figures—the central government invariably showing higher expenditures than states. In all cases we adopted the state figures that had the 'approval' of the concerned secretary. Many states (Assam, Haryana, and Kerala) had difficulties in understanding and analysing budget documents.
39. All in current prices.
40. The spending for Kerala was constructed by triangulating data. Since one-third of the budget is devolved to local bodies, the spending on primary care, in particular, may not be accurate. Though more work is needed, it does not change the assertion that the state has been withdrawing from the health sector in recent years. A document of the Kerala government shows the figure of spending on primary care to be 35 per cent (State Plan for Health, Government of Kerala, unpublished).
41. National Sample Survey, India: Household Consumer Expenditure (68th round), July 2011–June 2012, NSSO, GOI.
42. This is the most unfortunate aspect of cutting the fiscal deficit. Rather than resorting to mechanical cuts activity-wise across the board, a 10 per cent cut can be strategized in such a way that at least life-saving activities are not disrupted and people do not have to suffer.

43. In fact, for years NRHM funds were unauthorizedly diverted to the Aarogyasri Trust.
44. There is no clarity about post-2017 when the Twelfth Plan comes to an end. As of now, departments have been asked to prepare their plans until 2020 in order to synchronize the plan cycles with that of the Finance Commission, which is a good development.
45. With only 5 per cent of the NRHM funds, NACO had over a dozen people professionally trained in finance, on deputation, directly reporting to the director general, an additional secretary-level officer. Besides, NACO made it conditional for states to appoint a joint director on deputation in order to receive central grants worth more than Rs 1 billion. Additionally, it issued detailed operational guidelines on financing and audit, had finance officers at state and district levels trained periodically, and got accounts computerized and audit reports correlated before the release of grants, thereby resulting in higher absorption of funds.
46. It is unclear what will happen now with the disbandment of the Planning Commission.
47. A. Venkat Raman and J.W. Björkman, *Public-Private Partnerships in Health Care in India: Lessons for Developing Countries* (New Delhi: Routledge, 2009), p. 3.
48. Bhat and Jain, 'Analysis of Public and Private Healthcare Expenditures'.
49. My batchmate A. Ramaswamy was the secretary of cooperatives who designed this scheme with Devi Shetty. Shetty set up the Narayana Hrudayalaya with the mission of offering low-cost but high-quality treatment. But he did not find any takers for it. After meeting Ramaswamy, he went around the government offices for financial support to meet the costs of surgery.
50. I attended some of the meetings and could see Reddy's concern at the growing number of requests for financial aid for medical treatment from the CM Relief Fund. This was one of the reasons that drove him to innovate the RAS, in addition to the lobbying by the corporate industry that had made substantial investments in Hyderabad.
51. The whole population was 'insured' and the government made a lump-sum payment to the ICICI. Reports pointed towards huge profits made by the ICICI as the citizens were unaware of their entitlements and the documentation and procedures for getting reimbursement for their expenditures were impossible barriers to cross.

52. Sujatha Rao, 'For Public Health as Political Priority', *The Hindu*, 13 October 2014, available at http://www.thehindu.com/opinion/lead/for-public-health-as-political-priority/article6493944.ece (accessed on 23 June 2016).
53. I make a distinction between the private sector that invests in health for making profits as opposed to that private sector that makes profits and ploughs it back to improving patient care and reduce cost.
54. Rao and Choudhury, 'Health Care Financing Reforms in India'.
55. As per the 2004–5 prices, financial statistics, GOI, 2011–12.
56. Levying such cesses does not guarantee the availability of funds to the health sector. Such earmarked cesses should also have an automaticity of transfer to the concerned agency. Rs 14,000 billion of cesses collected over the past couple of years are reportedly lying unutilized (*The Times of India*, 26 December 2015).
57. Hart, *The Political Economy of Health Care*.
58. Todd G. Buchholz, *New Ideas from Dead Economists: An Introduction to Modern Economic Thought* (London: Penguin, 2007).

CHAPTER THREE

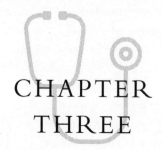

Governance: Impacting the Health System

The Setting

In February 2014, the union health secretary of the government of India was peremptorily transferred to another ministry. The same year in September, the cabinet minister for health was divested of his charge and given another portfolio. These shifts would have gone unnoticed but for the suddenness and so soon after their appointments. Also rumours (no one can ever know the reasons behind such exercise of administrative discretion) pointed to the hand of powerful interests that controlled the MCI.

Since 2000, the MCI witnessed stormy times when the duly elected council along with its president was set aside by a Supreme Court order. The council was restored in 2009 but again dissolved in April 2010 by a government ordinance. The elected council came back in 2013. A PIL[1] filed in the Supreme Court in 2014 alleged that the elections were rigged and nominees of Ketan Desai, the president of the MCI during 1998–2010, were appointed in all key positions of the MCI. Ketan Desai is not a member of the MCI. To nominate someone for the MCI membership, the Indian government has to issue a gazette notification. The notification for Desai is held up for want of advice of the law ministry as there are two cases of corruption against him awaiting trial in the courts of law. In the meanwhile, on 8 March 2016, taking suo moto cognizance of the functioning of the MCI, the parliamentary standing committee (PSC) on health submitted a scathing report to the two houses of Parliament. The PSC found severe deficiencies in the working of the MCI that ought to have resulted in its being set aside. Instead, the government appointed a three-member committee consisting of the vice chairperson and the secretary of the NITI Aayog and a senior official of the PMO. This committee was set up to once again examine options for action against the MCI. Sharp editorials in leading newspapers were written alongside letters from concerned citizens imploring the government to act. On 2 May 2016, the Supreme Court used its powers to constitute a three-member committee consisting of Justice Lodha, the former CAG, and the former MCI president to oversee the functioning of the MCI for a year or until such time as the government comes up with the proposal to revamp the MCI. That the MCI continues to function undeterred despite all this is a telling comment.

What is more disturbing is that even while the government's high-level committee (HLC) was submitting its report on revamping the MCI, the government sought to appoint the board members of the National Board of Education (NBE). It was alleged in a newspaper article that several members of the NBE were 'connected' to Ketan Desai and its president was a clinician of a little-known hospital in Gujarat with unknown academic credentials.[2] The NBE was established by a government order in 1975 for standardizing postgraduate medical education and conduct of examinations, giving rise to conflicts of jurisdiction between the board and the MCI on matters related to accrediting the diplomas awarded by the board. This conflict remains unresolved to this day. A part of the reform process of the MCI was to, inter alia, address these issues of jurisdiction as well.

What, then, does this say of governance in India, provoking a related question: can the health sector be insulated from the overall system of governance that prevails at any given time? It is widely believed that when systems of governance stifle questions related to propriety or encourage deviation from rules and procedures, it reflects three critical fault lines in its structure:

a) weakening of political resilience in face of pressures for differential treatment from politically powerful individuals and sectional interests to subvert rule-based systems, b) the diminished status of constitutional authorities in checking the abuse of power, and c) the moral void and corruption where political expediency seems to override adherence to the rule of law, public welfare, or propriety. These observations apply to the health sector as well.

If poor implementation of rules or weak functioning of regulatory bodies comprise one set of issues, yet another viewpoint of having no regulations or laws in the first place[3] also prevails and seems to be gaining ground. Such a viewpoint explains to a large extent the persistent silence on enacting laws to regulate healthcare providers, to the extent of caving in to the objections of the corporate sector, avoiding the appointment of an ombudsman for disposing peoples' grievances and instead supporting a governance model based on the principle of laissez-faire[4] irrespective of the welfare implications this may entail. I have heard several politicians and lawmakers explain away such abdication of their fundamental duty of enacting and enforcing laws on grounds of not allowing the re-entry of an 'inspector raj'. The same argument is also used to explain the overall reluctance to regulate the private sector in health, or the disinclination to implement laws related to tobacco control, or undertaking the revamp of the MCI despite the Supreme Court calling it a 'den of corruption'.

But then the state in India appearing to be under siege by sectional interests that have taken control of the instruments of governance is no exception. We find evidence of such situations in other countries as well, for instance, the influence of pharmaceutical companies, insurance companies, and medical associations over health policy in the US. Or, to cite yet another example, the ascending influence of the neo-liberal ideology on the privatization of the National Health Service in the UK.

Understanding health governance in India through the lens of the underlying factors mentioned previously help in differentiating between what is said and what is actually done and the shrinking space for independent action by any individual officer or a well-meaning minister. An understanding of these nuances then help explain the large governance deficit prevailing in the health sector, for example, the high levels of absenteeism in public facilities, lack of accountability of doctors (in public or private practice) for treatment outcomes, failure to procure and deliver drugs as well as essential consumables in a timely fashion or of good quality, and so on.

The Governance Deficit

The three key stakeholders in the health sector are the government, healthcare service providers, and patients or communities. The relative influence and levels of interaction among these three determine the nature of governance: open and democratic as against closed and inward-looking. In view of the extensive market failures in the health sector, the government's interventionist role assumes significance. Distortions creep in when governments let their guard down and allow regulatory oversight to favour individuals or interest groups for political expediency.

Given the centrality of governance in the realization of health goals, the World Bank and the WHO flagged 'good governance' as a critical determinant for health outcomes. Good governance improves efficiencies when based on rules, regulations, processes, and procedures that are transparent and fairly implemented. They become useful yardsticks to measure impact and explain failure.

This chapter is divided into two parts. The first part briefly touches upon the ideas that influenced the formulation of policies and the price of neglecting the importance of knowledge and evidence. It describes the functioning of the institutions of governance such as the parliamentarians, ministers, administrators, and technical bureaucracies that wield real power, exercise leadership, and oversee the implementation of policies.

The second part moves on to addressing critical challenges facing governance in health that need to be addressed for achieving positive health outcomes.

Source of Ideas: Influencing Health Policy

The exhaustive Joseph Bhore report of 1946 was a classic then and continues to be one even now. Bhore's blueprint for action has not been implemented on grounds of financial stringency.

Over the years, India's health system evolved without a clear direction and in an ad hoc fashion. Ideas and strategies emerged from the two dozen committees that the government periodically constituted to examine a wide array of issues that emerged from time to time—be it the revamping of the delivery system, reforming medical education, prioritization of comprehensive primary care, or ensuring access to essential drugs. In addition to these expert-committee reports, two national health policies were issued in 1983 and 2002. Besides, there were the plan documents, working-group reports prepared for the five-year plans, and the recommendations of the Central Council of Health and Family Welfare (CCHFW).[5] Of late, the Confederation of Indian Industry (CII) and the Federation of Indian Chambers of Commerce and Industry (FICCI) have emerged as thought leaders advocating policy reform that will benefit the industry. International accounting and consulting firms such as McKinsey, Ernst & Young, and PricewaterhouseCoopers (PWC) have followed in their wake and are rapidly occupying the policy space that once belonged to public health professionals, academicians, and activists in proposing strategies and designing policy interventions.

Donor organizations have been major stimulants of ideas and influencers in agenda-setting and determining priorities. At the time of Independence, India had no institutional capacity to handle many of the challenges it faced. The Rockefeller Foundation and the WHO helped India build capacity to reduce the incidence of malaria and eradicate smallpox. Over the years, donors, as a group, have exercised enormous influence on setting the agenda and shaping policy. For example, the imprint of the WHO, other UN organizations, bilateral and multilateral donors, and private foundations like the BMGF, the Rockefeller Foundation, and international summits is discernible on major policy initiatives of the central government. These initiatives include the abandoning of the Alma-Ata vision for comprehensive primary care and instead adopting the selective PHC approach[6] based on the verticalization of disease control programmes, prioritizing the polio pulse campaigns in 1995 over the country's universal immunization programme launched by Rajiv Gandhi as a technology mission in the late 1980s, closing down of three government vaccine-manufacturing facilities, according priority attention to HIV/AIDS control over other infectious diseases, broadening of family planning into a more comprehensive reproductive and child health (RCH) strategy, shift in policy attention to universal health coverage, increasing use of insurance and encouraging PPPs, the overriding focus on—and priority attention to—achieving the Millennium Development Goals (MDG), and so on.

Though donor organizations account for less than 2 per cent of the total health spending, their influence on setting priorities that are more aligned to international agendas has always been disproportionately high and continues to be so—the most recent example being the rapid expansion of the immunization programme or the swift adoption of policies that favour the privatization of the health sector. Apart from the commitments made under international agreements, the research, evidence, and high level of advocacy through thought leaders and the media that donors mobilize are the major reasons for such influence. While at one level such donor assistance helped build critical research and implementation capacity, at another level it fostered a culture of dependency and a loss of self-confidence.[7]

If low budgets increased vulnerability to donor grants, low investment in research and research institutions constrained India's ability to provide a counter narrative. As a consequence, public health experts rooted in Indian reality were often overlooked and many times health strategies shifted away from socialized medicine to biotechnological solutions, with one ear constantly seeking validation for actions and policies from foreign agencies. Not pursuing the objective of building a comprehensive primary healthcare system or the failure to prioritize the goal to eradicate polio and expand universal access to immunization within a comprehensive child health strategy as was done by Thailand or Sri Lanka, are two examples to illustrate this point.

The two times when India did decide to go with its own data and context, the outcomes exceeded expectations, be it the reversing of the HIV/AIDS epidemic when we went against international opinion and focused on prevention of high-risk behaviour, or overruling the initial reservations of donors to invest on community-based workers to revitalize primary healthcare under the NRHM. Again, as I can recall, the World Bank was keen on scaling up conventional surgery in outdoor camps under the National Programme for Control of Blindness, but we insisted on shifting to hospital-based IOL surgeries as it had better outcomes.

Despite such evidence of positive outcomes of policies grounded in our own realities, the influence of foreign advice or NRIs continues to dominate. The purport of this is not to sound xenophobic but to emphasize the point that health—unlike, say, IT—is grounded in social contexts. Examining evidence from within India and having policies that fit within the local contexts is more important than blindly transplanting ideas, suggestions, and policies of other countries without a critical evaluation of the feasibility of adapting them to the prevailing situations.

Need for Investing in Research

In systems of good governance, policymaking is participatory and inclusive. Research institutions are fostered to produce the required evidence and key stakeholders taken into confidence. This was seen when crafting policies for HIV/AIDS, where key population groups most vulnerable to HIV were included in all policymaking and implementation bodies at the NACO and state levels. But this was a rare example. By and large, policymakers have displayed a lack of conviction for such inclusion of the target groups and have neglected fostering and nurturing research institutions. Costly mistakes have been, and are still being, made such as disbanding malaria workers with multipurpose workers, reducing vigil and community-monitoring, neglecting primary care, opening up health markets without putting in place appropriate regulations,[8] prioritizing immunization over comprehensive child health or tackling the causal determinants of infectious diseases, and so on.

In the absence of research institutions, health ministries at the state and central levels largely depend upon consultative mechanisms to identify priorities and design interventions. Committees and expert groups are normally multidisciplinary consisting of academicians, activists, and experts. However, the limitation of this strategy is that the same individuals revolve around as members in all the committees.[9] Critics are sidelined rather than consulted for obtaining a consensus, giving rise to needless acrimony, suspicion, and litigation. At the state levels, even such limited engagement is halting with most policy being dictated by the department officers, politicians, lobbies, or individual doctors wired to the political party in power. Thus, for a large democratic and epidemiologically diverse country like India, participation in policymaking is confined to small groups of individuals and a few research institutions. Limited engagement robs policymaking of examining alternatives. Several public health experts, for example, believe that technological solutions like vaccines cannot substitute public health action and investments for building capacity for the same.

It is also not unusual for critical decisions to be taken hastily or even 'arbitrarily' at times. For example, in India a secretary is empowered to introduce a new vaccine, albeit on the advice of 'experts'. In a country like the US, however, such a decision would take over three years after complying with the processes laid down. The US constitutes technical committees and holds consultations with a range of people representing government agencies; health-related professional organizations and foundations; consumer bodies; and experts in infectious diseases, paediatrics, internal medicine, family medicine, virology, immunology, public health, preventive medicine, vaccine research and policy, economics and cost-effectiveness, geography, race and ethnicity, sex, disability, and so on. In all such committees membership is only for US nationals, a no-conflict-of-interest policy is strictly enforced, and all meetings are open to the public. In India, we have yet to establish a credible surveillance system for tracking child morbidity. In the absence of reliable data, we are dependent upon data provided by donors or donor-funded research.

Policymaking in the real world is not a straight path based on reason and data. It is often a sum of several distal factors related to the political economy such as the relative role and influence of stakeholders, strength and rigour of domestic data and research, political and administrative leadership's ability to take independent decisions, and the extent of transparency and public disclosure in policymaking.

Institutional Systems

The Indian Constitution lays down the norms, principles, and the institutional structures for governance—parliament, judiciary, permanent bureaucracy and the media—that together impact policy formulation profoundly. These institutions symbolize political equality, the rule of law, stability in governance, and freedom of expression and speech.

In such a framework, policymaking is not only complex but also highly dispersed over a number of institutional players such as the several parliamentary committees, the cabinet, the health ministry, the PMO, the Planning Commission, and other informal but powered groupings like the NAC or the Economic Advisory Council (during the UPA rule). Besides these bodies, there are also other constitutional entities like the CAG, the Central Vigilance Commissioner (CVC), and the hierarchy of courts and state governments. In addition to these, policy formulation also involves consultation with other related departments like finance, law, and so on as well as regulatory bodies like the MCI and groups outside the formal system—namely informal professional

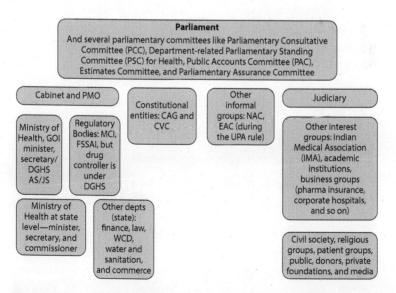

FIGURE 3.1 System of Health Governance in India
Source: Author

bodies like the IMA, academic institutions, business interests such as pharma companies, medical devices and insurance companies, corporate hospital chains, civil society, religious groups, patient groups, general public, international donors, private foundations, and the media.

Each constituent represents varied interests, biases, and influences that contribute to setting the agenda, formulating or stalling policymaking, influencing the nature and content of the policy, and shaping the character of its implementation, at times with no accountability to the final outcomes. In fact, such a system blurs accountability, contributes to delays in decision-making, diffuses ownership, and shifts responsibility.

As per business rules that govern work distribution among different ministries, the health ministry is expected to formulate the health policy and implement it. While doing so, it has no formal control over the direct causal determinants of disease—water, sanitation, nutrition, or environmental hygiene. Similarly, four ministries[10] adjudicate on matters related to drugs though the issue of affordable access to good-quality drugs has a direct bearing on health outcomes.

The key then lies in laying systems that ensure coordination and foster participation and an ethos of sharing responsibility. India has singularly failed in this regard. For over four decades and despite a plethora of joint letters between the secretaries of women and child welfare and health, it has been a herculean task to have the two front-line functionaries—the anganwadi worker and the ANM—work together. The NRHM has, however, sought to address this issue somewhat.

Multiplicity of institutions makes the policymaking process more arduous since coordination or convergence is difficult to ensure, especially in strictly hierarchical systems of governance as in India. A well-formulated policy involves consultations with interest groups for identifying key issues, formulating the design features, sequencing of implementation, mobilizing resources, and obtaining approvals of competent authorities that include the Planning Commission,[11] the finance departments, and the cabinet.

Structures of Governance

Parliament

Constitutionally, Parliament lays down policy and approves the budgets to be spent by the ministry and its constituents. It enforces accountability and oversight through its various subcommittees. The PSC is the most important body as it scrutinizes and approves the ministry's proposals for grants and critically reviews the implementation of programmes and policies and makes the bureaucracy accountable. There are times when an assertive PSC calls for frequent meetings and tends to 'interfere' with the functioning of policymaking which is the sole prerogative of the minister.

The PAC is chaired by a Member of Parliament (MP) from the main opposition party and is often considered to be the most powerful in making the government accountable for the utilization of money allocated to it. Its principal function is to scrutinize the audit reports of the ministry submitted by the controller of audit. The audit process is quite exhaustive. The final report is presented after several rounds of consultations with the concerned ministry that is given an opportunity to submit records and evidence to clarify or correct observations. Therefore, the report before the PAC is normally an agreed-upon document, making it more difficult to explain the omissions to the committee. This system of oversight, however, is flawed as the gap between the conduct of audit and actual scrutiny by the PAC could be as long as three years or more. Such a time lag makes it problematic to fix accountability as during this time period, the concerned officers may demit office, be transferred, or the policy context may change.

Rarely do these committees debate on larger issues such as the kind of health system India needs or introspect on the lack of regulation in this sector—an important omission given the fact that Parliament's fundamental role is to make laws and allocate resources to enhance public welfare and ensure their implementation. Lawmaking is arduous and it takes a minimum of two to four years on an average for a law to be enacted.

The most significant contribution of these committees is the reports they submit to Parliament after examining any legislation that the ministry may propose or on any issue of public importance.

These reports are often exhaustive, very well-researched, and balanced. The fault line in our system of governance is the absence of any accountability of the ministry to report action taken on recommendations made within a strict time limit. In the absence of such conventions and requirements, PSC reports could be waiting for action in the ministry for years. Parliamentary committees are valuable institutions and need to be strengthened by instituting mechanisms that help MPs understand key issues and provide guidance.

While Parliament cannot stop a policy from being formulated, the concerns of its committees are often taken into consideration. They have the ability to call attention to serious issues like their report recommending a revamp of the MCI or the drug regulator. They can also stall or delay policies they are not supportive of as, for example, in the case of the health ministry's initiative to introduce a graduate doctor (BSc in community health) in the sub-centre (see Box 3.1).

Ministry of Health

The health ministry has three centres of power and decision-making: the minister, the secretary as the administrative head, and the director general (DG) of health services as head of technical matters advising the secretary and the minister. While the minister is a politician, the secretary is a permanent civil servant, and the DG is invariably a medical doctor of the Central Health Service (CHS). Barring slight modifications, a similar structure of policy-making works at the state level too. This hierarchical structure and the staid, conservative culture provide predictability and stability. However, the scope for innovation is limited and changes, if any, are slow.

Ministers

As professional politicians, the health ministers are expected to provide the leadership for all health action. Health is not a much-sought-after ministry as it has measly resources, poor policy attention, and low priority in the eyes of the prime minister. This became evident when the coalition 'compulsions' of the NDA and

Box 3.1 Policy for Creating a Cadre of Doctor-Assistants

In 2010, the minister of health proposed the creation of a cadre of a three-year trained doctor stationed exclusively in sub-centres for every 5,000 people. The idea was prompted by the general reluctance of doctors to work in rural areas due to various reasons such as lack of professional growth, low salaries, poor working conditions, and urban orientation. To lend credibility and stature, the course was to be designed, accredited, and regulated by the MCI. This proposal was bitterly opposed by the IMA on specious grounds of providing substandard care to rural populations. Their argument carried no credibility as most private practice in rural areas is dependent upon referrals from untrained rural medical practitioners. The availability of a trained and qualified 'doctor' at the periphery would have reduced such referrals. The financial stakes were high.

On 12 April 2010, the MCI submitted the proposal to institute a degree of bachelor of rural healthcare to be conducted by the medical college attached to a district hospital and affiliated to the local university. An expert committee was constituted to examine it. The proposal was discussed on 31 May 2010 and on 25 June 2010 and approved by the minister on 5 July 2010. As observed on file (10 September 2010), approval of the CCHFW and all state chief ministers was also obtained by the minister. As the idea gained momentum, the IMA lobbied with MPs and the PSC swung into action to 'nip the proposal in the bud'. The PSC, in fact, had no jurisdiction to 'interfere' in this matter that was still 'work under progress'.[12] There was also an element of conflict of interest as some MPs were members of the IMA. On 24 November 2010, the prime minister held a review meeting in which the ministry was advised to drop the proposal and 'not perpetuate a dual system of healthcare'.

What makes this case interesting is that in the real world even a cabinet minister's policymaking space or a decision that may have the approval of relevant bodies or arrived at after extensive deliberations with related stakeholders can be so easily challenged by external institutions that have no direct responsibility to deliver services but have the power to stall and delay.

Source: Author

the UPA I led to bartering the health ministry in lieu of political support from the Pattali Makkal Katchi (PMK)—a small party of Tamil Nadu that had about six MPs. Consequently, from 1999 to 2009 the ministry was under the PMK, except for two years when the mantle passed on to BJP ministers. Neither of the first two ministers of the PMK (1999–2002) had any experience of governance at any level when they took over. A popular film star from the BJP succeeded them for a few months, followed by another high-profile minister under whose stewardship the ministry, for the first time after a decade, provided a semblance of governance and leadership to the health sector.

Under UPA I the health ministry was once again handed over to the PMK. Anbumani Ramadoss, the son of the founder of the party, learnt on the job rapidly and rose to become one of the effective health ministers India has had. Under him, the NRHM was introduced and scaled up, NACO revitalized, and the health profile within and outside India elevated.

Under UPA II, a very senior Congress leader was made the health minister. During his five-year stewardship of the ministry, he provided political leadership on issues of the ordinance setting aside the MCI's governing body, the long-pending legislations related to regulating private providers and clinical establishments and organ donation, the regulation of clinical trials, and conducting one common entrance examination for admission to medical colleges. He also focused on strengthening the public sector as the primary vehicle for health service delivery to the poor against the subtle pressures and overtures of the Planning Commission to privatize, finalizing the contracts and starting work on the six AIIMS-like institutions that had been tossing about since 2003 when the project was mooted, and so on. It is another matter that some of these important policy initiatives could not fructify[13] and little progress may have been achieved on any transformative reforms such as greater decentralization and involvement of the states, or providing autonomy to institutions by professionalizing their management, or revamping medical and nursing education and the regulatory councils, and a host of other issues.

Unlike most countries, ministers in India do not hold themselves accountable to the sector as a whole but only to the government-funded programmes, excluding the private sector from government oversight.

Likewise, hardly any leadership has been provided to expand and strengthen institutional development or take hard decisions to enforce discipline. Barring the first few decades, few institutions have been established in the last three decades. The focus has always been on medical education—not so much to improve but to sanction colleges or approve plans for undertaking civil works in the medical colleges.

At the state level, the attention of health ministers has been disproportionately focused on procurement and transfer of doctors and nurses. Most have sought to maintain status quo and been wary of fundamental changes, discouraged out-of-the-box thinking or radical solutions, and by and large followed the mantra of 'let sleeping dogs lie'.

While the health sector has been privatized by default, the ministers have also been relatively uninvolved in other developments in the field of drugs or technology, introduction of health insurance policies, or issuing of financial incentives to private providers—developments that have a profound impact on the nature of the health system. Nor have they taken proactive interest in ensuring the implementation of the social determinants that have a direct bearing on health outcomes. This is partly because of the fragmented nature of governance in India and in part due to the lack of an appreciation of the complexities of the health sector.[14]

Secretaries

In the system of governance laid down by the Constitution, the council of ministers is assisted by an executive consisting of the permanent civil service. Thus, the minister who is a politician functions through the bureaucracy that is headed by the secretary, who is responsible for providing policy advice to the minister, preparing briefs for the cabinet, formulating and implementing policy decisions, and defending the government policy in all parliamentary subcommittees. All along, the secretary functions on behalf of the minister but within and in accordance with the legal framework and principles laid down in the Constitution.

A second important function of the secretary is monitoring the various policies under implementation and giving guidance, resolving issues, and providing direction. This is critical as that which gets measured and flagged as important is what gets implemented. And when such monitoring includes travelling to states and the field, it is even more effective as it helps narrow the gap between the thoughts and ideas of the centre and the actual situation on the ground. Unfortunately, such field-level monitoring is becoming increasingly rare at the central and state levels. This distancing in part explains the several instances of policies and guidelines going beyond the levels of comprehension of ordinary district- and block-level medical officers and their capacity to implement.

Over the years, the institution of bureaucracy is beginning to show signs of weakening. With the emergence of interest groups, policy inputs are increasingly being sourced from 'extra-constitutional authorities', party intellectuals, lobbyists, or advisors such as their personal secretaries. As these groups are not accountable for the advice they render, the process of policymaking is becoming messy with the civil service losing its relational power with the ministers.[15] Under the Modi government, this aspect has been strengthened further as evidenced by, for example, the constitution of a committee consisting of three non-health persons—two from the NITI Aayog—and the additional secretary in the PMO to prepare the architecture of the MCI!

Policymaking at the state levels is, however, relatively easier and is dependent on the trust quotient between the secretary and the chief minister, who has the decisive voice. If that is high, decisions can be taken quickly and implemented with speed since the systems at the state level are less rigid and formal when compared to the central level.

Another critical aspect of governance is related to human resource management, such as posting of officers in the health ministry, record-maintenance systems, and documentation that help in keeping institutional memory that is necessary for continuity and stability of policies and reducing ad hocism. These aspects are also experiencing a strain. For example, given the growing complexity of the health sector, it would stand to reason that officers on deputation from the state government to the central health ministry have prior experience of the sector. Yet in my time as secretary, I witnessed officers with substantial experience of having worked in the health sector at the state level being randomly posted to other ministries such as Information and Broadcasting, textiles, Department of Personnel and Training (DoPT), and so on. These ministries did not require the skills these officers possessed, whereas the health ministry desperately needed them to implement the flagship programmes. Instead the health ministry would routinely be offered officers from the telecom department. For instance, it was hard to fathom the logic behind how a telecom engineer with no exposure to social issues and with the experience of having worked only in a telecom company could help rebuild the architecture of a battered health system.

Thus, the time has come to weigh merit and knowledge besides seniority in the deployment of officers to leadership positions. The administrative structure needs to be modernized to bring in greater professionalism and accountability on lines suggested in the various well-documented reports of the administrative commissions. Good governance is reflected most in systems' ability to foster a transparent system of reward and punishment and of promotions and postings, or of reviewing the impact of the officers' actions or omissions on the sector/policy or institution.

Contemporary principles of cadre management, appropriate placement of officers in accordance with their domain knowledge, and forward planning for building future leaders in key sectors need to be introduced. In other words, for example, the DoPT must have a system of spotting a potential list of half a dozen officers having the interest and aptitude for the health and education sectors as the future secretaries of health in 2025 and should be nurtured by exposure to these sectors from today. Thailand has such a nurturing policy for building leadership among the health professionals. The assumption that anyone can do any job is flawed and outdated. But it continues despite the fact that every sector today has multifarious demands and senior officers need to be more than just good officers.

Directorate General of Health Service (DGHS)

For technical matters, the DGHS, which is an attached office, assists the ministry. All senior posts in the DGHS belong to the CHS that is a 5,000-strong cadre. The CHS has four sub-cadres: public health, medical education, specialists, and non-specialists. As doctors, they are initially posted to the health facilities and hospitals owned by the central government and public health institutions like the National Tuberculosis Institute and the National Institute of Communicable Diseases where they gain exposure to field conditions, while the non-specialists work in the various CGHS facilities.

A majority of the CHS officers, however, could have worked all their life in Delhi-based hospitals with no experience of working in district hospitals or primary health facilities. Besides, the posting of technical officers also often does not nurture specialization in any particular area. Similar to IAS officers, they, too, could be rotating between different jobs that could range from being the doctor in charge of the airport health facility, to working in a leprosy unit and then be shifted to be in charge of immunization. With no system of training or service requirements upon entering government service to do so, the CHS officers virtually learn on the job. Not much has been invested on exposing them to training and specializing in international and national policies, nor are they sent abroad to study and acquire new skills. In other words, the technical skills are not utilized optimally.

In Thailand, for instance, a three-year service in provincial hospitals is a mandatory requirement for every doctor entering government service. This systemic weakness in the DGHS cadre management is responsible for the gradual decline of the institution with many of its functions being slowly taken over by the ministry, ranging from disease control programmes to the CGHS. This infirmity was known and recognized by several expert committees that suggested the revival of the Indian Medical Service. The reorganization[16] report and the NCMH (2005) strongly recommended the creation of the post of one more DG for public health based on open selection. None of these reports was ever considered or acted upon. Instead 12 posts of additional DG of the rank of additional secretary were created and the status quo strictly maintained. The DGHS is an important institution that needs to be revamped and reorganized to be able to provide critical advice to the ministry on areas that need new competencies such as health financing, costing, hospital management, and so on.

Judiciary and Media

The role of the judiciary and the media in the governance of the health sector has been profound. Among several other things, the media can be credited for helping the government in reducing stigma and discrimination against people infected with HIV/AIDS. It has also raised public awareness against Section 377 of the IPC that makes homosexuality an offence.

Similarly, judicial pronouncements disallowing multinational companies to extend their patent over life-saving drugs, ordering the illegality of Section 377, pushing the government to introduce treatment for HIV patients, and so on have impacted government policy. However, judicial interference as seen from the spate of judgments on admission of candidates into medical colleges, individual service matters, and the long-winding procedures with multiple courts having powers of adjudication on the same matter have undoubtedly affected governance.

But there have been times when court judgments have also diluted the government's capacity to govern and bring order on matters of great public importance, for example, the extremely important issue related to the National Entrance Examination Test (NEET). It was an attempt to control the commercialization of medical education in the country and promote merit. This was to be followed by an exit examination[17] that would have put pressure on medical colleges to abide by standards. Enforcement of an entry and exit examination would have taken the wind out of the sails of private colleges charging high capitation fees without necessarily providing quality education. This was not to be. The judgment striking down NEET on grounds that the MCI had no jurisdiction was unfortunate since the MCI is fully empowered to conduct such examinations and lay down any criteria required to ensure standards (see Box 3.2).

Box 3.2 NEET

In accordance with a direction to the MCI to investigate a media report of June 2009 stating that two well-known medical colleges were charging illegal fees, the three-member investigation team reported upon the travails of students—having to travel long distances, taking over 35 entrance tests for 412 colleges, overlapping examination dates, insufficient time for preparation, expenses, and so on—making it necessary to have one National Entrance Examination Test (NEET). The concept of entrance tests started with AIIMS, followed by some government and private colleges. Many states admitted students based on their class XII marks. As per a 1984 Supreme Court judgment, all government colleges were directed to set aside 30 per cent seats (later reduced to 15 per cent) for open admission on an all-India basis, giving birth to the annually held All India Pre-Medical Test (AIPMT).

In August 2009, the proposal for conducting one national examination was referred to the states for their views. In the meanwhile, a writ petition was filed in the Supreme Court for a single test, pursuant of which the MCI sent a proposal for consideration in February 2010 that got the minister's approval. In December 2010, the MCI issued a notification to conduct a common National Eligibility Cum Entrance Test (NEET) subjecting all admissions, even those under quota, to the ranking obtained in the examination. In light of some initial apprehensions, the MCI also revised the proposal to ensure that in adhering to merit, policies related to affirmative action that states extended for students from rural areas or backward communities would not in any way be compromised with.

Thus, with a view to standardize the process of admissions, reduce auctioning of medical seats, and get better-quality students to enter the profession, the MOHFW, in November 2011, approved the proposal for a fair and transparent selection based on merit and the concept of a single entrance test. But this decision was implemented only in May 2013. Ninety thousand students took the examination. However, in response to a PIL filed by 103 private medical colleges, a three-judge bench of the Supreme Court stayed the test on 18 July 2013—a day before Chief Justice Atlamas Kabir demitted office—on the grounds that the MCI had no jurisdiction to conduct such an examination. The judgment was delivered with one dissenting note. The government of India appealed against this order.

The NEET, however, continued to be held for the all-India seats and those states and private colleges that opted to use this list for their admissions. Recently on 11 April 2016, a five-judge bench of the Supreme Court admitted that its earlier order on NEET was faulty and recalled the 2013 judgment. As a special case, it permitted the national test to be held in two phases for the current year—one on 1 May and the next on July 24. This order invited adverse reactions from the media and several states, namely Tamil Nadu that, by law, has no entrance tests.

In response to the media hype and reservations expressed by some states that a centralized examination conducted by the CBSE would be disadvantageous to the students from rural areas who, by implication, had a lower standard of education, the government, on 24 May 2016, issued an ordinance making admissions through the NEET ranking only for the management quota of private colleges. States were also given the option to adopt the NEET ranking for admission to the government medical colleges and for filling the government quota in private colleges. This ordinance will last for a one-year period.

The three reasons that have compelled the instituting of NEET are: multiple examinations often held on overlapping dates; rampant malpractice in admissions where merit is of little consequence; and the abysmally poor standards of knowledge, particularly in science subjects, largely reflective of the mediocre standards of the country's high-school education system. The bottom line is that medical profession is a tough one that deals with human lives and is dependent on doctors' knowledge and basic competencies. Thus it is important to ensure that standards are not diluted for any reasons. The government should instead focus on improving the standards of science education in high schools—public and private—an area that is neglected by our politicians. A high-standard examination for NEET will compel state governments to focus on high-school education. NEET will, therefore, have a beneficial spillover effect. Yet, as seen from above, policy changes that affect commercial interests are difficult. Seven years on, there is still no political will to provide a fair opportunity for merit and standards in the medical profession.

Source: Author.

The judiciary and the media have a critical role to play in safeguarding patient interests and in making the government, the providers of care, and the private sector as such accountable to patient welfare. These are the only institutions with that capacity.

Need for Institutional Reform

The current system of policymaking at the centre, or for that matter the states as well, is systemically flawed as key policymakers could have weak domain knowledge of the subjects they are to make policies upon, a situation that is further exacerbated by instability in tenures. For example, during the period from 2011 to 2016, there have been six health secretaries. Over the years, the health ministry has also developed the culture of 'a closed system',[18] partly on account of the rapid developments in its external environment outpacing its capacity to respond to, and cope with, them. This has affected agenda-setting and policies continue to be formulated with little discussion and unreliable data.[19] When pushed, the tendency is to either 'leave it to the states'—which in the immediate term implies abdication since the states' capacity to plan, analyse, and design policy is limited and weak—or to postpone indefinitely by constituting committees. A general fatigue has set in the system making one wonder if the stimulation for change will have to come from elsewhere.

While so, the situation is getting blurred. Under the new government, things have worsened with the ministry's central role in policymaking and agenda-setting being severely compromised due to the strong interventionist role of the PMO and the NITI Aayog. The manner in which the ministry was virtually sidelined with regard to an important reform issue like the revamping of the MCI is disturbing. So is the unilateral manner in which the Ministry of Finance in the 2016 budget announced two intitiatives entailing substantive policy and fiscal implications. Such overlapping of institutional jurisdictions and lack of clarity are further weakening the ministry at a time when it needs to be strengthened to coordinate an increasingly complex environment.

Notwithstanding the aforementioned, even within the limited scope of the ministry, the technical and administrative bureaucracies are far too powerfully entrenched. Situated at the apex of formulating health policies for the country, they enjoy an influence and power vastly disproportionate to the resources they transfer to states or are held accountable for. It is a piquant situation where the centre has power without responsibility and the states have responsibility without resources, and both are mutually dependent. The current policy of shifting the responsibility to states under 'cooperative federalism' is also likely to be problematic due to the absence of required capacities within ministries or institutions and weak civil society engagement at the state and district levels.

Yet the trend is in the right direction. Over time, cooperative federalism operating on the principle of decentralization in policy formulation and implementation will help build those capacities within the states. Such a reversal of roles will also require the centre to leverage its convening power to mobilize the financial and human resources to help states build such capacities and steer the process of change. This is elaborated further in Chapter 6.

Institutions are designed for a specific purpose. They mutate, get discarded, or new ones are created when objectives change or new challenges emerge. Unlike in the early years of Independence, the state is neither the only provider of care nor the only payer. The private sector has become dominant and the financing of health highly complex. There is a chaotic condition since its growth has been unregulated. Bringing in a semblance of order would require expertise and knowledge of how markets function. Gauging the impact of incentives on human behaviour is an important capacity. Designing contracts and enforcing them are critical abilities that also require to be backed by institutions for redressal of grievances and punitive action against deviation or misdemeanour. Transparency and public information are essential attributes.

The capacity to bring change is limited. Transitioning from a welfare state to a market-dominated system should 'involve experimentation and learning by a number of actors and the gradual development of appropriate rules, behavioural norms and mutual expectations. The Chinese use a compelling metaphor to describe their management of multiple transitions as "crossing the river while feeling for the stones".'[20] While Thailand took 30 years of reform before announcing its universal health policy in 2002, China underwent extensive experimentation for almost a decade before pronouncing its intention to implement the UHC.

However, unlike the Thais and the Chinese, India has not worked out a strategy of building such capacities and skills based on reforming institutions and learning from doing. Instead most policies have emerged by default and as a reaction to address an emergency situation.

Recognizing the urgency and importance of institutional reform, the NCMH (2005) as well as the report of the HLEG (2012) recommended the establishment of institutional mechanisms and autonomous regulatory bodies for handling the special needs for drugs, medical devices, health insurance, procurement, quality assurance, human resources for health, disease surveillance, and public information. But anxious not to increase the non-Plan expenditures, these vitally needed instruments of governance are not being constituted. Instead the trend is to burden the ministry with more responsibilities of implementation. For example, building AIIMS-like institutions and running them in a centralized fashion, or managing insurance programmes like the RSBY that require a host of new skill sets and competencies are not the way to address key issues facing the sector. Appointing inexperienced persons as consultants, outsourcing or contracting private accounting firms like Ernst & Young or PWC to design policy, or using information technology is akin to simplifying issues to the extreme and will prove to be counterproductive.

Establishing a Department of Public Health

An important omission in health policy has been the reluctance to create a department of public health to bring the much-needed focus on public health. The training, curriculum, and requirements of a nurse and a doctor working in a primary health setting are vastly different from those working in hospitals. The system of having a family doctor can enable effective gatekeeping and checking needless hospital visits.

With the emergence of new infections and drug-resistant forms of infections, there is a need to focus on having specialization in infectious diseases, family medicine, and public health. Tackling chronic illnesses and geriatric care require counsellors, physiotherapists, and home-based palliative care.

Public health managers need abilities to integrate and converge health with other social determinants, community surveillance of diseases, building an environment of public participation, and a capability to enforce public health laws, while effective monitoring requires skills in data management and data analysis. Training institutions need to be built and civil society organizations partnered with for training, capacity-building, information dissemination among caregivers as well as community stakeholders, and conducting social audits for greater accountability. The mindset for this kind of work is different from the concerns and requirements of the complex hospital environments treating and managing institution-based, diagnostic, and specialist dependent care that again requires a host of new skills the tradition-bound ministries lack and urgently require.

Managing the process of transition from a welfare state to one dictated by market laws is complex. It requires an enormous understanding of the system of governance prevailing in the country in order to design the best-suited framework to fit the varied landscape in the country—the disparities, inequities, unevenness and variations in expectations and aspirations. There simply cannot be a one-size-fits-all formula for health governance. The first step, then, is to understand the issues and challenges. Based on my understanding of this sector, I have listed seven broad areas as detailed in the following paragraphs.

Issues and Challenges

While funding is of critical and foundational importance, its mere increase is not a sufficient condition. Spending of money to achieve technical and allocative efficiencies and health outcomes should be accompanied by systemic reforms.

There are 10 key challenges corresponding with seven underlying elements of good governance that have been listed further.

a. Strategic vision, participation, and consensus orientation
   (i) Centralized policymaking
   (ii) Lack of coordination and social determinants
   (iii) Weakened public health capacity
b. Equity and inclusiveness
   (iv) Inequities in health access
c. Responsiveness, transparency, effectiveness, and efficiency
   (v) Inadequate human resources and weak incentive structures for optimal functioning
   (vi) Poor procurement systems
d. Rule of law
   (vii) Weak regulatory environment
   (viii) Absence of a coherent policy for partnering with private sector providers and markets for drugs and medical devices
e. Intelligence and information
   (ix) Poor supervision and monitoring systems
f. Accountability
   (x) Governing the private sector
g. Ethics and Corruption

Addressing these challenges requires careful planning based on a comprehensive understanding of evidence and undertaking institutional reforms at all levels of policy formulation and implementation.

Strategic Vision, Participation, and Consensus

Centralized Policymaking

Despite a federal polity, the centre has always set the agenda for the country as a whole. In the early 1950s, the focus was on primary care and the control of infectious diseases, particularly malaria. In the 1960s and 1970s, family planning was emphasized until it got suspended after the disastrous political fallout post the Emergency. In the 1980s, the Universal Immunization Programme was implemented as a technology mission monitored by the PMO. The central focus in the 1990s was the verticalization of disease control programmes with the World Bank funding. A reproductive child health strategy focused on promoting institutional deliveries as central to the NRHM has been the priority from 2005 onwards—all designed by the centre and implemented by the states in vertical silos. Every decade had one idea and a set of schemes on which the entire machinery focused its resources and energies.

The two national health policies of 1984 and 2002 had spelt out several strategies of reform that were not followed up. The Planning Commission reports continued to repeat more of what had gone before. They never evaluated reasons for not realizing the targets or why goals kept shifting from year to year. Also, health has never been considered important enough to be discussed in the NDC meetings.

Centralization means setting goals, priorities, policy frameworks, and operational guidelines. Planned down to the last detail, these guidelines leave little flexibility for states to modify policies in accordance with the local conditions. During its initial two years, the NRHM flirted with flexibility as a concept that soon collapsed as the accompanying effort of building analytical capacity at state and district levels was not undertaken. Before long, the NRHM lapsed back into the traditional system of centralized planning where the states are required to submit their plans consisting of 65 activities and a score of budget lines with the help of consultants deputed by the centre and not by the states or the affected communities.

Centralization has meant predetermining those aspects that could be left to the community and for local action. By definition then, local bodies or communities are not engaged in deciding matters that concern them such as the location of the sub-centre, selection and monitoring of community health workers, organization of house-spraying of insecticides for malaria protection, and a host of maternal and child-care issues. Though such involvement would enhance the quality of implementation and enable the convergence of efforts and processes, reduce leakages, and be cost-effective in the long run, it has always been found more convenient to make communities passive recipients of government services delivered at defined centres. Talking to people, engaging with them, and letting go of some of the authority to decide for others are things considered a 'vast inconvenience'.[21]

Over the years, the status of states has been reduced to that of a recipient with little opportunity to present their difficulties to contest the goals and strategies proposed by the rigid central system. Venkatraman, an HR specialist of Delhi University, notes, 'The NRHM has actually made states voiceless and health has become more a central subject now.... The NRHM director wields more power than any other official; in some states NRHM funds are to the tune of 65 per cent or more of the state health budget, giving more scope to the centre to "arm twist".'[22]

Under the NRHM, decentralization was affected by bringing in some institutional changes in the form of the state and district health societies, hospital advisory committees, village health and nutrition societies at community levels (see Chapter 5 on the NRHM in Part II). The primary intention was to bring all programmes under one head for better coordination, avoiding duplication, and enabling prioritization in accordance with the community needs. But this did not happen. In several states the directorates of health continued to administer disease control programmes while the state health societies under the MD of the NRHM reported to the commissioner of family welfare that handled RCH programmes.

The issue of centralized policymaking as articulated by Vineet Chaudhary, a state health secretary, reflects the growing gap between the centre and the states.

> For sure it [NRHM] has placed enhanced financial resources at the disposal of the states. However, all these resources are linked to conditions driven by a one-size-fits-all approach. States are told what they should do and what they should not do. In short, the approach has been very prescriptive. An analysis would reveal that most expenditure is being incurred by states on ambulance services, followed by doles for institutional deliveries and cataract operations. Every year there is the drill of PIP [Programme Implementation Plans] approvals whereby states are instructed about the limits within which they must operate.... Could states not choose from a basket of programmes and implement programmes

of their choice without their resource envelope being affected? For the national government, the focus has to be on achieving the MDGs. States need to be assisted to strategize for achieving these goals. States don't have to be told what they have to do and when and how.[23]

Standardization helps scaling up with speed while ensuring uniformity in quality and outcomes. The centre understood the importance of this relationship and in that context norms for standardizing the establishment of health delivery facilities across the country were set up as an important policy step. But such standardization works only when the unit of implementation is uniform, such as diagnosing or treating AIDS or TB patients or immunization schedules. But in matters like health service delivery, the differentials are extensive: varied disease burdens, geographical contexts, functional needs, population densities, peoples' preferences, or affordability. While one of the five principles under the NRHM was flexibility, the central government further tightened the norms under the Indian Public Health Standards (IPHS)[24] without any reference to the fiscal implications or availability of human resources. Worse, having prescribed the norms, the central government reneged on putting in place complementary policies—money and appropriately trained personnel on which it has control. No state took the initiative to set up their own priorities or service delivery mechanisms either, though they were constitutionally entitled to do so.[25]

The already fiscally burdened states are thus overweighed with a model they can ill afford. With no funds for capital expenditures, the backlog has accumulated and the states are unable to cope with the expanding agendas. With the adoption of ad hoc approaches, the delivery system has developed without regard to spatial or epidemiological considerations or, more importantly, financial affordability.

For a federal country like India, the processes of standardization have been disastrous on two counts: they have stifled innovation and disincentivized the states and communities to examine more feasible and affordable alternatives and local solutions. Basically, the centre never got it right and, over time, lost the trust and confidence of people who ultimately made their own arrangements at the local level for addressing their everyday needs—often resorting to unqualified practitioners or even quacks.

However, attempts to decentralize and provide a measure of autonomy were made from time to time. In 1993, Parliament enacted the 73rd and 74th amendments to the Constitution that sought to decentralize funds, functionaries, and functions to the locally elected bodies. But this did not happen in the manner envisaged. Kerala is possibly the only state that sought to implement the provisions of the Act by releasing funds to the gram panchayats. Intensive training of elected leaders preceded the actual decentralization. However, in the health sector, such decentralization may not necessarily have a positive impact as it fragments the budgets. For example, in several states the sub-centre serves five panchayats or a community health centre serves a hundred panchayats making divisibility of the budget sanctioned to the facility difficult. Besides, diseases do not occur and spread uniformly. Such factors place limitations on the concept of decentralization of budgets to the panchayat level. Notwithstanding that, involving panchayats and placing a small health fund as was done under the NRHM do enable drawing in people and raising public awareness. It is a positive step forward.

However, besides the need for inclusiveness in policy planning and implementation, there are several who view panchayats as consolidating feudal power structures and being positively discriminatory to the marginalized sections. Secondly, in an electoral polity yielding control over the grassroots is equivalent to losing power[26] since local issues tend to dominate voting patterns. This is the main reason for the increasing trend towards formulating CSS named after political leaders despite the lack of constitutional jurisdiction.

But India has no option. The community and other stakeholders have to be made active participants in setting priorities and implementation processes. A greater investment of money and trust in the abilities of the locally elected leaders, training and building their capacity, and using their energies to achieve health goals related to prevention and promotion of healthy lifestyles are essential. Surveillance systems, disease, and facility-mapping should be decentralized to the community level to enable policy formulations and interventions in accordance with disease prevalence, morbidity patterns, and people's preferences. This also implies making the community and local bodies accountable for results and linking funding to evidence of achievements towards enhancing well-being and reducing ill health. Likewise, it is equally essential to establish systems of social audit and make the delivery system accountable to the people. The panic and fear that was created during the dengue outbreak in Delhi in 2015 is a clear example of the impossibility of controlling outbreaks without the involvement of the local authorities and the community.[27]

Need for Coordination and Focus on Social Determinants

India has a huge disease burden. It has failed to transit from pre-development diseases, commonly referred to as diseases of poverty, to post-development diseases known as lifestyle diseases that are disproportionately higher among the affluent. India is saddled with a high burden of diseases at both ends of the development scale. On the one hand, it has to combat communicable diseases that it cannot ignore because of the huge health implications for the population. Nor can it focus its entire energy on combating non-communicable and chronic diseases that are expensive to treat and impoverish households that seek treatment. Most conditions can, however, be largely prevented with access to public goods and lifestyle modifications. Besides, nearly 90 per cent of all morbidity can be handled at community-embedded primary care facilities.

Almost all countries—developed, and many developing like Sri Lanka, Thailand, and Turkey—recognized early enough the connections between environment, behavioural changes, and early access to diagnosis and treatment. They focused on building a healthcare system that guaranteed all their citizens access to basic goods. Such a focus was based on evidence that environmental hygiene and healthy habits reduced diarrhoea more effectively than drugs or doctors.

In light of Table 3.1, inter-sectoral coordination has always been cited as a cornerstone of a policy aimed at improving health and well-being. In fact, Guinea worm eradication is a good example of the beneficial impact of coordination between the health and

TABLE 3.1 Social Determinants of U5MR among the Top-three and Bottom-three States

States	% Population Covered with Piped Water		% Population Covered with Toilets		% Children Malnourished under 6 Years (by Weight)	U5MR/1,000 Live Births
	Rural	Urban	Rural	Urban		
Top 3						
Tamil Nadu	79	80	23	75	30	25
Kerala	24	35	93	97	23	13
Punjab	35	76	70	93	25	38
Bottom 3						
Bihar	3	20	18	69	56	59
Uttar Pradesh	20	52	22	83	42	77
Madhya Pradesh	10	62	13	79	60	73
All India	31 (71)		31 (81)			
All India Total	44		47		42	55
China	45 (95)		56 (74)			15

Source: Census 2011 for water and sanitation, National Family Health Survey (NFHS) III for nutrition, and MOHFW, GOI, for U5MR (2011).

water-supply departments at the ground level. Yet in the absence of administrative mechanisms to coordinate these different factors that are under the purview of different ministries, India's record has been patchy at the policy level and virtually non-existent at the community level. It is such a lack of coordination and convergence of activities at the community level that explains the persistence of malnutrition, poor coverage under immunization, waterborne infections, and a host of other such diseases.

As coordination in rigid hierarchical structures does not happen automatically, two mechanisms were put in place: the Planning Commission and the Mission Steering Group (MSG) under the NRHM consisting of ministers and secretaries representing all the related departments. Both failed. The Planning Commission never ensured that resource allocations and the pace of implementation of these underlying determinants are in tandem with health action. It, therefore, rapidly lost its relevance and ability to provide the leadership to position health within the larger development context. The MSG, on the other hand, was an ineffective body that met once a year for a couple of hours to discuss the agenda put up by the NRHM office that never really paid much attention to inter-sectoral issues.

In 2010, an opportunity arose with the Planning Commission taking the lead on the issue of malnutrition. The prime minister was the chair of a high-level committee (HLC) on nutrition that had not met since its constitution in 2009. The PM desired to convene a meeting, triggering a series of meetings by the Planning Commission with activists, corporate honchos, and the health and women and child development (WCD) departments. The health and WCD departments were asked to prepare a joint paper. The paper highlighted the shortcomings of the Integrated Child Development Scheme (ICDS) on account of various operational reasons and pointed out the gaps. One glaring flaw in public policy was the non-inclusion of infants in the age band of 0–2 years—the age when the brain and other cognitive abilities of a child actually develop.

In a supplementary note submitted to the member-in-charge of health, it was also suggested that at the proposed meeting with the PM only two or three major policy issues be taken up for a decision, namely policy for covering the critical age band and creating a department of nutrition within the WCD or separately under the direct oversight of the PM since malnutrition was a major public health problem that could not be implemented by a poorly funded ICDS monitored by a joint secretary. A parallel was drawn with NACO that had over 150 people working in its office. The example of Thailand was also cited where nutrition counsellors worked at the community level with families and their advice on healthy diets was linked to local foods. For smooth and seamless functioning, Thailand was divided into agricultural and nutritional zones.

The meeting of the HLC was held on 25 November 2010 but it was yet another ritual. The prevalence of malnutrition continues unabated with 68 per cent of women being anaemic and over a third of children stunted or underweight. Malnutrition is the cause of preventable deaths and morbidity in India and this condition cannot be resolved simply by a free supply of rice as promised under the food law. Is this situation a result of miscalculation or indifference?

A cardinal principle of good governance is accountability. Be it in patient care or in large organizations, implementation is effective only when every actor is aware of what they will be held accountable for. But in the health sector, health outcomes are the result of coordinated action of different individuals working as a team. In Andhra Pradesh, a policy that aimed to converge self-help groups with nutrition under the ICDS, primary health, primary education, and the Mahatma Gandhi National Rural Employment Guarantee Scheme (MNREGS) never took off as bureaucrats of individual ministries feared loss of control. Lack of convergence, the absence of institutional mechanisms to coordinate, and a systemic failure to envision the overall interdependence of the several elements that contribute to health and well-being continue to plague the system of health governance in India.

Weakened Public Health Capacity

The weakening of public health in India has attracted policy attention for some time. Large public health institutions that had helped India reduce its burden of infectious diseases—namely the National Institute of Health and Family Welfare (NIHFW), the State Institute of Health and Family Welfare (SIHFW), the National Institute of Communicable Diseases (NICD), the National Institute of Cholera and Enteric Diseases (NICED), the Tuberculosis Research Centre (TRC), the National Institute of Nutrition (NIN), the National Institute of Epidemiology (NIE)—have slipped into a leadership crisis. The public health cadres at the central and state levels have reduced in numbers with the merger of medical and public health cadres except in Tamil Nadu. None of the various recommendations related to changes in medical curricula and early exposure of medical students to work in rural areas on population health problems have been implemented. Nor have recommendations for filling senior technical management posts in the ministry through open recruitment, or giving preference to candidates with work experience in the field of public health been considered.

Budgetary constraints combined with a higher priority for RCH resulted in a large number of unfilled vacancies of male multipurpose workers, mainly responsible for disease-control programmes. Training schools fell into disuse so much so that when the ministry did agree to provide financial support for salaries of about 53,000 male workers in 2010, there was a major problem in finding trained workers or adequate number of training schools capable of providing quality training to new recruits.

The significance of the issue is now being recognized as the scaling up of interventions does not have the desired speed. Malaria is still responsible for 30,000–50,000 deaths a year,[28] TB continues with an increasing curve towards multidrug resistance MDR, leprosy is back, and HIV/AIDS is indicating a plateau while the occurrence of seasonal infections is spiralling out of control. The issue of improving public health capacity continues to challenge our imagination.

Several urgent steps need to be taken to arrest any further decline. The first is to expand the list of notifiable diseases and strengthen community surveillance. The second is to institute laws to strengthen the persuasive power of the state in enforcing them. Infectious diseases affect all alike. Just as hospitals and doctors have to be held accountable for the inappropriate disposal of dangerous toxic waste and prescribing antibiotics when not required, so should households and individuals be held accountable for allowing water stagnation providing breeding grounds for mosquitoes. Third, it is essential that central assistance be made conditional to the states earmarking and filling up public health posts with trained personnel and strengthening public health institutions. Fourth, payment systems for primary healthcare doctors should be competitive with clinical disciplines and raise the stature of public health specialization. Such measures need to be taken urgently, starting with the creation of the department of public health in the first instance. Exhortations cannot substitute institutions or legal frameworks that are the cornerstone of good governance.

Strengthening health capacity for public health management is also critical for ensuring health security against risks like swine flu, H1N1, Ebola, or pandemic flu. Such outbreaks can devastate economies as we saw it happen in China during the SARS outbreak in 2002–4 and West Africa due to Ebola in 2014. A study to find out risk preparedness in united Andhra Pradesh showed how dismal the situation was despite the implementation of a well-funded World Bank project for disease surveillance. It found that there was poor interdepartmental coordination; low involvement of the private sector despite it being the main provider of health services; poor training of district cadres and no supportive supervision; weak capacities for outbreak investigations, epidemiological data analysis, reporting and documentation; and that only 17 per cent of laboratories had the capacity to undertake tests of all the listed diseases.[29] What, however, is a positive development is the manner in which the national universal immunization programme has been built at the national level with huge monitoring and capacity-building capabilities. With nearly 300 people working with the government providing it the technical support for implementing the programme, India today has created a critical mass of trained people to face any outbreak. Its strength, however, has yet to be tested.

Equity and Inclusiveness

Disparities Undermine Equity

Ensuring equity would require systems having clear rules, regulations, directions, and instructions on how to achieve that objective.

Health status in India has wide socio-economic and gender differentials, besides disparities between rural and urban populations and substantial inequities in the distribution of ill health across geographical, caste, wealth, gender, and educational strata.[30]

Variance in the quality of services and the denial of care on grounds of prejudice, affordability, or geographical distances are reported in the media with disturbing frequency. While the major fault lines are inadequate resources and poor planning, a more important reason is the absence of a commitment to equity as central to all policymaking. As per law, all departments are required to earmark 22 per cent of the budgets for interventions benefitting scheduled caste and scheduled tribe population groups. Health is the only sector that does this notionally.[31]

Health inequities reflect the fissures that are embedded within India's social system. The impact of health inequities on health outcomes is often not understood or factored in policy formulation. Many a time one wonders why Kerala or Tamil Nadu have better health indicators than Uttar Pradesh or Bihar. Per capita incomes, general economic conditions, levels of literacy, easier access to health facilities, and awareness are certainly some valid explanations.

A closer analysis, however, reveals the importance of another variable: social inequality. In the early twentieth century, both Kerala and Tamil Nadu experienced social movements that demanded equality of education, questioning the Brahminical monopoly over it. Since education was the main vehicle for opportunity and upward mobility, its democratization was vital. Caste barriers were ruptured. Uttar Pradesh and Bihar, on the other hand, have had no such social upheavals. When Mayawati and her caste-based party formed the government in Uttar Pradesh, it was hoped that policies would be geared towards enhancing access and empowerment of the scheduled castes and other marginalized groups. This did not happen and both states continue to have highly stratified societies. This stratification is so rigid that a health worker had no compunction in telling me that she does not enter the locality where the low castes live! The fact that it is these very 'low castes' that have low immunization coverage or high maternal and child deaths was of no concern to the health worker. Caste issues often triumph over their jobs and duties as health workers. There is enough evidence to prove that such systematic denial of services due to social prejudices, be they based on caste or sexual orientation, is endemic. Resolving disparities and ensuring equity in a fractured social community requires an understanding of society. But such indicators are not factored in our monitoring formats.[32]

Alongside caste, gender is yet another social barrier. Gender discrimination is a major social issue in India where in some parts of the country female foetuses are aborted and if born, denied equal access to health services. Gender discrimination is practised at all levels of society and explains to a large extent the higher proportion of female deaths among children under five. An all-India survey conducted by the Indian Institute of Population Sciences (IIPS) in 2012 showed high mortality of 70,000 girls among the under-five age group. This is against global trends that do not necessarily have such wide gender disparities among children.

Even in flagship programmes like RCH, the focus is on delivery. Post-partum care is a neglected area. If the mother dies, she becomes a statistic; if alive, attention shifts to the infant. Post-partum visits for treating any morbidities are yet to be factored in our programmes, though it is believed that for every case of maternal mortality, there would be 20 cases of maternal morbidity.[33] Likewise, when I joined as secretary, transportation of a pregnant woman was reimbursed only for one way—to the institution for delivery. The return ride of the mother and the newborn was left to the family. Signs of our gender-insensitive and discriminatory system are everywhere from hospitals where women lie on dirty floors to sterilization operations that are conducted in camps without any privacy. Further, India has yet to develop a comprehensive policy dealing with all aspects of women's health—from birth to old age, to her mental and physical well-being in an environment that is non-discriminatory, non-stigmatizing, and not stressful. In other words, being a woman in a poor rural family or being a homosexual can have real consequences for accessing healthcare services.

Finally, there are differentials that exist between the urban and rural areas and the rich and poorer classes. The rural–urban or rich–poor divide is nowhere more apparent than in the health system. More than three quarters of facilities and doctors are in urban areas. Though the rich are able to afford private care, they also consume almost 30 per cent of subsidized or free care. Absenteeism in public facilities, particularly those located in rural areas, is high. In over 174 of the poorest districts of the country, several sub-centres are located more than 3 km away from the village making access problematic. In fact, almost 78 per cent of the rural population or about 50 per cent of all Indians live in settlements that are located at a distance of 5 km or more from the nearest town.[34]

In 2012, sub-centres had a population range from 1,009 to 10,227 against the norm of 5,000, while several CHCs catered to over 131,000 people against a norm of 100,000. While barely 742 CHCs, 3,633 PHCs, and 23,940 sub-centres conform to the standards laid down by the government,[35] over 65 per cent sub-centres do not have the complementary male worker, 10.3 per cent PHCs have no doctors, and there is a 69.7 per cent overall shortage of specialists in CHCs. Under each of these indicators—adequacy of facilities, infrastructure, and personnel—the worst performers are the high-focus states of Jharkhand, Chhattisgarh, Bihar, and Uttar Pradesh. Such spatial disparities are responsible for lower institutional deliveries and higher levels of maternal, infant, and child mortality with a worse situation among the lowest socio-economic quintiles.[36]

Unmindful of these supply-side deficiencies, governments sought to expand access to the poor with government-paid insurance schemes. Such measures, it was felt, would enable the less well-off to have access to hospitals, public or private, as per need. But that does not happen as seen in the case of Andhra Pradesh which showed that demand-side instruments like insurance can be beneficial, particularly for the poor, only if there is a demand–supply equilibrium. Inequitable distribution of, and gross deficiencies in, the availability of services make access difficult and unaffordable for the poorest living in underserved areas. Thus, the wide discrepancies in the equitable spread of facilities within states and districts need attention on priority. About or less than half the districts in the country, particularly in states like Uttar Pradesh, have a delivery system, public or private. Neglecting this aspect and providing insurance cards to all is no substitute and will only widen disparities and inequities even further.

The rich-poor disparities are not just about access to services but also the structure of demand. Be it malnutrition or disease burden, the poor tend to have a higher load of communicable diseases and a disproportionately lower incidence of non-communicable diseases. This epidemiological divide is, however, narrowing with the improvement in access to essential services for treating infectious diseases. Yet fevers, body pains, weakness, snake bites, injuries, and waterborne and airborne diseases predominate among the poor, while the richer sections suffer more on account of lifestyle diseases like diabetes and hypertension. Most data also seems to suggest higher morbidities on account of domestic violence, alcoholism, and tobacco, substance abuse, and sexually transmitted diseases among urban populations as compared to rural populations. For example, HIV infections are concentrated among the urban and semi-urban populations living in relatively more affluent regions of the country. Such data sets make it necessary to craft differential policies based on epidemiological data and redesign the delivery system accordingly. In other words, equity is not guaranteed by merely promoting a narrowly defined universal health coverage that is focused on hospitalization of secondary and tertiary services. Instead, it demands a more comprehensive health system designed to address each according to his needs. It is for this reason that the promotion of comprehensive primary care is considered to have a far greater impact on equity and fairness.

Responsiveness, Transparency, Effectiveness, and Efficiency

Human Resources

Management of human resources calls for clarity and transparency in the processes related to education, recruitment, retention, promotion, professional development, and payment systems.

Medical Education[37]

Privatization of medical education, as also nursing and allied services, grew exponentially since 1993 on account of three factors, namely liberalization of the economy without putting in place the rules and attendant laws; fiscal crises; and the insertion of Clause 10(a) to the Medical Council Act of 1956 that centralized all powers for the sanction of colleges, determining student strength, and introduction of courses in the health ministry. This reduced the role of the MCI to that of an advisory body. This amendment was made at the instance of the then prime minister Narasimha Rao to stall the proposal of the Andhra Pradesh CM to sanction seven private medical colleges.[38] Ironically, this amendment initiated to limit political influence on medical education had the opposite effect. It hastened the emergence of the nexus between the political system and financial investors, who in many cases were connected to politicians as relatives, proxies, or funders for their elections.

The rapid privatization of medical education in an 'unregulated' manner has profoundly impacted the availability of doctors, treatment practices of physicians, motivation levels, and value systems that together affect the cost of healthcare and health outcomes. India failed to see these connections between the processes adopted in 'making' a doctor[39] and the consequential impact on the kind of care provided to patients.

Apart from money, the lack of appropriately trained human resources is the biggest barrier to achieving health goals. India's failures in this respect have been two: one, in not assessing the emerging demand for doctors, nurses, and allied staff on account of the shifts in disease burden and epidemiology; and two, in not establishing institutional arrangements to ensure that the production of human resources keeps up with the need—both in terms of the numbers and geographical availability as well as in terms of competencies and skill sets. Such an absence of linkage between requirement and availability is one reason for the acute shortage of human resources in India. In the UK, it is the government that indicates the annual speciality-specific requirements to the British Medical Council. In India, the MCI makes these decisions based on factors like the availability of faculty positions in the institution. This is a critical area of concern that needs a policy review and a stronger interventionist role from the ministry. Since human resources form the fulcrum around which the health sector revolves, the biggest policy challenge is revamping the regulatory councils and the government exercising a greater vigil on their functioning. Chapter 6 elaborates further on this issue.

Issues related to the crisis facing medical education in India are not only corruption and weak value systems associated with it, but also inadequate numbers insufficiently trained, outdated curricula and teaching systems, inequitable availability of training colleges and trained doctors, and varied quality. Of concern is the mismatch between the type of training the medical graduates receive and the nature of work they are expected to do. Taught in tertiary environments, their knowledge and understanding of primary care is weak.[40]

Recruitment

Most state government systems are abysmally deficient. Recruitment processes for public employment are carried out through the public service commissions that have very elaborate procedures. In India, the Union Public Service Commission (UPSC) takes almost three years to recruit doctors by which time the capable candidates usually move on. Haryana alone recognized the problem and suspended the recruitment of doctors and specialists by the public service commission replacing it altogether with a system of walk-in interviews, alongside increased remuneration, deployment policies, hardship allowances, and quicker decision-making. With this, Haryana was able to recruit 825 doctors including 525 specialists in one year and had no further vacancies.[41] Besides, while recruitment is based on qualifications obtained rather than aptitude for public service, there is also no system of pre-service training where the gaps, if any, in skills or understanding can be filled.[42]

Basically, public employment of doctors and nurses never kept pace with need. The burgeoning and recurring budgets stymied attempts by most states to create and fill up public health posts. To ease the pressure, sometimes the central government would sanction the creation of posts under the CSS with no liability to the states. This, too, was not helpful as the states continued to be reluctant for fear of the liability falling on them after the plan period. To overcome this problem, some states resorted to appointing personnel on contract. Even this was not successful since the policy was ad hoc; in almost all cases the contractual employees sought court intervention to regularize their services. As contractual ad hoc appointees sought parity with those recruited through the regular process, the situation was further exacerbated and created additional litigation that pushed governments to keep the posts vacant.

The Sixth Pay Commission formalized the concept of contracting personnel as a public policy option. This provided flexibility to the central government to approve payment of salaries from its grants. States recruited nearly 175,000 personnel based on an advertisement or walk-in interviews under the NRHM within a short space of time—a procedure that would have taken over a decade in normal circumstances.

While the policy of recruiting personnel on contract alleviated the immediate problem of shortages and vacancies, as a policy it was flawed for three reasons: a) high attrition; b) being contractual, recruits were not subject to training; and c) recruits were not given any responsibilities. Due to the contractual nature of their employment, they were not considered 'government' employees and therefore not held accountable as their contracts were non-specific. More importantly, the appointments sanctioned were not calibrated with the fiscal impact on state finances with the cessation of central grants. In other words, the continuance of the contractuals in several states was contingent upon the availability of grants from the central government.

Overall, the policy of appointing personnel on annual contracts does not provide a sound basis for building a value-based health system. Moreover, good-quality care is premised on the two principles of continuity of care and trust. Both these aspects are compromised when the contractual appointee is seen as a stopgap arrangement. Short-term contractual appointments have been a suboptimal solution to the problems of restructuring the process of recruitment and placement of appropriately trained personnel in the system. Essentially, there is no escaping the simple fact that governments have to spend more, create and fill posts, and necessarily improve the processes for recruitment.

Transfer Policies

Once recruited, employees seek a fair salary, a just system of postings and transfers, and a good working environment with clarity in goals and outcomes. As a rule, transfer policies are non-transparent and arbitrary and constitute the most lucrative source of rent-seeking. A rule-minded doctor posted to a tough, environmentally hostile area is left there for years until he can bribe his way to the main line. In some states, the concept of counselling was resorted to as a means of imparting transparency to the process. But here again, there were allegations that the 'good' posts were reserved for 'favourites'.

A major problem has been vacancies of specialists despite the availability of good infrastructure—operation theatres, labour rooms, and wards left unused as the gynaecologist and anaesthetist are often not posted together. These are deliberate games motivated to enable the specialists to continue with their private practice resulting in lopsided deployment of doctors to facilities. Mismatches also occur when two or more of the same speciality are appointed in one facility or without any reference to patient load. In 2010, the central government requested states to formulate policies that would ensure that transfers of gynaecologists and anaesthetists would be within those facilities where infrastructure of operation theatres and so on had been built and to ensure no two specialists are appointed to the same facility unless justified on grounds of patient load. None did. Posting of personnel is an administrative matter that is most difficult to implement.

Postings and transfers are lucrative, a source of power and patronage and control over doctors besides being the biggest source of indiscipline in the department. Postings are often politically motivated and the formulation of a sound and transparent HR policy continues to be a challenge. Even the Planning Commission was wary of considering the suggestion to make central grants to states conditional to putting in place a transparent transfer policy.

Retention of doctors in rural areas is yet another challenge. But to be fair, who would want to work in a facility with no accommodation to set up a family, no schools for children, no social life, no phone, no vehicle, no drugs, and no diagnostic equipment. These deprivations preclude job satisfaction and there are no monetary compensations either. Appropriate incentive structures need to be institutionalized to motivate personnel to work in such conditions. Until then, they are obliged to maintain two residences and do 'up-and-down', as it is called, and constantly look out for posting to areas where they can converge their personal and professional lives. In 2010, a mapping of 'backward' areas was undertaken by the National Health Systems Resource Centre (NHSRC) to address this issue. The idea was to evolve a better policy for personnel working in 'hardship' areas. But nothing much emerged and the effort was lost.

Or, for example, working in tribal areas can be difficult. In the tribal areas of Adilabad in Telangana, the jurisdiction of the sub-centre spans over 200 km. Due to a low density of population and lack of transport, this distance has to be largely covered by foot. This resulted in the health workers outsourcing some of their responsibilities to local persons against a small remuneration out of their salary, severely undermining their motivation to work. The district authorities were aware of this matter and sought to alleviate the problem by instituting the cadre of community health workers, a precursor to the accredited social health activists (ASHAs). Central guidelines are at times complex, difficult to understand, and impossible to implement.

Professional Development

More than salaries and perks, most doctors and nurses value professional satisfaction: a clean work environment where they are able to discharge their duties to the best of their abilities and also acquire new skills and knowledge. Good-quality training, therefore, acquires great significance. It becomes even more important as the initial training of doctors in medical colleges does not prepare them to work in primary settings or district hospitals where they may have to handle patients on their own. The 1973 Kartar Singh Committee recognized that these doctors with no formal training in infectious-disease control, surveillance systems, data management, and community health-related problems were ill-equipped to do their jobs. They were also not imparted leadership and communication skills, exposed to the rural environment and its social dynamics, or trained to manage a facility and a team, draw up budget estimates, account for expenditures, and so on. Today's doctor, the committee noted, is a misfit in primary healthcare facilities.

> It was also felt that the medical education that he receives has hardly any relevance to the conditions in which he would be required to work either in the state run health programme or even in private practice.... Since medical education in this country is based almost entirely on the Western model, he is more suitable for the conditions that prevail in Western countries than in his own.[43]

The poor quality of institutionalized training is a matter of great concern. Evidence seems to suggest minor differences between 'trained' doctors and the untrained quacks in diagnosis and treatment. In a study in Madhya Pradesh, it was found that 41.2 per cent of providers interviewed gave partly correct answers to their questionnaire while 32.6 per cent could not even answer the questions.[44] Several of our colleges suffer serious crisis of credibility that the government and policymakers cannot afford to ignore any longer.

In-service training is equally poor and the overall work culture is not motivating enough due to various factors. Another weak area is career development. Compare this government policy with new private initiatives in primary care that are beginning to dot the landscape particularly in urban cities, such as NationWide in Bangalore and Health Springs in Mumbai. In the same country, they have developed innovative approaches to attract, retain, and inspire higher productivity from their employees and have, at their core, continuous medical education. NationWide has a mandatory four hours of training every week and then after 18 months the doctors are encouraged to take UK's PG diploma examination in family medicine. On-site mentoring and close supervision of performance in terms of health outcomes being linked to earnings beyond the base salary have resulted in less than 15 per cent attrition in a highly competitive environment like Bangalore.

Payment Systems

India has one uniform system of paying its doctors: salaries as fixed by the pay commissions constituted by the central and state governments respectively. Often the states seek to provide a modicum of parity with central scales that does have a major impact on their finances. The pay scales are set irrespective of the work done and not combined with systems of punishing non-performance or rewarding good work. The motivation to work is dependent on the basic integrity of the individual. A weak supervisory system, the virtual absence of monitoring for outcomes, and no means of fixing accountability make it is easy to get by with doing a minimal amount of work. The manner of rewarding or recognizing the value of the work done has different impacts on the way in which the providers and caregivers respond.

Government salaries are pegged to other government functionaries. This means that even an outstanding surgeon with a formidable reputation of having performed maximum surgeries will receive remuneration in accordance with his date of recruitment into government service where his seniority is fixed. The pay bands of the hierarchy of posts—say, in a medical college with an assistant professor, associate professor, and a professor—are made comparable to similar positions in the civil service and other academic institutions like the IITs. This is not the optimal way of handling the medical profession. A civil servant may be substitutable but a good surgeon is not since he has years of specialized education, training, and practice. These factors need to be taken into account.

Similarly, doctors are also not comparable to college professors. Doctors have no fixed hours: they teach, perform surgeries, run outpatient departments, take rounds in the wards, do research, and have to be available 24/7. This issue came to a head when the Sixth Pay Commission gave lower pay scales to the AIIMS faculty as compared to the IIT professors and the issue had to be resolved in favour of AIIMS at the level of the cabinet secretary. It is for this reason that the payment systems for the medical profession need to be handled differently. Compared to the private sector, the government, for some categories, is a poor paymaster. Yet several join the government for job and pension security, the social prestige it carries, and the satisfaction of helping the poor and most vulnerable sections.[45]

To overcome the issue of low salaries, most state governments permitted private practice, a privilege that no other government employee enjoys but one that has created a serious conflict of interest and has been instrumental in undermining the public health system and giving rise to corruption. Not only does private-sector practice take the doctors away from their legitimate duties, but, reportedly, also results in siphoning off government supplies to private patients.[46] There has been adequate documentation regarding the differences in the quality of care provided in government facilities and the private practice by the same doctor, forcing people to visit the private chambers. With parallel practice and huge earnings, doctors are known to grease the pipeline to get the desired place of posting or be absent from their place of duty. Finally, at some levels and in some states, payment to health functionaries is quite comparable and good. Yet outcomes are poor and absenteeism high, once again pointing out the need to establish accountability frameworks in tandem with pay scales.

A major lacuna in the governance system is weak supervision and enforcement of rules and standards. Additionally, there is a near absence of accountability frameworks—accountability to policies, target set, patients, or community. What is desperately needed is a cadre of highly trained and motivated supervisors equipped with the skills to support, review, and monitor outcomes; to enforce accountability at all levels of functionaries; and a more extensive use of IT platforms and metrics to identify errant behaviour.

Effective supervision does not mean checking every case but demanding accountability and, if necessary, punishing those who do not measure up; it means building competencies and motivating higher performances rather than fault-finding and constantly threatening dire action. The practice of suspending doctors—a punishment often disproportionate to the error or mishap—is disconcerting. In the absence of accountability protocols, the tendency is to hold the chief medical officers or the doctors on duty responsible for instances that are not perhaps of their making. The reinstatement and exonerations later do not compensate for the humiliation and demoralization they undergo. The failure of public systems is not reflected just in the absence of supervisory systems but also in developing a positive work culture and an encouraging and stimulating work environment.

However, while systems do need to improve, it is equally true that the basic issue that runs through the public sector is one of indiscipline. Human workforce ranging from sweepers to doctors has become highly unionized and politicized making any governance a very serious challenge. In a study of the two states of Madhya Pradesh and Delhi, Sheikh, Saligram, and Hort pointed out how most laws, rules, and regulations are not or inadequately implemented and, more seriously, the absence of a system of disciplinary action in case of violation of rules and a sense of accountability. Punishment, if any, is not only absent most of the times but also of a very low order.[47] The reasons behind such poor governance were the interference of medical associations, lobbying power of hospital owners, social pressures, political influence, and the weak functioning of consumer courts.

Training and Capacity Building

Two assumptions dominate our HR policies—one, that any doctor can handle any clinical condition; and two, that the management does not need any training. Delinking disease burden with the required skills has created a mismatch resulting in the systems' inability to achieve results commensurate to expenditures. It has also created a real and a notional shortage. While multi-skilling has been one option to cope with the problem of shortages, it cannot be an adequate response to the demands of a full scale-up of interventions throughout the country.

Mismanagement per se is the second major concern. Doctors are not trained in managing accounts, reading financial statements and budgets, procurement procedures, or in monitoring and data analysis and supervision techniques explaining in part why government hospitals and primary facilities are so badly managed. In the private sector, efficiencies are achieved by separating accounts and management from clinical work. What is surprising is that the observations of the 1973 Kartar Singh Committee report hold good even today after 40 years:

> It is indeed ironical that whereas a doctor is said to be a leader of the team consisting of nursing and para-medical staff, no training is imparted to him to enable him to discharge such a function... not a single hour is devoted to develop managerial skills, checking of accounts, supervision of his juniors and other duties expected of a leader.... [N]ot only does he have a feeling of technical insecurity but he also feels shaky ...[48]

The NRHM tried to resolve this issue by appointing accountants and those with MBA degrees at the district level and in block health facilities. But because these personnel are not trained in health management or public accounts, the impact has been limited. However, what needs to be recognized is that health delivery requires multiple skill sets.

Deteriorating standards in the quality of training has been a major concern. The amount incurred on training is less than 1 per cent as against a minimum of 6 per cent that should be incurred. The focus is also more on the numbers trained than the outcome. Due to years of underfunding and policy neglect, training institutions have decayed. Most of these training institutions provide substandard and uninspired training with a faculty that is itself in dire need of professional development. The incremental value of training is marginal due to the institutionalized structures of training that have no feedback loops for the purpose of providing additional training to those in need. Training is also not linked with the acquisition of advanced skills, promotions, better emoluments, training abroad, privileged admission into other courses, paid leave to study further, and research grants.[49] Without any such accompanying policies, mere training in skills has been of little value. This condition finds resonance in the Kartar Singh report cited previously where it is observed:

> [T]he trainees are sent to the training institution less on their own initiative and more on administrative orders. Promotion is not linked with training ... moreover stipend paid to the trainee is low ... he is reluctant to come for training.... This vicious cycle of training, unrelated to job performance, underutilization of woeful inadequate training facilities, high expenditures and poor results need to be broken....

Four decades later we are standing at the crossroads again reposing the same questions regarding training. India has a vast network of training institutions that consists of state institutes of training, over 47 regional institutes, district training centres in the World Bank-assisted IPP-VII project states, ANM, and nursing schools. Yet most function suboptimally due to the lack of funds required for appropriate infrastructure and trained faculty. Most of these underperforming institutes are grim reminders of the value that the government accords to building its own capabilities to confront challenging times.

Procurement Systems

As a system, procurement procedures are quite well-designed. The process starts with laying down specifications of the product to be procured, issuing advertisements inviting bids, and then evaluating them in a two-step process—technical and financial. As a rule, the one quoting the lowest price, providing detailed justifications for any deviation, and obtaining the prior approval of the CVC in certain instances comes out on top. The proposal is then sent to the finance division and secretary for approval and if it is above an amount of Rs 100 million in value, they obtain the approval of the minister. Such a process enables transparency and fairness and helps the government procure the technically best product and at the most competitive rate.

As a system it is fairly soundproof, yet allegations of bias keep emerging in matters related to the laying down of specifications, pre-qualification criteria, and so on. In the absence of a system of close analysis of performance data, setting the standard and defining quality becomes problematic. Similarly, close monitoring is required to ensure that the quality of the product delivered to the consignee is similar to the sample provided.

Government procurement is a highly contested area as several objectives are sought to be achieved together: transparency, competition, high quality, low price, speed of execution, and integrity. This is one important area that needs professionalizing and streamlining. Since 1998, the ministry sought to establish a centralized procurement agency as an autonomous body along the lines of the Tamil Nadu Medical Supplies Corporation (TNMSC) that not only achieved the objectives listed above but also worked as a sustained model. The TNMSC is an autonomous body that centralizes all procurement of drugs, vaccines, and consumables for government health facilities. Such centralization helped in the standardization of procedures, timely procurement, and supply of good-quality drugs and consumables at cheaper cost. A vast network of warehouses and a computerized inventory system with trained people were put in place. But its success lies not so much in the hardware but in building systems of transparency, timeliness and reliability of payments, and fair play.[50] This encouraged the participation of many good companies and also helped to bring down prices due to competition. The central government sought to replicate this model and the idea was first mooted and discussed at length in 2002 and finally got approved in 2010–11. It is still to become fully functional; the delays reveal the strength of vested interests in the ministry who do not want to 'let go'.

The central government has been exhorting states to do their own procurement given the fact that the most common drugs and supplies such as cotton gauze or a Paracetamol were locally available in most states. Under the NRHM, financial support was also assured to incentivize states to establish autonomous bodies but with little success. Shortage of IAS officers or non-availability of qualified persons in the open market is a serious barrier, while outsourcing management or recruiting a person from outside the state in such a sensitive post is politically unacceptable.

Some states like Haryana and Rajasthan tried different ways of expanding access to drugs and medicines by procuring only generic drugs and making them freely available, while states like West Bengal outsourced the pharmacy shops in hospitals based on prices quoted. Prices fell by over 40 per cent and in Andhra Pradesh the shops were handed over to self-help groups to manage. Such experimentation of alternative procurement processes has been helpful and attempts to streamline the processes have been encouraging. Yet timely procurement continues to be an issue and stock-outs of drugs, diagnostic kits, and consumables under the national programmes continue to dog several states. The failure to establish sound and rigorous quality-assurance systems and the absence of infrastructure account for the tardy implementation of the policy of supplying free drugs in all public health facilities announced in the Second Plan document. Considering that three quarters of the out-of-pocket expenditures are incurred on drugs and diagnostics, sorting out procurement systems can have a major impact on reducing impoverishment.

Procurement processes take almost six to nine months in the best-case scenario. Despite all the 'transparency' and elaborate procurement procedures and manuals, the scope for corruption is wide, be it at the central or state levels. The poor success rate of the ministry in this regard is an issue that requires careful thinking, innovative approaches, and sound management practices.

Rule of Law

Regulation

The fundamental tenet of good governance is having sound laws that ensure public safety and clarity on the rules and regulations to be followed. Some important laws in the context of health systems are characterized in Box 3.3.

Box 3.3 Regulations Required in the Health Sector

Category of Regulation	Examples
Public safety	a. Standards for food hygiene, purity of drugs
	b. Licensing of physicians, nurses, and pharmacists
	c. Accreditation of laboratories, hospitals
	d. Labelling
Rules of the game	a. Advertisement restrictions
	b. Negligence and malpractice liabilities
	c. Property rights protection and patents
	d. Solvency and bankruptcy laws for health service institutions
	e. Patients' rights
	f. Professional ethics
Equity promotion	a. Assignment of new medical graduates to serve in underserved areas
	b. Patients' rights to emergency services
Market failures correction	
i) Manpower	a. Limits on training slots and 'billing' numbers
	b. Foreign medical school graduates entry restrictions
ii) Capital investment	a. Adoption/construction of new technology/facility approvals
iii) Information disclosure	a. Conflicts of interest disclosure
	b. Advertisement restrictions
iv) Monopoly	a. Anti-trust laws
v) Quality	a. Practice guidelines
	b. Standard-quality report cards
vi) Price	a. Price schedule for services
	b. Reference prices for drugs

Source: Hsiao, 'What Is a Health System?'

India's poor record of health indicators, varied quality of care, and high prices are the result of the absence of a regulatory environment, laying down of rules, and transparent processes. Despite a plethora of laws regulating things such as organ donation, furnishing of data for notifiable diseases, establishing medical or nursing colleges, disposal of biodegradable waste and the like, setting up a hospital or a nursing home requires no approvals from any authorities except the municipality, that too for the approval of building plans and not necessarily the appropriateness of the location. Further, there are no laws to determine what services a provider can provide—an MBBS doctor may be half-trained but is, by law, licensed to practice. To address this chaos, the Clinical Establishment Act of 2010 did seek to mandate the registration of clinical establishments. However, its main criticisms are that it failed to separate the enforcement of the Act from the executive authorities, does not provide adequate grievance redressal mechanisms, and had a limited scope for stakeholder involvement. The standards prescribed are also critiqued to be high, affecting the small, more accessible, and affordable health facilities while helping the bigger and corporate hospitals.

Absence of regulations governing location could be part of the reason for the crowding of hospitals in cities and towns. Such certificates of need should also be required for locating diagnostic facilities and expensive diagnostics like MRI. Providers should be made accountable and regulations are needed to enforce and penalize for deviations from standards and expected outcomes. Without such regulatory systems in place, merely contracting private sector cannot alleviate the problem since in the long run it is the government that gets shortchanged. Information about tests done, prices charged for different procedures and outcomes, and other information should be in the public domain. The concept of choice can have some relevance only when there is transparency and full disclosure of such vital information.

Finally, the bane of governance in India is the non-implementation of most laws whether against sex determination, quality of drugs, or education. Strong and effective implementation requires hundreds of people to be employed for supervision and monitoring to check for deviations and ensure accountability. Good governance is dependent on the ability of the state to enforce its regulatory power.

Regulating Medical Education: MCI

The British constituted the MCI in 1934 vide the Medical Council Act of 1933, as an elected body, for maintaining the medical register and providing ethical oversight, with no specific role in medical education that lay in the realm of the universities. The Amendment of 1956, however, mandated the MCI 'to maintain uniform standards of medical education, both under graduate and postgraduate; recommend for recognition/de-recognition of medical qualifications of medical institutions of India or foreign countries; accord permanent registration/provisional registration of doctors with recognized medical qualifications; and ensure reciprocity with foreign countries in the matter of mutual recognition of medical qualifications'.

The second amendment to the Act was in 1993, at a time when there was a new-found enthusiasm for private colleges. Under this amendment, the role of the MCI was reduced to that of an advisory body with the three critical functions of sanctioning medical colleges, approving the student intake and further expansion, and approving new courses necessitating prior consent of the MOHFW. The MCI is governed by an elected body of doctors.

The MCI is largely responsible for the deterioration in the standards of medical education and the enormous corruption associated with it. This was not due to the policy of privatization introduced post 1993 but because of the failure in putting appropriate checks and balances, in laying down rules and regulations and ensuring their strict implementation. There has also been a gross failure in not revamping the MCI with the skills and competencies required to handle private markets and advances in knowledge as well as in building accountability systems. A major failure was in not seeing the deep conflicts of interest inherent in the process of election of the members to the regulatory body. The requirement of inspecting a medical college 25 times over a five-year period before the final approval is accorded provides a huge scope for corruption, calling for a revamp of the Act and the processes of sanctions. This, undoubtedly, was—and continues to be—a major contributory factor for the crisis we witness in the medical education sector.

The government's response to the credibility crisis of the MCI has been generally weak and ambivalent. It took some action in setting aside the elected body of the MCI through an ordinance on 15 May 2010. A six-member board of governors consisting of eminent persons known for their integrity and scholarship was nominated. The ordinance was to be in effect for a year by when the government was to bring in a law revamping the regulatory system replacing it with the National Commission for Human Resources in Health (NCHRH). Under this structure, the elected body of the MCI was to be confined to the registration of doctors and regulating physician practice, while curriculum, setting of standards, systems of accreditation, and quality-assurance and related matters were to be handled by different autonomous bodies consisting of experts who were to be nominated by the government.

The draft law for the NCHRH aimed to provide for an overarching body in order to bring under its ambit all disciplines of medicine and allied services so that there could be better coordination between them. It was prepared after widespread consultations and introduced in Parliament on 22 December 2011. The PSC had 13 sittings and returned the draft bill in October 2012 to re-examine three major concerns: (a) the states' autonomy and potential violation of federal principles, (b) excessive bureaucratization and centralization, and (c) faulty selection procedure of regulators, providing scope for abuse. There was political support for this initiative with the prime minister announcing the constitution of the NCHRH in his Independence Day speech in 2009. Instead of quickly revising the draft by taking into consideration the standing committee's observations, the ministry constituted yet another expert committee that was subsequently shelved. The moment was lost as after extending the ordinance for two more years, an election was ordered in 2013 for reconstituting the MCI. The reconstituted MCI took office in December 2013 restoring the pre-2010 status quo.

When the NDA government took over, the minister established an expert committee under the chairpersonship of Ranjit Roy Chaudhury to review the architecture of the MCI. This committee submitted its report in February 2015. In the meanwhile, the PSC related to health took up a suo moto examination of the MCI and submitted its report to the Rajya Sabha on 8 March 2016. It was an exhaustive report that was scathing in its observations of the MCI. It virtually accepted all the recommendations of the Ranjit Roy Chaudhury Committee.

Among the many and wide-sweeping recommendations, the PSC recommended that the architecture of the MCI be revamped to make it more in tune with the needs and requirement of the rapidly changing health sector in India. It recommended the establishment of four independent boards for curriculum development, teacher training, and standard-setting for a) undergraduate education; b) postgraduate education; c) accreditation and assessment processes of colleges and courses for ensuring uniformity in standards; and d) the registration of doctors, licensing, and overseeing adherence to ethical standards. These boards should be coordinated and supervised by a national medical commission (NMC) responsible for setting policy and planning of human resources based on geographical and epidemiological needs. It is to be assisted by a national advisory council (NAC).

The government's response has been tepid. A three-member committee was constituted. Some of us wrote to the PM suggesting that the existing MCI be replaced by a transition team and that the committee be asked to focus on how to operationalize the recommendations, not to review them once again. The Medical Council Act provided the government adequate powers to do so.

On 7 August, the committee's report was released. While the terms of reference were to provide options for the way forward and study the regulatory systems in other countries, the report instead submitted a draft bill. Not unexpectedly, it has invited strong comments since the manner in which it has been currently drafted, it will only further the commercialization of medical education and make it more non-accountable to the patients (see Chapter 6).

Medical education in India is in a mess. Commercialization of medical education can be traced back to the policy of admissions to medical colleges. Under this policy, admission to government colleges and 50 per cent of the seats in private colleges is required to be in accordance with the rank obtained in an entrance examination conducted by the respective state governments. For example, in Andhra Pradesh, students are admitted under three categories. The A grade students are those who have passed an open examination and are admitted in the 50 per cent government quota. These students pay Rs 50,000 per year. Grade B students are those that fit in the 35 per cent of the management quota where the students pay Rs 1.25 million a year. These students are supposed to be selected in accordance with the merit list prepared by the college authorities based on an internal examination conducted by them. Needless to say, manipulation of these lists is routine. The remaining 15 per cent of the management quota is for NRIs who have to pay five to six times of what is paid by Grade B students. With this, the investment made is recovered in five years. In such a scheme of things, merit is irrelevant. The rates differ between graduate and postgraduate courses. Various contrary judgments of the Supreme Court in response to individual petitions have added to the confusion that prevails in the process of admission to medical colleges.

The practice of levying capitation fees is the first step in corrupting the profession as it compromises the value systems and contributes to the moral void prevailing in the medical profession. Ill-trained graduates under pressure and anxious to recover the money incurred in getting the degree tend to resort to unethical practices, such as prescribing unnecessary diagnostic tests. Laboratory reports are a good substitute to clinical competence, besides providing the scope to make money through kickbacks and commissions towards referrals.

Standards in medical education are routinely compromised with, and often in, collusion between the MCI and private investors establishing medical colleges. Supervision or enforcement of standards is farcical as is clear from the several anecdotal accounts of how patients, faculty, and libraries are created overnight. Most colleges have a serious problem of faculty. There are also about 10 to 15 colleges with deemed university status that empowers the college authorities to admit students, set the examination, and also award degrees, leaving ample scope for manipulation, non-transparency, and corrupt practices. The result has been a serious dilution of standards, worsened by scandals such as the Vyapam[51] scam where impersonators have taken examinations and the system of professional education and public employment subverted in a cynical manner. The quality of education is a serious issue in some government and most private colleges.

What is important to note is that despite the government having extensive powers under the Medical Council Act, the recommendations of the MCI on policy and technical matters are rarely questioned. In other words, the ministry's oversight of its regulator is ambivalent and its ability to make it more accountable circumscribed due to factors related to political economy. For example, the MCI issued a circular dated 16 February 2016 that enables setting up of private medical colleges by taking over 300-bed public hospitals on a 33-year or 99-year lease from the government under an MoU. This notification could not have been released without the approval of the ministry. Yet no one questioned the propriety of a regulator adjudicating on government hospitals that are being strengthened by another wing of the ministry. The long-term fiscal implications also do not seem to have been studied, nor the fact that all the previous attempts to hand over public assets to private bodies have been ridden with conflicts and compromised the interests of the poor.

Over 25 years ago, the Manipal group took over the district hospital at Mangalore. Even today most of its students do their internships in medical colleges of other states. Manipal also promised Sikkim to provide specialist care and PG seats to Sikkimese citizens. It did neither even after taking over valuable assets. The citizens of Sikkim still go out of the state for specialist care besides losing the seats reserved for NE states for PG education. In 2006, the government hospital in Bhuj was handed over to the Adani group. There are still two PILs in the state high court alleging that patients are being denied access to free care. After protracted difficulty, the government of Karnataka had to take back its hospital in Raichur from the Apollo group. In Andhra Pradesh, the Chittoor district hospital spread over 9.23 acres of land has been handed over to Apollo on a five-year lease that has since been extended to

33 years. This is despite the fact that there are three other medical colleges in that district. The conditions imposed are to provide free care in a revamped-to-international-standards district hospital, build a medical college with a capacity to accommodate over 250 students, and leave without seeking any remuneration after the cessation of the lease period. No redressal mechanisms have been provided nor are there any processes to adjudicate the violation of conditions, if any. In each case, contracting has been biased with the government taking all the risks and no safeguards ensured.

The unquestioned manner in which the MCI has pushed the privatization agenda in a partisan way is indicative of the low oversight by the government or Parliament. Bestowing so much autonomy and power in the hands of a body that carries low moral authority and professional competence is the primary reason for the ills that plague India's health sector. This is a critical time to see how powerful and deep are the tentacles of vested interests and how strong and committed is the government in safeguarding the interests of the public in general and the patients in particular.

Drugs and Medical Devices

Two key reasons for the spiralling costs in the health sector are drugs and technology—the more advanced they are, the greater their cost. New drugs and scientific advances in technology have saved lives but have also driven up the cost of care. In fact, drugs and diagnostics account for 70 per cent of the out-of-pocket expenditures incurred by Indian households.

Presently, the Indian pharmaceutical market accounts for USD 30 billion with about half coming from exports to over 200 countries. The sector is expected to grow at 12–13 per cent to reach USD 45 billion in 2020. Medical devices and cosmetics account for Rs 150 billion and Rs 80 billion respectively while clinical trials contribute about Rs 20 billion. In order to ensure competition, drug-manufacturing was opened up and liberalized resulting in about 10,000 drug-manufacturing units in the country and 800,000 retail/wholesale outlets. However, about 100 companies manufacture 95 per cent of the drugs. Most production by these big companies is through contract manufacturing—principal to principal—minimizing their role to that of mere wholesalers but extracting brand premium from the consumer. Injeti Srinivas, the chairman of the National Pharmaceutical Pricing Authority (NPPA), says:

> Although there is nothing wrong with outsourcing, the problem is that big manufacturers are openly circumventing the Drugs and Cosmetics Act to escape the primary responsibility of maintaining quality, safety, and efficacy. As per the Act, they should take a loan licence—that is, hire the manufacturing facility—in which case the onus of supervision and quality would lie with them as the manufacturer. This is both illegal and unethical.[52]

The health ministry is concerned with the quality, safety, and efficacy of the drugs being manufactured or imported into the country for sale. This is regulated under the provisions of Drugs and Cosmetics Act of 1940 and the rules made thereunder. Under this Act, while the regulatory control over products imported into the country lies with the central government and is exercised by the Central Drugs Standard Control Organization (CDSCO) headed by the drug controller general (India), the manufacture, sale, and distribution fall under the jurisdiction of the state drug control authorities. Such fragmentation of regulatory functions and the non-uniformity in implementation of the existing regulatory requirements and policies are among the main reasons for their weak implementation. To rectify the situation, the centre tried several times to make drug administration a central subject by amending the constitution but ended up facing a stout resistance from the states for obvious reasons. Besides infirmities in the existing law and the poor enforcement of even these regulations, the availability of assured standardized drugs throughout the country continues to be an issue.

The CDSCO is a poorly manned organization working under the administrative control of the DGHS. The sanctioned strength of 111 posts in 2008 was increased to 474 in 2013—of which, as of today, only 223 posts have been filled up. The cumbersome procedures involved in framing the recruitment rules and the process of recruitment by the UPSC/Staff Selection commissions are largely responsible for the delay in filling these vacancies. The problem is clear and has been recognized; the system as a whole, however, appears to be reluctant to change even though the lack of critical staff has adverse implications on this very sensitive issue. Besides, like other health sectors, the CDSCO does not have adequately trained and skilled manpower. The non-availability of in-house experts for review of dossiers, approval of clinical trials and new drugs—especially in the emerging therapeutic areas like gene therapy, stem-cell therapy, and other therapies—is a serious handicap.

The Drugs and Cosmetics Act of 1940 is also grossly inadequate as it has no provisions for the regulation of the safety and efficacy of medical devices or the conducting of clinical trials or penal measures in case of violations. In fact, these shortcomings were recognized long ago. The Act was accordingly amended and referred to the PSC in 2008 that returned it in 2009, suggesting over 80 amendments. On 29 August 2013, the MOHFW introduced the Drugs and Cosmetics (Amendment) Bill (2013) in the Rajya Sabha providing for the creation of a central drug authority headed by the secretary of the Department of Health and Family Welfare and the introduction of a new schedule under the Act, containing the list of drugs for which the Central Licensing Authority would be empowered to issue manufacturing licences. The bill also contained separate chapters on clinical trials and regulation of medical devices in the country. It was referred to the PSC that made some further recommendations.

Due to concerns raised by the medical device industry, the ministry proposed to reintroduce the Drugs and Cosmetics (Amendment) Bill in 2015. The latest amendment bill seeks to separate drugs from medical devices. Medical devices comprise numerous devices ranging from an MRI machine to a drug-eluting stent. Although all devices cannot be treated as drugs, some such as a drug-eluting stent must be included in that category because it is both a drug and a device. Moreover, some devices are absorbed by the body after some time. Hence, this issue needs to be studied more carefully. Even if we separate medical devices from drugs, some of them need to remain under price control by suitably amending the Essential Commodities Act. A study done by NHSRC (2015) showed that in several cases the MRP of imported stents is four times its landed cost.[53] There is certainly no great value addition in the supply chain to extract such huge margins.

The glacial speed and meandering ways in which such an important issue has been handled compels one to wonder whether such inordinate delays are indeed due to bureaucratic lethargy or to help vested interests who benefit from the status quo.

Availability of drugs at affordable prices is yet another issue for the Indian population, especially the poorer sections of society. India's pharma market is essentially dominated by the production of generic drugs that has enabled access to good-quality drugs at affordable prices. This is now under threat. The amendment to the Patent Act of 2005 provided for safeguards against the abuse of evergreening that is 'the practice whereby pharmaceutical firms extend the patent life of a drug by obtaining additional 20-year patents for minor reformulations or other iterations of the drug, without necessarily increasing the therapeutic efficacy'.[54] Under Section 3(d), unless there is demonstrable improvement in the therapeutic value of the drug, the mere addition or change of the chemical composition of the existing drug cannot lead to its being treated as a new drug for the purposes of awarding a patent. In other words, multinational companies make minor changes in the chemical composition of a drug and claim it as a new discovery extending their monopoly for another 20 years. In two cases filed in the Supreme Court by Novartis and Gilead, the ruling went against them, provoking a sharp reaction from the European and the American governments. The pressure on India to drop this clause has been relentless with rising apprehensions about whether this market-friendly government will yield to pressures from Western pharma companies or stand by its own domestic industry and consumers.

Patented drugs cost four to ten times more than their generic variants. But overpricing of branded generics is also a vital issue. The NPPA, under the purview of the Ministry of Pharmaceuticals, fixes prices of drugs that are listed as essential.

The Twelfth Five Year Plan provided for the free supply of essential drugs in all government facilities. In pursuance of that policy in 2013, the NPPA issued the Drug (Price Control) Order (DPCO 2013) expanding the span of its control from 74 to 348 drugs translating into 680 formulations across 27 therapeutic groups. However, it accounts for a net of about 628 drugs as some appear in more than one therapeutic group. The NPPA has so far (mid-2015) fixed prices and notified them for 509 drugs and also the ceiling prices of 106 anti-hypertensive and anti-diabetic formulations. Out of the remaining 119 drugs, 17 are common to both DPCOs of 1995 and 2013 and are not yet due. The prices of the remaining 102 formulations are not fixed because there is insignificant movement in the retail market with most being sold to institutions.

> The market-based price is simple average and not weighted average. We are really not controlling the supply-chain margins. The 16 per cent retail margin is merely notional and is added to the price to retailer to derive the ceiling price. It is common to see more than 70–80 per cent retailer margins in trade generics (of course, not in branded generics). In fact keeping unrealistic MRPs not only deceives the consumer but also distorts the moderated price.[55]

The changing methodology of price-fixing and control from cost-based to market-based pricing rested on taking the weighted average price of all brands in a segment with more than 1 per cent market share by volume. The change resulted in halving the profit margin for retailers and stockists from 20 per cent to 10 per cent and 16 per cent to 8 per cent respectively. Further, the DPCO stipulated that prior permission of the NPPA was necessary for launching any new formulation by combining a drug with another drug or changing the strength or dosages of the same drug as listed in the National List of Essential Medicines (NLEM and, under extraordinary circumstances, the right to fix the ceiling price or retail price of any drug.

While the market has witnessed a double-digit growth since the past five years, there was a decline from 16 per cent to 8 per cent in 2013, largely on account of the implementation of the DPCO in 2013. While activists wish more drugs to be controlled, the long-run benefit also needs to be kept in mind. It is important to balance the need to ensure availability of drugs at reasonable prices alongside the need to incentivize innovation and growth.

Similarly, the implementation was tightened in response to the PSC's stringent criticism of the functioning of the CDSCO and adverse media reports about the unethical conduct of clinical trials and payment of compensation indicating the lackadaisical manner in which approvals were granted for clinical trials and new drugs, mainly combination drugs without local trials. Recently in March 2016, the government banned 337 combination drugs based on the report of an expert committee. All these drugs had been approved by the state drug controllers but concurrence, as required by law, had not been taken from the central drug controller. These combination drugs were believed to have increased resistance to antibiotics and have also been found to have side effects and issues with efficacy. Some of these banned drugs (also banned abroad) were manufactured by leading MNCs like Pfizer.

In matters related to clinical trials that also drew significant media attention, 12 new drug advisory committees and six medical device advisory committees comprising medical experts from government medical colleges/institutions were constituted in 2011 for advising the drugs controller general (India) to evaluate applications of new drugs, clinical trials, and medical devices. Similarly, in order to strengthen the regulation of clinical trials in the country, the government introduced provisions for examination of reports of serious adverse events (SAEs) and payment of compensation in case of injury or death in clinical trials, guidelines and requirements for registration of ethics committees, and taking regulatory action in case of non-compliance such as debarment of the sponsor and/or their representative investigators from conducting clinical trials in future.

Interestingly, the mere implementation of these routine checks jolted the industry to react. Accordingly, approvals for new drugs and clinical trials slowed down: against 65 new drug molecules approved in 2010, the number dropped to only five in 2013 and against 237 global clinical trials approved in 2010, only 17 global clinical trials were approved in 2013. The industry also alleged lack of clarity with regard to the roles and responsibilities of advisory committees and timelines for approval and a lack of transparency and predictability in the system.

The conflicts of interest are most evident in the area of drugs and vaccines making it the most political too. The question that then arises is: why is governance so weak? While some of it can be blamed on the general environment where governance per se is poor, in the health sector the issue has been compounded to some extent due to the multiplicity of institutions and poor leadership.

The issues of drugs are far more complex than what has been explained here. It is a very critical and important area. Drugs, vaccines, diagnostic machines, devices, and consumables are critically required and are an integral element of the health system. Unfortunately, this is one area that is poorly governed, partly because of the huge vested interests involved. But that is not an adequate explanation, for it must be admitted that there has been administrative oversight or indifference. Raising the educational criteria for personnel, amending recruitment rules, improving the career management issues by timely recruitment, promotions, and so on, or sanctioning adequate workforce that is skilled and competent are all administrative matters where there is no political interference. This is an omission. In other words, this area should be listed as priority and given its due importance. The Constitution must be amended and drugs brought under central control, stricter guidelines should be laid down, and investments should be made to strengthen the office of the regulator with qualified and well-trained personnel by amending archaic laws.

Intelligence and Information

Poor Supervision and Monitoring Systems

An important aspect of governance is monitoring for outcomes. If data management is a complex issue, making sense of it is indispensable in order to understand whether the programme is being implemented in the intended direction and for the timely identification of areas for corrective action. Monitoring by integrating financial expenditures aligned with physical outputs and the established processes is the only way to minimize corruption or the routine deviations from standards that are today the biggest challenges in the health sector.

The health ministry uses two types of data: internal data from the programme and external data from surveys. The internal data generated by the programme includes the Health Management Information System (HMIS) that monitors almost 140 indicators, facility-wise, from all the states and the Mother and Child Tracking System (MCTS) started in 2010 that provides a line-listing of mothers and children along with information on services delivered. It also includes the parallel data that individual programmes collect from the implementing units at state levels.

While the HMIS and MCTS are important initiatives to improve data availability, problems of reliability and errors, incompleteness, quality, and a lack of clarity in indicator definitions contributing to inconsistencies in recording continue to persist and are being addressed.

The external data includes information from multiple agencies: first, the SRS of the registrar general of India that provides reliable estimates of birth and death rates as well as infant mortality rates for rural and urban areas. The sample size is of 4,433 rural and 3,164 urban areas and this data is collected annually. Second, the NFHS is conducted by the IIPS, Mumbai, which is the nodal agency for the survey. Since 1992, three rounds have been conducted and the fourth has just been completed. The sample size is 109,041 households in 29 states and costs about USD 13.6 million. Third, the District Level Household Survey (DLHS), a combination of facility and household survey, collects information on a variety of indicators and thereby provides a good evaluation of programme impact. Here, too, four rounds have been completed. The DLHS covers about 720,000 households and costs Rs 520 million. Finally, the Annual Health Survey (AHS) launched in 2010 was carried out by the registrar general of India in 284 districts of the nine northern states for three years (2011–13) covering a sample size of 3.6 million households. Over 110 people were specially appointed for this purpose and Rs 3.34 billion incurred. The focus of this survey and its value lay in being able to obtain district-level estimates for maternal, under-five, and infant mortality rates as well as fertility rates.

Different data sources and definitions are not triangulated to provide the narrative and, therefore, give rise to different perceptions of performance. While the external surveys have a sound and rigorous system of data collection and validation, preceded by the training of investigators, the HMIS and other internal programme data do not have any systems of data verification. Most of the information originates from the ANMs (in today's context, they probably rely on ASHAs) who generally lack an understanding of the system or the potential utility of the data for their work. This (mis)information is furnished to the PHC from where it reaches the district authorities—state and then centre. At every level of aggregation, data is smoothened to reflect higher performance against targets.

The low priority accorded to data management or honing the departmental capacity with analytical skills is responsible for a weak culture of using or valuing data. Such confusion exists partly because data is collected largely for the purpose of quantifying the achievements made. Such focus on quantifying data was determined by the system that constantly badgered about progress reports. Since programme data is vital for activity planning, its collection and analysis have since improved.

The lack of standard protocols for organizing and analysing data leads to paralysis in programme management, often reducing monthly meetings for punitive actions rather than as an opportunity to identify and solve problems. In such a system, plans are made on the basis of 'previous performances' instead of what is 'needed'. Figure 3.2 summarizes the problems of poor usage of data in decision-making.

Moving from NACO to the ministry, where data collection and monitoring was a high priority, I found two major flaws in the NRHM approach. The first was the low priority being accorded to data analysis and the second was not using a denominator for analysis. As we had no denominator, we were unable to intervene appropriately. For example, in Uttar Pradesh there were about

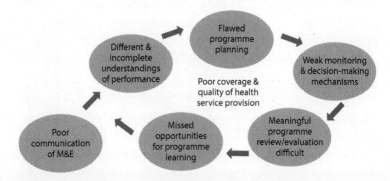

Figure 3.2 Problems of Poor Data in Decision-making
Source: University of Manitoba and India Health Action Trust, UP state TSU, RMNCH+A dashboards.

50 per cent home deliveries and yet there were no interventions designed to address the problem as only institutional deliveries were being monitored. Programmatically, this was a major omission as inability to come to the institutions for delivery despite the cash incentives was indicative of two possibilities: the lack of facilities (a supply-side barrier) or low demand necessitating more efforts towards behaviour change and raising awareness. Besides, not monitoring home deliveries also implied the non-implementation of the Supreme Court's directive of providing every pregnant woman, irrespective of the place of birth, an incentive of Rs 500.

Another example of not using evidence is the absence of priority attention towards the 170-odd districts in the country that account for over two-thirds of all MMR, IMR, U5MR, and total fertility rate (TFR). These were the districts that have weak health delivery systems, high levels of poverty and illiteracy, low access to social determinants, and so on. The programme ought to have developed differential plans and interventions to go on an 'attack' mode in these districts, providing a substantially higher quantity of resources and policy attention. Such programmatic errors arise when data collection, analysis, and linkage with programme implementation is uneven and weak. In 2010, the first task was to develop the institutional capacity for data management by bringing the statistical wing to the centre stage on data management and simultaneously launching three interventions: the identification of 20,000 RCH centres where deliveries take place that led to the formulation of the Janani Shishu Suraksha Karyakram (JSSK); the computerized MCTS under which up to 25 million pregnant women are to be registered every year and tracked individually; and the AHS.

Besides the issues of quality, reliability, accuracy, and regularity, the main problem with the ministry data is the lack of clarity with regard to the 'why' question: what purpose does it serve? Why are we collecting this data, for whom, and for what reason? What are we monitoring? For example, the guidelines issued to donors for providing support to implementing agencies to achieve the RMNCH+A[56] programme covered block monitoring, supportive supervision, HMIS dashboards, gap analysis, and so on. The BMGF that is providing such support for implementing the programme in 25 high-priority districts of Uttar Pradesh, instead focuses on mentoring ASHA—the caregiver on site—PIP tracking, concurrent monitoring, ICT support for data collection for the HMIS and the MCTS, and so on. In other words, broad outlines are of little value. What is needed is that specific attention be given to the processes that address the 'how to' part of the equation that needs to be watched over.

Likewise, dashboards are valuable only if they are relevant to programme managers at various levels—national, state, district, and block—enabling them to gauge critical performance indicators and drill down to communities and health facilities to plan programme activities and monitor implementation gaps for corrective action and reviews to create feedback loops to guide future planning.

Data and evidence are the key to the success of a programme and good management. But our goal-setting has been irrational and not based on any biostatistical projections or modelling. The need to have metrics to monitor the processes and outputs at periodic intervals through internal assessments is the key and needs to be given much more attention than is currently the case. Besides, there is also a need to get information from diverse sources to establish a measure of reliability. In the private sector, such monitoring is easier as it has the reliable measure of revenues earned to reflect the impact of its service delivery. The money earned gives information on patient preferences and enables course correction. Clear metrics and the ability to utilize and analyse large quantitative and qualitative data is required to effectively monitor providers, particularly as the policy to co-opt private players gets underway.

Accountability

Governance in the Private Sector

Profit and loss can be powerful motivations to determine entrepreneurial behaviour and guide investment decisions—where and on what to invest and how to sustain it. But an equal motivation can be saving a life and serving those in need. Entrepreneurs look for markets and beat competition with innovation. But the service-minded go where the need is and also compete with the for-profit sector on cost as well as quality. A perfect example of such a socially motivated practice that is also competitive with regard to price and standards is Aravind Eye of Madurai. This is one of the best practices that serve the poor for free or at rates they can afford while providing a quality of care that can be benchmarked against global standards.

Today's hospital chains accord higher priority to profitable areas. Revenue-maximization approaches guide investment decisions. The latest technology is accompanied by efforts to induce utilization irrespective of need in order to recover the investment. Patient outcomes are secondary. Maximization of patient satisfaction, on the other hand, implies reducing the financial and physical stress on patients, getting them well at the earliest and at the lowest cost. Common to both is the reputational factor as footfalls are based on the trust and confidence that enterprises generate.

Governance styles vary between the two faces of the private sector. The for-profit sector in India has brought in technology, new markers for quality, and aggressive treatment styles. They are highly competitive and capital is mobilized from the markets at high rates of interest.

The not-for-profit sector operates through its own funds, has a more limited vision, pays reasonable salaries, and sustains itself through equitable user fees, cross-subsidizing between the poor and better-off patients, and making profits to cover costs by increasing the volume of patients.

Two different objectives (revenue maximization versus service), two different approaches (aggression versus patient satisfaction), and two different clientele (the better-off versus the poor) are influencing the style and ethos of the management culture adopted in the two types of private sectors.

The barrier to the expansion of the private sector is the shortage of well-trained professionals. Domestic and global demand exceeds supply. The better-known doctors do not migrate alone—they take their team and patients along. Many specialist hospitals have gone into financial losses as a result of such migrations. An unintended fallout of such shortages coupled with a weak regulatory environment is the employment of Ayush practitioners and ANM's compromising quality and safety of patients.

While the remuneration packages offered is an important variable, others like career progression, opportunities for skill acquisition, and a hassle-free work environment also impact career choices. Contrary to general perception, a majority of doctors, if given an opportunity, would like to work in the government or not-for-profit sector, provided the work conditions are reasonable. Security of tenure, opportunities for research, a measure of autonomy, and freedom from the tension of revenue generation are factors that have been strong incentives for doctors and nurses working in public hospitals like AIIMS, PGI Chandigarh, JIPMER or CMC Vellore, where doctors have not migrated despite unattractive financial remunerations.

Social enterprise models are a new entry in the health landscape and are getting visible in the urban areas. Catering largely to the middle classes, such social enterprise models are based on the broad principles of the GP system as prevailing in the UK, with focus on the concept of a family doctor. Family is the unit and gatekeeping a critical function. Interesting payment systems and disincentives have been experimented with. It has been found that concepts such as outcome-linked payment systems, professional development through training and on-site mentoring, a team approach with accountability frameworks, and so on have increased motivation and resulted in high levels of retention. Pioneers in setting up such coordinated care models on scale are NationWide in Bangalore and LifeSpring in Mumbai. They are being aggressively followed up by new entrants like Shiv Nadar and others. Several NGOs are working among the poor on a smaller scale.

Malpractice in a government facility could lead to suspension and punishment. Government employees are subject to oversight by multiple bodies: the department, the Comptroller and Auditor General (CAG), the Central Bureau of Investigation (CBI), the Anti Corruption Bureau (ACB), parliamentary committees, and finally the courts. They can be charged under various Acts—the CrPC, the IPC, and anti-corruption Act, and so on. For private providers or hospital management, the only disciplining authority is the MCI. With no fraud or malpractice laws, it is only the MCI that can de-license a doctor or enquire into the wrongdoings of a private hospital if found guilty of any serious misdemeanour. The fact that until today the MCI has not punished in any significant measure deviant, unethical, or negligent behaviour speaks volumes about the efficacy of the regulator.

In the context of PPPs, the government is particularly handicapped as the lack of systems prevents the punishing of a private doctor or an agency acting in bad faith. Government options are to abrogate the contract, file a case, and get into long litigation. If a doctor's actions have killed a patient, he can be charged for murder under the IPC by filing an FIR and leading evidence. All this is time-intensive and most governments are short of staff hands to follow up each such case in police stations and courts of law.

The patients, too, are equally at a disadvantage. Until recently, they were not even allowed access to medical records to file cases in consumer courts or law courts. The results of consumer courts have also been disappointing as after years of litigation, the compensation amounts are pitifully low, making the whole exercise not worthwhile.[57] Besides, collegial solidarity often means that rarely do we get to see panels comprising doctors finding a colleague guilty of negligence or careless conduct. If found guilty, the aggrieved doctor can appeal to a whole chain of civil courts, making a mockery of the system of redressal. India lacks systems of accountability, quick and ready justice, and compensation to the aggrieved. To alleviate this issue, recommendations to appoint an ombudsman and have grievance redressal committees were made several times. But these reforms are constantly scuttled.[58]

Ethics and Corruption

The market failures inherent in the health sector place limitations on regulatory powers. The sector is rife with conflicts of interest at every level of its functioning. In most countries standard protocols, intensive monitoring and supervisory systems, grievance redressal mechanisms, and a strong judiciary contain such conflicts of interest. In the absence of such instruments, it is difficult to detect, prove, and handle corrupt practices when they occur.

In 2013, Transparency International declared that as per a survey conducted in 17 countries, 70 per cent of the households interviewed felt that the health sector was the most corrupt. It was estimated that of the USD 7 trillion global health spending, corruption in government procurement accounted for about 10 to 25 per cent and about 5.6 per cent was lost to fraud. It is undoubtedly a lucrative sector registering a 22.7 per cent growth rate during the years 2007–10 when the global economy was reportedly facing a recession.

Corruption has been defined 'as the abuse of entrusted power for private gain'.[59] Corruption in the health sector takes several forms and is widely prevalent in both the government and the private sectors. It is of two kinds: siphoning off money as we saw happen in Uttar Pradesh, where the NRHM funds were swindled resulting in the murder of five people,[60] the imprisonment of the health secretary, and the resignation of the minister. At another level, there is a more insidious type of intellectual and moral corruption in the form of foreign assignments, memberships, honours, and awards.

In the government sector, corruption is mainly in human resource management and it is systemic. Bribes are often required to be paid at every step of one's career, starting with getting admission into a medical college to recruitment, postings, transfers, release of salary or travelling allowance bills, promotions—all the way to clearing the papers for award of pensions.

As stated earlier, the policy of giving government doctors the right of private practice has vitiated and undermined the delivery system in the public sector. Absenteeism is high as doctors are busy in their private nursing homes, treatment in public facilities is abrupt and unkind where patients are pushed to avail of services in the doctors' private clinics, equipment and drugs meant for the poor are diverted to their clinics, while in hospitals expensive equipment are deliberately spoilt so as to force the patients to go to their preferred diagnostic centres, making the creeping privatization of the public system inevitable.

There are rules to punish deviant behaviour, starting with suspension from service. What is interesting is how even this is circumvented by paying bribes to the supervising officers, an array of politicians, and clerical staff for not 'putting up the file' or adopting dilatory tactics. Such delays in settling the matter enable the doctor to carry on with his private practice and after a while, at the time of promotion, get back to service, invariably with strictures from the courts for the inordinate delay in settling the case, 'inflicting mental agony', and justifying payment of all salary and perks with retrospective effect! Likewise, there are several instances of doctors going abroad for work while continuing to take salaries against the place of posting; with the post 'filled' the absence cannot be redressed with a new incumbent and the government money is 'spent' without public benefit.

Corruption is prevalent in procurement of services; building contracts; purchase of equipment, drugs, and consumables, including the release of dead bodies from the mortuary and issuance of death certificates. And so, until corruption is not eliminated through appropriate checks and balances, no matter what the government does, provides, and aspires for, the public health systems will remain in a crisis with the poor who rely on it continuing to incur huge expenses in seeking private care.

The private sector, however, is no better—only less crude and more sophisticated. In the name of tie-ups, cut practice and kickbacks have become a fine art. In the majority of cases, ordering of tests, drugs, referrals, line of treatment, and so on entail economic benefit. Corporate hospitals give targets for revenue mobilization to their doctors as a precondition for employment that translates to the number of expensive tests ordered or surgeries recommended. The government has had to face issues of fraudulent billing by corporate hospitals under the CGHS. Insurance companies collude with providers—individual specialists or hospital managements—in fixing package rates and settling bills. In fact, it is known that city-based hospitals send money on a regular basis to a satellite of primary care units for referrals to their hospitals. It is this environment of shady incentives that makes it inadvisable to allow corporate or profit-based hospitals an entry into primary healthcare markets, as profits lie in the number of referrals for treatment, particularly diagnostic tests, rather than in averting disease which is the main purpose of primary care. The manner in which pharma companies offer inducements to specialists and doctors to prescribe banned or expensive drugs that have profit margins, manipulate the tender system to buy cheap drugs from the lowest bidder, and do not check the quality supplied—thereby allowing counterfeit and falsified drug markets to flourish—is well known.

Corruption and fraud is not peculiar to India and is prevalent even in highly regulated countries like the US—its nature is possibly different based on the local conditions. Such distorted responses occur when an unmeasurable and complex product like health is subjected to the play of market forces based on choice and competition.

Policymaking is politics and an arena of huge conflicts of interest. It is the elites who run medical and nursing colleges or private nursing homes. The rent-seeking behaviour of the powerful ensures that laws are neither enacted nor enforced. I often despair[61] that the biggest subsidy the government has extended to the health industry as a whole is not having regulations or ensuring weak enforcement with shamefully low conviction rates and no grievance redressal mechanisms to ensure accountability.

In such a context, where the patient's welfare is of secondary concern, systems of governance—rules, laws, and processes—are weak for want of clarity and enforcement. We will have a fair health system when, and if, we have a government that has the political incentive to put in place a system that has zero tolerance to corruption—intellectual, moral, or monetary.

In democratic societies, governments are incentivized only when people become aware and demand greater transparency and public disclosure, when citizens recognize dedicated doctors and make them role models for inspiring the next generation, and when doctors' associations insist upon greater accountability to restore the growing trust deficit in the relationship between the doctor and the patient. This struggle for integrity and high ethical standards in the medical profession is thus the responsibility of all the three stakeholders—the government, the people, and the caregivers.

⁂

India has few options and cannot continue to evade improving governance in the health sector. In keeping with the current realities, the style and substance of governance will need to change from a state-dominated, regulated, and centralized system to a state-dominated, regulated but decentralized system. Engagement with the private sector—commercial or non-profit—would require specifying accountability. This, then, requires undertaking several deep reforms. In this chapter, several suggestions have been made with regard to what needs to be done and how. The following paragraphs seek to recapture some of the important ones.

First, there is a need to move away from centralized approaches towards cooperative federalism where the centre and the states will have to work together towards ensuring that all citizens access guarantees provided in the Constitution for their well-being. For ensuring an equitable and balanced development, the central government should develop differential policies: decentralizing resources in some cases and directly taking responsibility in others—controlling at first and gradually decentralizing as the capacity and systems develop. This is necessary as it is the poorer areas that have weak capacities. So the mere release of funds to states is no solution. States have to be provided additional help with technical support for the weak areas. For bridging disparities and promoting equity, more money has to be accompanied with human capital and management systems.

Similarly, for optimizing the available resources, earmarking boundaries for interventions between different providers is necessary—services that have to be assured by the government and those that can be left to the private sector and those that need to be implemented by the private sector but tightly monitored by the government. For instance, in most parts of the country, the public sector is poised to deliver good-quality primary care in rural areas. The gaps need to be filled and in areas where government provisioning is weak, the charitable sector and the not-for-profit NGO sector can be incentivized. But in urban areas, given the highly competitive environment, it may be a better option to incentivize social enterprises to set up practice.

Public systems need to focus on ensuring universal access to comprehensive primary care that must include access to social determinants. Time has also come to give prominence to public health specialization and constitute a department of public health in the centre and states. This recommendation has been elaborated in Chapter 6.

Second, the governments at the centre and states should focus on data management and evaluation systems as the basis for financial support, since the first principle of good management is 'what is not measured is not monitored and what is not monitored is not managed'.[62] Evaluations are useful in helping policy correction but data monitoring by third parties on a daily basis or IT-enabled data flows and direct contact with the beneficiaries through call centres, for example, are some of the measures that should be strengthened. Besides, health is a knowledge activity. For too long the government has ignored investing in operational research, so much so that India barely has a handful of institutions of some calibre in the area of operational research for health policy development, though given the country's size there ought to be more than a dozen.

Third, providers, whether private or public, need to be regulated and held accountable for outcomes. Payment systems and performance evaluations should be based on norms and principles such as non-denial of care, non-charging of user fees alongside patient outcomes. These quantitative and qualitative targets will then need to be monitored through surveys, patient satisfaction feedback forms, medical records, and surveillance data to assess compliance.

Fourth, the long-pending recommendations for institutional reforms made in several reports by the NCMH, the HLEG, and so on should be taken up and implemented. Without institutions, the health system does not have the implementation capacity to deliver its mandate. Likewise, quality assurance, encouraging innovation, and laying down procurement systems to lower prices will need to be internalized and financial reforms to ensure greater predictability, reliability, and auditing of funds alongside delegation for decision-making ensured.

Fifth, IT is the future. It has a great potential to bridge distances, monitor closely, and ensure better health outcomes at lower costs. So far its potential has not been fully utilized. If used well, it can make information available to lay public. Corruption in the system can be contained by transparency. IT and social media are tools with the power to make the governments and caregivers accountable in a manner no statutes or courts of law can.

Finally, ensuring the rule of law, revamping the medical and other professional councils and the drug regulatory authority, developing human resource management systems on principles of fairness and transparency, building supervisory structures and the capacity to monitor the private sector alongside building systems to reduce, if not eliminate, corruption are all measures that should be implemented. How these reforms have to implemented is known, just as it is also known that no one can substitute the government in doing what it has to. It is time that policies are not made on an ad hoc basis or to satisfy lobbyists but on hard evidence. It all boils down to political will and health being made a priority.

Notes and References

1. Kunal Saha, *People for Better Treatment thru its President* v. *Union of India & Ors,* public interest litigation petition, WP (C) No/2014.
2. Rema Nagarajan, 'Curtains for MCI, Actors Get New Role', *The Times of India*, 4 July 2016, available at http://timesofindia.indiatimes.com/India/Curtains-for-MCI-actors-get-new-role/articleshow/53037645.cms?from=mdr (accessed on 12 July 2016).
3. As the story goes, such thinking originated when the French finance minister Colbert asked Le Gendre, a businessman, how best the government could help commerce. The businessman replied, 'Let us do what we want to do.'
4. Laissez-faire is an economic system in which transactions between private parties are free from government interference such as regulations, privileges, tariffs, and subsidies (Wikipedia).
5. The CCHFW is a body constituted under Article 246 of the Constitution. Its membership consists of all state health ministers and a few experts nominated by the central government. It is chaired by the Union Minister for Health.
6. The Alma-Ata Conference of 1976, of which India was a signatory, resolved to implement a comprehensive primary care approach that would include preventive and curative services and social determinants. For want of funds to implement such a comprehensive vision, the concept of selective primary care emerged for low-income countries. Under this approach public funds were spent on diseases that had maximum impact on population health like TB, malaria, leprosy, and so on, resulting in verticalizing the system instead of following the comprehensive horizontal approach of Alma-Ata.
7. For example, the DOTS strategy for controlling TB was an innovation of the TRC, Chennai, but India adopted it only when it was endorsed and promoted by the WHO 10 years later.

8. In 1998, an international consultation was held in which top experts warned India of the irreversible consequences of allowing the private sector without any regulations. We did not listen then and still do not.
9. See the composition of the various committees constituted under the NRHM.
10. The Ministry of Commerce negotiates with the WTO on matters related to patents, the Ministry of Industrial Policy and Promotion grants patents, the NPPA under the Department of Pharmaceuticals fixes prices, and the health ministry is responsible for regulating the quality and availability of drugs.
11. With the abolition of the Planning Commission, the procedure is unclear now.
12. The standing committee in its 65th report dated 19 March 2013 recommended not to go ahead with the proposed BSc in community health course.
13. Before he demitted office, the MCI was restored to its pre-ordinance status and the NEET examination was overturned by the Supreme Court. Additionally, the BSc doctor has not seen the light of day, the public sector continues to flounder, and the efforts to reform AIIMS have been wrapped.
14. Such a situation, however, is not peculiar to India. The HSPH runs a Ministerial Leadership in Health Program under which, since its inception in 2012, over 94 ministers of health from developing countries and a large number of finance ministers have been exposed to issues concerning the health sector in order to improve decision-making and governance for achieving better outcomes.
15. See Chapter 5 on the NRHM for a greater amplification of this issue.
16. This report was prepared in 1995 by the Administrative Staff College of India, Hyderabad.
17. A nationally conducted exit examination implied that for practising on an all-India basis or for going abroad, the student would have to take the MCI test. The idea was to have a standardized 'Indian doctor'.
18. It refers to a theoretical system that does not interact with the environment and is not influenced by it. Only the components within such a system are significant. For example, nothing enters or exits a sealed jar but whatever is inside may interact. It is an isolated system that has no interaction with its external environment.

19. An example is the policy to push in a UHC in three districts of each state without understanding the delivery system, fiscal implications, or the constraints on human resources for implementing the proposed benefit package and the ability of the district authorities to regulate adherence to rules.
20. See the chapter 'Conclusions: Making Health Markets Work Better for Poor People', in Gerald Bloom, Barun Kanjilal, Henry Lucas, and David H. Peters (eds), *Transforming Health Markets in Asia and Africa: Improving Quality and Access for the Poor* (New Delhi: Routledge: 2013).
21. Peter Hennessey, *Whitehall* (New York: Free Press, 1989).
22. Personal communication with Venkatraman (February 2014).
23. Personal communication with Vineet Chaudhary, health secretary, Himachal Pradesh (March 2015).
24. The IPHS are developed by DGHS and consist of the physical infrastructure, equipment, drugs, and personnel that should be available at all times in facilities ranging from sub-centres to district hospitals.
25. When the health secretary of Andhra Pradesh was suggested to review the architecture of the primary health system to make it functionally useful and more cost-effective, he indicated his inability to do so on grounds that the central government would not agree. This was so even when primary care falls fully within the ambit of the state government.
26. At the state level, most politicians do not favour Panchayati Raj. Decentralization of power to lower levels made a chief minister ask, 'Then what am I for?'
27. *The Indian Express*, 'The Wrong Response to Dengue', 6 October 2015, available on http://indianexpress.com/article/opinion/columns/the-wrong-response-to-dengue/ (accessed on 3 June 2016).
28. Neeraj Dhingra, Prabhat Jha, Vinod P. Sharma, Alan A. Cohen, Raju M. Jotkar et al., 2010, 'Adult and Child Malaria Mortality in India: A Nationally Representative Mortality Survey, *The Lancet*, 376, DOI:10.1016/S0140- 6736(10)60831-8. They estimated deaths due to malaria to be around 205,000 (below the age of 70). The plausible lower and upper range was 125,000–277,000 that was reduced to 30,000–50,000 by the ministry's expert committee. The health ministry continues to use old estimates that indicate absurdly low number of malaria deaths.
29. Suresh K., 2008, 'Integrated Diseases Surveillance Project (IDSP) through a Consultant's Lens', *Indian Journal of Public Health*, 52(3): 136–43.

30. Y. Balarajan, S. Selvaraj, and S.V. Subramanian, 2011, 'India: Towards Universal Health Coverage—Health Care and Equity in India', *The Lancet*, 377(12): 505–15, published online on 12 January 2011, DOI:10.1016/S0140- 6736(10)61894-6.
31. It is there in the budget books but no activity plan is prepared that exclusively focuses on the specific needs of these groups. In such a situation, money spent on malaria could well be counted as having met the ST target as the disease is most prevalent in tribal areas.
32. I recall an incident when on a visit to Tamil Nadu, I insisted that the reports being furnished on cataract surgeries must contain two more columns to include women and SC/ST. The state official flatly refused. I declined to release any further grants until they complied with this constitutional provision. In India, caste clearly overlaps poverty and gender. Factoring in caste and gender in monitoring statistics would have ensured that the programme was reaching the poorest. It is noteworthy that if this was the reaction of a progressive state, what must be the condition in other states? After I left, this requirement was quietly dropped.
33. Karen Hardee, Jill Gay, and Ann K. Blanc, 2012, 'Maternal Morbidity: Neglected Dimension of Safe Motherhood in the Developing World', *Global Public Health*, 7(6): 603–17.
34. Anirudh Krishna and Kripa Ananth Pur, 2013, 'Globalization, Distance and Disease: Spatial Health Disparities in Rural India', *Millennial Asia*, 4(1): 3–25, DOI:10.1177/0976399613480879.
35. Rural Health Statistics, MOHFW, GOI, 2011.
36. District-level Household Survey (2011), IIPS.
37. Similar is the situation with the other two regulatory bodies—the Indian Nursing Council and the Dental Council of India—which, too, require a massive reform.
38. This information was gathered from an interview with Shailaja Chandra who was joint secretary, Medical Education, during the 1990s.
39. In the UK, they follow the concept of a 'UK doctor' to suggest that a doctor licensed by the British Medical Council is guaranteed to be having the minimum standards of knowledge and competencies. In India, we have no such concept of an 'Indian doctor', for example, the skills and knowledge of a person qualifying from a private college of any state could vary from those qualifying from AIIMS or CMC Vellore, and the like. Quality varies from institution to institution, including value systems. Almost half of the medical

colleges—public and private—could be found wanting in terms of the quality of education being imparted.

40. Raman Kumar, 2012, 'Medical Education Reform in India', *Journal of Family Medicine and Primary Care*, 1(1): 1–2.
41. T. Sundaraman, 2009, 'Case Study: Improving Work Force Management Practices in Haryana State to Attract and Retain Medical Professionals in Rural Public Health Service', NHSRC (internal note).
42. Venkat Raman, 2015, 'From Ideology to Impact: Exploring the "What", "Why" and "How" of Public-Private Partnerships in India', Expert Insight#1, Health Systems Hub, available at http://health-systemshub.org/interview s/3 (accessed on 25 August 2016). In fact, during the mid-1980s, in order to contain fiscal deficit, Andhra Pradesh banned recruitment except in primary care. Due to the urgent need for specialists in district hospitals and medical colleges, specialists were recruited for primary care and posted to work in hospitals. Such lopsided policies had a very deleterious impact on building cadres trained for the jobs they were recruited for.
43. Kartar Singh Committee, 1973, *Report of the Committee on Multipurpose Workers under the Health & Family Welfare Programmes*, GOI.
44. Jishnu Das, Alaka Holla, Veena Das, Manoj Mohanan, Diana Tabak, and Brian Chan, 2012, 'In Urban and Rural India: A Standardized Patient Study Showed Low Levels of Provider Training and Huge Quality Gaps', *Health Affairs*, 21(12): 2774–84.
45. For a majority of doctors, this is more important. Many doctors dislike the pressures put on them by private managements to prescribe tests and procedures even if not required as they find such practices unethical and an abuse of power.
46. In Thailand and the UK, government doctors can do private practice—but they are regulated. In the UK, such practice can only be within government premises and fees are split. The issue is that for such arrangements, there must be a basic level of integrity. Sadly, this is missing in India.
47. K. Sheikh, P.S. Saligram, and K. Hort, 2013, 'What Explains Regulatory Failure? Analysing the Architecture of Health Care Regulation in Two Indian States', *Health Policy and Planning*, 30(1): 1–17.
48. Kartar Singh Committee, *Report of the Committee on Multipurpose Workers*.
49. Under the blindness control programme, doctors were sent to Aravind Eye in Madurai and such institutes of excellence. It cost the

government five times more but it was worthwhile as not only did the doctors willingly go for the three-month training as they saw a huge value addition to their skill base but shift to IOL surgeries also became easier and scaled up rapidly thereafter.

50. This information was gathered from a conversation with Purnalingam, the first MD of TNMSC, New Delhi, 2011.
51. Vyapam—Vyavsayik Pareeksha Mandal—is a professional examination board established in Madhya Pradesh in 1982. This agency conducts entrance examinations required for recruiting personnel for government service and admission to professional colleges. It has been wrought with allegations of wrongdoing and corruption.
52. Private communication with Injeti Srinivas (2015).
53. 'Capping Cardiac Stents Gets NHSRC Backing', 12 August 2015, *The Economic Times*, available at http://articles.economictimes.indiatimes.com/2015-08-12/news/65490470_1_bare-metal-stents-drug-eluting-stents-drug-eluting-stents (accessed on 6 July 2016).
54. R. Sushmita, 'Ever Greening: An Abuse of the Patent System', 16 January 2015, available at http://www.lawctopus.com/academike/evergreening-an-abuse-of-the-patent-system/ (accessed on 6 July 2016).
55. Private communication with Injeti Srinivas (2015).
56. The RMNCH+A programme covers reproductive, maternal, newborn, child, and adolescent health.
57. Last year, the Kolkata High Court awarded Rs 0.12 billion as compensation to a woman who died in a private hospital, shocking the industry. The matter is under appeal. In the meanwhile, the private sector is seeking a law putting a cap on the compensation to be paid as is the case in the US. This may need to be examined as one reason for the high cost of care in the US is malpractice suits.
58. It is rumoured that the health minister of a state wants to appoint an ombudsman but a powerful corporate entity is mounting pressure on him not to. While in NACO, I, too, tried to build a system of having an ombudsman in every state. The whole scheme was worked out but the file never came back from the minister. This is a contentious area.
59. See Transparency International, available at http://www.transparency.org/what-is-corruption/ (accessed on 19 November 2015).
60. In 2011, the health ministry sent an audit party to review the financial spending of the NRHM funds in Uttar Pradesh. The report revealed gross irregularities: fraudulent bills, vouchers, siphoning of

funds, and so on. The matter was referred to the CBI for investigation. The Minister of Health was sacked, the health secretary imprisoned, and about five people—potential witnesses—murdered. The trial is on. The amounts involved ran into over Rs 50 billion.

61. I had two direct experiences in this regard. During the three months in 2005 when I was special secretary of Health in Andhra Pradesh, I notified the rules for the Clinical Establishments Act passed by the legislature in 2002. Yet the Act stays on the shelf. In 2010, when I was a union secretary, I faced a great amount of difficulty in getting the relatively toothless Clinical Establishments Act that had been pending in the ministry for close to five years tabled and enacted. Its lax enforcement is a more telling comment.

62. At times attributed to the management guru Peter Drucker. But in a post in athinkingperson.com, dated 2 December 2012, the following is noted:

    [T]he most likely source of this idea ... is William Thomson, the Scottish physicist also known as Lord Kelvin. According to the *Encyclopaedia of Occupational Health and Safety*, by Jeanne Mager Stellman (page 1992), Kelvin said in his May 3, 1883 lecture on 'Electrical Units of Measurement' (*Popular Lectures*, Vol. 1, page 73): 'I often say that when you can measure what you are speaking about, and express it in numbers, you know something about it; but when you cannot express it in numbers, your knowledge is of a meagre and unsatisfactory kind; it may be the beginning of knowledge, but you have scarcely, in your thoughts, advanced to the stage of science, whatever the matter may be'. That might be the best we can do in tracking down the source of this bit of management wisdom.

PART II
Implementing Policy: Successes, Failures, and the Road Ahead

This part contains a detailed exposition of two high-profile public health programmes that were given substantial political support in 2005, namely the National AIDS Control Project (NACP, Phase III) and the NRHM. Under the NACP III, the struggle to contain and reverse the HIV epidemic that was spreading at an alarming pace matured. With a fivefold increase in resources and the rapid scaling up of the programme's interventions, India achieved a 57 per cent reduction in incidence that was recorded as the highest in the world. This scale-up happened directly under my watch. How the policies were formulated, strategies crafted, and implementation ensured is explained ahead.

Around the same time, the central government launched the NRHM. The objective of this mission was to scale up the implementation of strategies aimed at revitalizing the primary healthcare system in rural areas. A threefold increase in resources helped it to design several policy interventions that strengthened the capacity to escalate the reductions under infant, child, and maternal mortalities. How the policy evolved; what ideas were deliberated upon; and what impact did individual players have on the content, shape, and ultimately the nature of policy and its eventual outcomes are elaborated further.

In narrating the events that led to the formulation of the programmes, the intention is to document the thinking, debates, and ideas that went into shaping policy. I also seek to explain how agendas are actually set, how the system responds, and how personal perceptions of those in power influence the evolution of policy with time. In both instances, it was the perception of an unfolding crisis that provided the stimulus for change.

Both programmes were launched around the same time and had the same political and social contexts, systems of governance, and financial constraints. But there were important dissimilarities. Conceptually, the HIV/AIDS programme was a global priority and a top-down programme singularly focused on HIV, fully designed, funded, and monitored by the central government. On the other hand, the NRHM contained multiple strategies and interventions to meet a wider variety of objectives. Significantly, the key constraint for a full scale-up of both programmes was the weak health system. Deficiencies in human resources, financial resources, and infrastructure were serious impediments for a full-blown response, highlighting the fact that a well-functioning health system is the key to achieving health outcomes. In other words, when the health system is battered and broken, increased financial resources are necessary but inadequate.

The wide differences in the evolution, history, and the environment in which the two programmes took shape make comparisons difficult. Yet what is important is the fact that the underlying policy formulation and its implementation are certain basic principles of management. At the conclusion of the chapter on the NRHM, a brief comparative analysis of the two programmes has been provided that would prove useful for those interested in issues related to policy implementation.

Besides, since both programmes were essentially aimed at scaling up known strategies, it is also instructive to understand what 'scaling up' means. Lisa Hirschhorn and others[1] assessed different definitions of scaling up that ranged from the simplest implying a quantitative expansion of interventions to 'the widespread achievement of impact at affordable cost' with impact 'serving as a function of coverage, effectiveness, efficiency, local ownership promoting sustainability, and equity'. Their article, written specifically in the context of HIV/AIDS, identified 10 domains as important for a successful scaling up and for the sustainability of programmes:

'fiscal support; political support; community involvement, integration, buy-in, and depth; partnerships; balancing flexibility/adaptability and standardization; supportive policy, regulatory, and legal environment; building and sustaining strong organizational capacity; transferring ownership; decentralization; and ongoing focus on sustainability'. They identified one additionally important potential domain for programmes sustaining delivery at scale: 'emphasizing equity'.

The quoted definition is insightful. It helps in identifying the relative importance of each of these domains in the scaling up of the two programmes and for ensuring sustainability. My practical experience would lead me to add two more domains: one of leadership that cannot be included under 'strong organizational capacity' and the other of ideas or innovation. Organizational capacity can be strong on fundamentals in terms of systems and the processes laid down and yet there may be non-performance for want of leadership at all levels of implementation.

Likewise, large public health programmes can never be cast in stone. Causal factors make them fluctuate in accordance with the shifts in the terrain, requiring ideas and innovative approaches to sustain the momentum. In other words, no scale-up can be based on one design since each policy design addresses a particular reality. When that reality moves on to another plane, partly as a result of the interventions and in part due to changes in the objective conditions, the design has to change too, or else the strategy becomes rigid and loses its relevance over time.

The plateauing we witness today in the NRHM and HIV programmes can be attributed to such a development, where the domain of ideas and innovation failed to keep pace with the changes in the context. If a diminished political support, reduced budgets, and a withdrawn civil society form one aspect of the changed context, the other aspect is accounted for by the shifts in expectations and aspirations calling for a broadening of the agenda, new solutions, and a reconfiguration of responses and actors.

No policy, no matter how well-thought-out, can be valid for all times. Every policy that sets out to solve one crisis creates conditions for the emergence of a new one. Such constant change and cycles of instability are inevitable and need to be managed.

While providing balance and continuity, a new round of policy also needs to generate ideas, solutions, and the platform to resolve the demands for change. Staying focused on the ultimate goal and anchored on evidence are the only ways to manage such contradictions.

Reference

1. Lisa R. Hirschhorn, J.R. Talbot, A.C. Irwin, M.A. May et al., 2013, 'From Scaling Up to Sustainability in HIV: Potential Lessons for Moving Forward', *Globalization and Health*, 9(1): 57–65.

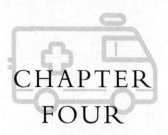

CHAPTER FOUR

Scaling Up to Reverse the HIV/AIDS Epidemic

The Background

Within the two decades prior to 2005, the world witnessed over 70 million young people infected with, and over 10 million dying due to, HIV/AIDS. The scale of this disaster evoked a political, social, economic, and moral upheaval and an unprecedented global response. In an exceptional display of cross-country partnerships and a unity of purpose cutting across all geographical boundaries and social barriers, global attention to this disease on which an amount of more than USD 25 billion was spent over a 25-year period ranging from 1990 to 2015 helped bring down new infections by 33 per cent and AIDS-related mortality by 29 per cent, and increased access to free treatment for those in need by over 40 per cent.

India was a part of this success story. Accounting for the third-largest number of the infected, by 2012 India achieved a 57 per cent reduction in new infections—the highest in the world—and provided access to treatment for 75 per cent of those identified as infected. Around 0.15 million people are estimated to have been saved from premature death and over 0.6 million prevented from getting infected. These were no mean achievements given that health was accorded a low political priority, was chronically underfunded, and had weak organizational capabilities, feeble structures of community participation, and conservative societal values.

Though the first case of HIV infection was detected in 1986, the programmatic response came only in the summer of 1992. For India, with only 96 reported AIDS cases (13 of them were foreigners) and 5,879 people infected, HIV was not a priority. Seeking a World Bank loan for HIV/AIDS made no sense. But circumstances were compelling. Media reports of discrimination and social boycott of HIV patients, denial of treatment by hospitals, suicides driven by fear and shame, abandoned dead bodies with no one willing to cremate them, and the handcuffing and jailing of drug addicts in Manipur created panic and disbelief.

In 1992, the government signed an agreement for an International Development Association (IDA) loan of USD 84 million from the World Bank and upon the WHO's insistence, a dedicated division within the health ministry was established. NACO was headed by a project director of the rank of additional secretary but assigned the powers of a secretary.

With an institutional mechanism in place, the NACP I (1993–8) strategy focused on five activities: establishing 80 sentinel surveillance sites, improving blood safety, raising awareness about HIV, treatment for sexually transmitted diseases (STDs), and strengthening programme management. Evidence showed that while contaminated blood was responsible for 15 per cent of the transmission of HIV, the dominant route was heterosexual behaviour. For want of clarity on how to address these highly vulnerable groups and the absence of NGOs willing to work with them due to the association of stigma and social ostracism, NACO, with the help of WHO consultants, focused on raising general awareness, hoping that social education and information would lead to a decline in the demand for unprotected sex.

By the end of the century, it was clear that 90 per cent of the infections were being transmitted by people having multipartner sexual relations, also known as high-risk sexual behaviour. This understanding formed the basis of the strategy crafted for the NACP II (2000–5) that was launched with a World Bank loan of USD 191 million.

> **Box 4.1** Lack of Experience
>
> We had little understanding of how to 'communicate' a sensitive subject like the use of condom to a conservative society. Simplistic deductions guided strategy. Since sex workers were perceived as the 'reservoirs' of HIV infection, people needed to be forewarned and motivated to stay monogamous or desist from visiting sex workers. The condom was the firewall and billboards would scream out 'sex causes HIV which has no cure'. Since that made no sense and was not entirely true, it was changed to 'have safe sex, use the condom always'. This drew protests from the moral brigades accusing NACO of promoting sexual promiscuity, while the more sober rightly wondered what would happen to procreation if condoms were to be used 'always'!
>
> *Source*: Author.

The NACP II provided the road map. This phase was important for the strategic decisions that were taken, namely shifting from general awareness to focused intervention among groups practising high-risk behaviour (normally referred to in the programme as high-risk groups (HRGs)/key populations), bringing back STDs into focus, expanding testing, introducing treatment on a pilot basis, undertaking substantial advocacy with the media, and establishing the State AIDS Control Societies (SACS) as autonomous bodies.

A patchy civil society engagement, inadequate funds, and low priority accorded to the programme made it difficult to implement the strategy. Stimulating states' commitment to HIV-related work generally failed resulting in an uneven response, particularly among those with high incidence and weak health systems. For example, in 2002 even though the epidemic was raging in Andhra Pradesh that had the highest HIV prevalence of 1.45 per cent against 0.83 per cent in the neighbouring Tamil Nadu, and data showed that 19.2 per cent men were having sex with non-regular partners with more than half of them not using the condom, the government was preoccupied with promoting family planning. Like most politicians, the chief minister of Andhra Pradesh,

Chandrababu Naidu, accorded a limited priority to health. To contain the epidemic, it was vital to get Andhra Pradesh on board and thus it became essential to mobilize the services of the president of the World Bank. The message was not lost. Nine years after establishing the State AIDS Control Cell/Society, Andhra Pradesh began to pay attention to the programme. It was, however, too little, too late since thousands had by then contracted the infection and many had succumbed to the disease.

Sensing the unfolding crisis in the North East, Prime Minister Atal Bihari Vajpayee proactively called for a meeting of the state chief ministers from the North East to pay attention to HIV/AIDS implementation. Apart from that one isolated instance, political leadership was, on the whole, non-existent until Sushma Swaraj took over as the health minister in 2003. Though she vehemently opposed condom advertisements being aired on TV during prime time except 'after 11 pm when the children have slept', her unexpected announcement on the World AIDS Day on 1 December 2003 to provide free antiretroviral treatment, overruling bureaucratic objections and apprehensions, significantly impacted the course of the epidemic. Enhancing access to medical treatment reduced transmission, lessened stigma, and saved lives. In April 2004, the highly active antiretroviral therapy (HAART) was launched on a pilot basis in 25 centres.

NACP III (2007–12)

When I joined as the DG in 2006, NACO had about 30 employees. Though new challenges were emerging, the organizational structure designed during the NACP I was unchanged. NACO was also a divided house with doctors on one side and the non-medical professionals on the other.

At the state level AIDS cells had been established under the NACP I. Since AIDS control was a low priority, most states posted 'disinterested' people as project officers. The meagre funding was mostly spent on printing diaries and posters. Under the NACP II, the departmental AIDS cells were registered as autonomous societies under the Societies Act and provided with a modest staff.

During the period 1993–2005, NACO had seven project directors. Around 1997, the project director shifted the office to the main ministry that meant additional responsibilities and a shift in focus with the post renamed as additional secretary and project director (renamed again in 2004 as director general).

HIV/AIDS was a donor-led programme. By 2006, there were 29 donors—small and big, largely coordinated by the United Nations Development Programme (UNDP) and UNAIDS. While the UNAIDS was the point agency for HIV/AIDS, the United Nations Population Fund (UNFPA), an organization essentially meant to focus on population stabilization and promote family planning, was ironically allocated the work of sex workers who were promiscuous due to the nature of their profession. A technical support unit (TSU) funded by, and accountable to, the Department for International Development (DFID) under a bilateral agreement was earmarked for NACO. A big player was Avahan, an agency funded by the BMGF, with a budget of USD 250 million, for AIDS control programme activities in 85 key districts accounting for half of the HIV infected. It had a weak working relationship with NACO.

Clearly, there were three tasks at hand: one, to further fine-tune the strategy with better design features for the upcoming NACP III; two, strengthen NACO and its organizational capacity on an immediate basis to quickly scale up implementation; and three, to assert the leadership of NACO and channelize donor efforts to provide a united response.

Designing the Strategy

India had a sound evidence-based strategy that required to be scaled up. With the NACP II coming to a closure, there was an opportunity to review, consolidate, and expand under the NACP III.

A design team consisting largely of people with no ground-level experience of the health sector had been constituted for preparing the NACP III document. It necessitated a reconfiguration with health economists for preparing a costed plan based on a more rigorous standard of data analysis. A steering committee consisting of all donors was also constituted that met monthly on an informal basis to review the drafts.

To gain a better understanding of the programme, field visits were undertaken and extensive interactions held with a wide cross section of people at risk. Such interactions generated ideas that were later incorporated into the formulation of the NACP III. Early visits to Andhra Pradesh, Karnataka, sex worker collectives in Bangalore, Mysore (now Mysuru), and Bagalkot as well as discussions with the staff at SACS and several experts like Jana, Sundar, Dr D.C.S. Reddy, and Ashok Rao Kavi exposed NACO to field-level problems. Donor organizations also contributed with their research and participation of people with years of experience on the issues facing the HIV strategy, such as Suneeta Singh from the World Bank, Sudhakar from the Centers for Disease Control and Prevention (CDC), Vidya Ganesh from UNICEF, Po Lin from the WHO, Ashok Alexander and his team from Avahan, and Denis Broun from UNAIDS. Members of civil society, people living with HIV/AIDS (PLHA) groups, and implementing agencies provided insights and shared evidence.

The visits and interactions shaped the trajectory of the NACP III—be it the adoption of a target of 50 per cent for community-based organizations (CBOs), costing data for a targeted intervention (TI) from NGOs and the Bangalore-based Ashodaya that was a CBO, fixing the size of a 1,000-member TI based on a cost-effective study done by the London School of Hygiene and Tropical Medicine, or the three-tiered structure of a TI consisting of peer educators (PEs), outreach workers, and the project director taken from the Sonagachi experience, or the idea of link workers and its costing adopted from the Karnataka Health Promotion Trust that had implemented such a scheme in Bagalkot, or the shift from voluntary testing centres to integrated counselling and testing centres and the scale-up to primary health centres from the Tamil Nadu State AIDS Control Society (TANSACS), or antiretroviral treatment (ART) and treatment challenges from the CDC-funded Tambaram ART centre in Tamil Nadu, or the focus on monitoring and evaluation (M&E) and programme strengthening from Avahan. What NACO was attempting during that period is today referred to as 'implementation science'—defined as the study of methods to promote the integration of research findings and evidence into healthcare policy and practice.[1]

In May 2007, the NACP III was launched. It reflected NACO's audaciously ambitious plan that envisioned a fivefold increase in funding from USD 500 million under NACP II to USD 2.5 billion and a universal coverage under all programme activities to be provided free. The objective was to reverse the epidemic by reducing new infections by half within the five-year period.

Reflection, thinking, and understanding paved the way for the next step that was planning and implementation. A robust institutional base was essential to knit together all the different strands of opinions, views, fears, apprehensions, aspirations, agendas, and motivations to face this huge challenge.

Gathering Evidence

NACO's strategy was based on evidence gathered from a wide variety of sources: sentinel surveillance, behavioural surveys, mapping, household surveys, operational research, programme evaluations, and so on. This evidence was collected by reaching out to consultants, experts, donors, academicians, research institutions, civil society activists, affected groups through technical resource groups, review meetings, consultations, field trips, tour notes, and the monthly programme data. These constituted the leitmotif for understanding the nature of the virus, its modes of transmission, and led to designing of appropriate strategies. These strategies are briefly described in Box 4.2.

The sentinel surveillance[2] system was the bedrock of NACO's strategies. Under this system, every year during a fixed time period—August to October—at a fixed facility, a fixed number of blood samples (400 from antenatal clinics and 250 from high-risk locations) from the same category of people were taken in a consecutive sequence. And to ensure no bias, information on residence, education, occupation, age, and parity helped profile the infected persons and construct the infection's anatomy.

The focus in the initial years was on STDs as HIV was considered an STD. Later pregnant women were also considered to be

Box 4.2 Early Years of the Epidemic

A dominantly held view is that in 1984, Jacob John, the head of the Department of Virology, CMC, Vellore, acquired an ELISA machine from Sweden. Erik Somoese, a paediatrician working in Goa, and a trainee fellow at the National Institutes of Health (USA) brought back reagents for about a thousand sera. Since 300 blood samples from people undergoing blood transfusion were negative and identifying a homosexual rare, a hypothesis of examining sex workers was proposed. Taking the help of the state minister of health, 100 blood samples from the inmates of remand homes in Chennai, Salem, Trichi, and Vellore were drawn. Analysis showed 14 to be positive—3 from Madurai, 1 from Vellore, 10 from Chennai—and were confirmed with Western blot test. Soon thereafter, the National Institute of Virology (NIV), Pune, diagnosed the first two AIDS patients: one infected by blood transfusion and the other following Factor VIII transfusion in the US.

In 1986–7, the Indian Council for Medical Research (ICMR) established an HIV task force to conduct serological and clinical surveillance. Focusing on obtaining seroprevalence data was against the official advice of the WHO and world opinion because it was seen as chasing AIDS cases. In 1987, the NICED established an HIV surveillance centre in Imphal and in 1988, the CMC in Vellore established a department of virology and initiated blood screening, not without being adversely commented upon as both unethical and unnecessary by the WHO and experts like Jonathan Mann.

By 1991, the surveillance system had tested over 0.6 million blood samples that showed over 15 per cent HIV infections due to contaminated blood; nearly 50 per cent of these were on account of heterosexual behaviour and the high susceptibility of injectable drug users to HIV. The relationship between HIV and TB, HIV and STDs, HIV and pregnancy, and vertical transmission and paediatric AIDS was clear. Further, based on this data, population groups were categorized according to behaviour as high-risk, intermediate, and low-risk. India initiated HIV Sentinel Surveillance (HSS) in 1992 and formalized its annual rounds from 1998 onwards.

Source: Author.

a sensitive and reliable indicator and proxy for the general population as they were young and sexually active, while pregnancy, being a physiological condition, reduced bias. Further, India's cultural context of comparatively lower levels of extramarital sexual relationships among married women made them the end point of the transmission chain. Besides, it was argued that if men as clients of sex workers, drug addicts, or as partners of other men contracted the virus, it would show up in the blood stream of their wives or partners.

Since blood tests were the only means of diagnosing the HIV infection, expansion of surveillance centres to track the spread of the epidemic was critical. In 2006, the sites were increased from 397 to 704,[3] and further to 1,359 in 2010–11. Likewise, surveillance sites among HRG populations also increased from 59 in 2003 to 487 in 2011. Legal and social barriers made expansion of such centres among HRGs a challenge: sex workers were disorganized, hostile, and had negligible contact with the formal health system, while the conservative and positively discriminatory environment made it impossible for gays to come out or seek healthcare services from the public system.

The quality of surveillance data was accorded a high priority. Prior to 2006, timeliness, inspections, and validations were hardly reviewed and there were barely 22 supervisory teams in the country. The year 2007 saw a major overhaul and by the end of the NACP III in 2012, the surveillance system comprised an expansive network of regional institutes, namely AIIMS, the National AIDS Research Institute (NARI), the PGI, the National Institute of Epidemiology (NIE), and the All India Institute of Hygiene and Public Health (AIIHPH). Furthermore, the National Institute of Medical Science (NIMS) and the NIHFW were provided with teams consisting of data entry operators, epidemiologists, and research analysts: 70 members constituting the central government and institute teams, 95 people working in the SACS, 540 sentinel staff in the centres, 117 laboratories, and 13 national reference laboratories.[4]

Sample checks of the sentinel sites during the initial years were alarming. There were no lab technicians and those who were there were poorly trained raising questions about the reliability of data.

Issues such as vacancies, non-supply of kits, and poor supervision led to a tendency to fudge data. Site-wise deficiencies were documented, training workshops held, state surveillance teams constituted, checklists prepared, and reviews held to follow up the action taken to rectify the errors. Similarly, before proposing a site, a prevalidation visit was made mandatory. Guidelines and protocols were developed, training given, and a four-tier supervisory structure for supportive supervisions introduced.

Getting the Numbers Right

Sentinel surveillance data was also used to estimate prevalence levels. In 2006, the NFHS data provided state-level estimations of HIV prevalence in the six high-prevalence states of Tamil Nadu, Andhra Pradesh, Maharashtra, Karnataka, Manipur, and Nagaland as well as a national estimate. Lalit Dandona, an epidemiologist from the Administrative Staff College of India, a Hyderabad-based institute, analysed the blood samples collected in the NFHS for Guntur district of Andhra Pradesh and concluded that HIV prevalence could not be more than 0.3 per cent that translated to about 2.3 million, halving the official estimate of 5.2 million. When further triangulated with multiple data sources—Integrated Bio-Behavioural Assessments (IBBA), Integrated Testing and Counselling Centres (ICTCs), and sentinel surveillance—these figures provided ample scope to replace mere assumptions with evidence-based values. This was an explosive piece of news not without political fallouts.

Aware that any unilateral announcement of a reduced number would invite instant criticism from donors and since donor perceptions mattered to the government and the media, a strategic decision was taken to place raw data for external inspection by prestigious institutions such as CDC (Atlanta), Imperial College (London), the WHO, UNAIDS, and others—an approach that raised NACO's reputational standing. Analysis of the 2007 sentinel data with the revised methodology confirmed Dandona's estimations resulting in the reduction in global estimates of AIDS from 30 million to about 25 million and in India from 5.2 million to 2.3 million.

Integrated Bio-Behavioural Assessments (IBBA) and Mapping

NACO also actively used data made available from other sources such as the IBBA, an innovation of the AIDS Prevention and Control Project (APAC) funded by the United States Agency for International Development (USAID) that was under implementation in Tamil Nadu. The IBBA consisted of household surveys to assess the behavioural responses towards safe-sex practices, namely the use of condoms and an understanding of how HIV spreads among HRGs.[5] Besides, NACO used the snowballing effect to gain information about the hidden populations based on oral evidence given by the people in the trade or group that helped determine key transmission arteries such as the sex routes, truck routes, drug routes, and migrant destinations. Such mapping was done by professional organizations with data validation by the IIPS, Mumbai. Mapping was also undertaken in villages to identify hidden risky behaviour, including that of transgenders. Such mapping exercises provided evidence of the size and spread of people practising high-risk behaviour that further helped NACO make appropriate budget allocations, locating and scaling up the siting of interventions.

Operational Research

The fourth source of information was operational research and studies conducted by various institutions and organizations on a wide variety of aspects ranging from migrant behaviour and practices to the access and utilization of ART services, ethical practices of physicians, impact of drugs, quality of testing in laboratories and counselling services in ICTC, the functioning of blood banks, quality of the implementation of the TI by NGOs, and later the evaluation of NACO strategies to assess impact. NACO used the NARI and other government research institutions on a concurrent basis to provide insights, information, and data to guide policy.

Differential Planning

Surveillance data provided the prevalence levels of HIV and STDs. India was, and continues to be, a concentrated epidemic with

TABLE 4.1 Prevalence Levels of HIV Infection among Different Key Population Groups (in Percentage Points)

Category	2003	2007	2012	2015
General Population (antenatal care)	0.8	0.49	0.35	0.29
Sex Workers	10.33	5.06	2.67	2.2
MSM	8.47	7.41	4.43	4.3
Injectable Drug Users	13.15	7.23	7.14	9.9

Source: NACO; surveillance data over the years.

higher prevalence among certain groups of people and geographically concentrated in six states that accounted for 70 per cent of the HIV-infected. The prevalence levels among different population groups have been provided in Table 4.1.

Based on the prevalence of antenatal care (ANC), six states in India were identified as high-prevalence states (having more than 1.0 per cent HIV prevalence in the general population), three states as moderate-prevalence states (concentrated epidemic with more than 5 per cent HIV prevalence in high-risk populations), and the rest as low-prevalence states.

Categorizing Districts for Differential Programme Planning

Triangulation and analysis of all sources of data helped NACO undertake differential planning efforts simultaneously on two fronts: among subpopulation groups versus general population and in some states and districts versus others in geographic terms. Given the heterogeneity of the epidemic and the wide variance in HIV prevalence between districts and intra-districts, the data from HIV sentinel surveillance centres and Voluntary Counselling and Testing Centres (VCTCs), and assessing risk and vulnerability, NACO classified the 584 districts in the country into four categories, namely A, B, C, and D. While a majority of districts were located within the low-prevalence states, further vulnerability factors such as migration, size of the population, and weak health infrastructures were utilized to identify the 'highly vulnerable' among the low-prevalence states/UTs (Table 4.2).

TABLE 4.2 Categories of Districts, 2007

	Category of Districts	
1.	More than 1% ANC/Prevention of Parent to Child Transmission (PPTCT) prevalence in districts at any time in any of the sites in the last three years	A (6 states, 156 districts)
2.	Less than 1% ANC/PPTCT prevalence in all the sites during the last three years associated with more than 5% prevalence in any HRG (STD/CSW/MSM/IDU)	B (3 states, 39 districts)
3.	Less than 1% ANC prevalence in all sites during the last three years with less than 5% in all STD clinic attendees or any HRG with known hotspots (migrants, truckers, large aggregation of factory workers, tourists, and so on)	C (278 districts)
4.	Less than 1% ANC prevalence in all sites during the last three years with less than 5% in all STD clinic attendees or any HRG or no or poor HIV data with no known hotspots/unknown	D (111 districts)

Source: NACO (2007).

The A and B districts received preferential treatment in resource distribution, higher policy attention, stronger managerial capacity and organizational structures at the SACS, tighter monitoring, and more frequent visits from NACO. Further, with the increase in programme activities, District AIDS Prevention and Control Units (DAPCUs) were established in these districts, functioning under the overall supervision of the district administration, to enable closer monitoring and better convergence of service delivery activities into the health system under the NRHM and across other sectors. Besides, surveillance data was also used to identify intra-district differentials for locating the ICTC and ART centres, while mapping data was used to identify the hotspots for locating the TIs and closely reviewing the sexual networks prevailing in that area to identify the factors that were fuelling the epidemic.

Organizational strengthening at NACO and SACS followed programme strategies that were packaged into three broad categories for easier comprehension of the linkages among them: a) prevention; b) treatment, care, and support; and c) reduction in discrimination and creating an enabling environment. The divisions for administration, finance, training, monitoring, and evaluation cut across all sectors. Each programmatic intervention was drilled down into activities and each activity had unit costs that were then multiplied with the target number to be achieved during that year for arriving at the total budget to be provided for the intervention—state- and district-wise.

The poor capacity at state levels necessitated that programme officers and consultants be sent to the states and workshops held in Delhi, Jaipur, and Agra to learn how to use evidence to prepare plans, how to assess the needs of vulnerable populations, and how to interlink the activities and prepare the budgets. After two years of intense effort, the states developed their own capacity reducing their dependence on outside help, even as the formats became less complex and more standardized.

Planning is a continuous dynamic. Gathering and analysing evidence was given much importance. For example, analysis showed that prior to the NACP III, TI projects were often granted not according to need but on the basis of where a 'good' NGO was working. In fact, data in Tamil Nadu demonstrated how blocks with very high prevalence rates had no interventions while those that were on the roadside and had good NGOs were provided grants. Evidence helped even out such distortions.

Differential planning by the categorization of districts to determine implementation was a unique contribution of NACO. It led to a more efficient use of scarce resources and narrowing of the focus areas for close monitoring rather than spreading attention thinly over a wide canvas.

Organizational Strengthening

Ideas and strategies might be sound. The difficult and often neglected part is the building of systems and institutional mechanisms to implement them. Often, institutional design is ignored and guidelines or government orders treated as adequate substitutes. NACO was perceived as confused, weak, and ineffective—a perception that had to be corrected. NACO's organization was accordingly restructured and revamped to be able to lead the country's response and be respected.

NACO's programme needs emerged from the evaluation data that was collected. HIV was one infection but had subsidiary disciplines like STD or blood safety and expanding access to these services was hindered by a host of social and behavioural issues like poverty, stigma, ostracism, and many others. Each focus area was a complex field with specific needs for human resources and skills: STD, for example, required specialists in virology, while blood safety needed haematologists, microbiologists, and laboratory scientists. PPTCT needed paediatricians and gynaecologists, ART required specialists in medicine, TIs required social scientists, while Information, Education and Communication (IEC) needed expertise in communication, programme management needed epidemiologists and statisticians, and finance required people who understood public finance. Based on an understanding of these needs, nine principal areas that needed priority attention were mapped out: TIs to refer to the programmes among HRG (also known as key populations), STD control, integrated counselling and testing, blood safety, treatment, IEC, surveillance, HMIS, administration/HR and Finance.

To ensure accountability and flow of responsibility it is critical to create structures and hierarchies with clear job functions and reporting lines. The organizational restructuring thus consisted of divisions comprising a team led by a joint director that consisted of one or more programme officers, two or more technical officers, and a statistician for M&E. The joint directors were senior government officers selected to ensure continuity, stability, and accountability.[6] Division heads defined their goals and targets, obtained and analysed data independent of NACO's information system for corrective action, and were accountable to the DG.

Constitution of teams and building a team approach was given emphasis to foster a certain work culture. To get the right people with the right skills, campus recruitments were made from reputed institutions like the Tata Institute of Social Sciences (TISS) and the Institute of Rural Management Anand (IRMA), medical schools, and schools of public health like the Indian Institute of Health Management Research (IIHMR). Selected candidates were provided with orientation on the NACP III strategy in general and their area of work in particular and were encouraged to visit project sites. For example, in the TI division, the Gates Foundation took the responsibility of providing the division with technical support by recruiting experienced hands to work within NACO so as to train, mentor, and guide the TI team on a daily basis. Likewise, the ART team was handheld by the CDC as well as the WHO.

A transparent HR policy was formulated and remuneration was linked to market rates by monetizing the health, transport, and housing benefits that government employees obtained in kind. They were given the title of programme officer or technical officer as the case may be and made accountable to NACO. This engendered a feeling of belonging, accountability, and responsibility as well as liberty to work.

A national technical support unit (NTSU) was also envisaged so that capacity-building could be a continuous process under the watchful eye of a mentor rather than by short-term trainings elsewhere. So the TSU funded by the DFID was replaced by an NTSU consisting of full-time consultants to work with divisional teams. But that was easier said than done. Experienced and well-qualified people were not easily available and certainly not at the salaries that the government could afford to pay. The need was most acutely felt in the TI division as the experts in this field were very few. And even those few had been mopped up by the Gates Foundation and other international NGOs and UN agencies that paid huge salaries. The irony of the situation was evident: while NACO was charged with the responsibility of reversing the epidemic, the donors had all the expertise to give NACO advice!

Since reversing the epidemic was dependent on scaling up the organizational capabilities of NACO, donors had to work with and not in competition with the government. This meant building the implementation capacity of NACO by appointing experienced consultants to work with the programme heads and integrating donor plans with NACO's annual plans for ensuring India's response to HIV. An understanding was also arrived at with donors that no one from NACO would be poached to work in their organizations. Accordingly, divisions were partnered with donors, for instance, TI, STD, and IEC were the responsibility of the World Bank, the Gates Foundation, and the DFID while the ART division was that of the WHO, the CDC, and so on. Donors helped recruit personnel, provide training, conduct workshops, organize site visits, and so on. Similar technical support was established in the high-priority states and regional directors were appointed to closely monitor the roll-out of the ART programme. For building surveillance capacity, NACO consultants were given training on surveillance methods, data management, epidemiology, and some were even sent for training abroad.

Such a collaborative arrangement helped in aligning the efforts of donors and NACO and reduced duplication. For example, five modules for doctors, three for counsellors, and masses of IEC materials—all of high quality—were found lying around unused. NACO simply took permission of the donors and printed the material for use with a joint logo and acknowledgements, thereby saving almost a year in developing teaching/learning materials. NACO also included the donors in all technical resource groups. Such partnerships ensured all worked together as a team and in an atmosphere of trust.

State AIDS Control Societies (SACS)

SACS were similarly strengthened with an organizational structure and further expanded with additional posts. Posts were fixed in accordance with the disease burden of the state and the consequent workload. However, strengthening SACS proved more challenging as in many states it was difficult to find qualified and suitable people with the right skills. Human resources were a major challenge, particularly in the area of targeted interventions and condom promotion. This weakness had to be addressed on a priority basis as both these formed the core of the strategy.

The DFID and USAID had demonstrated interesting models and innovations in governance. APAC, a USAID-funded body in Chennai, was located within the Voluntary Health Services, an NGO, but chaired by the secretary of health with a representative of NACO as a member. Likewise, under its Partnerships of Sexual Health (PSH) Project, the DFID established State Management Agencies (SMAs) and Regional Management Units (RMUs) consisting of qualified and experienced professionals from management, social sciences, and public health to work on the specialized aspects of HIV. The governance structure of these SMAs consisted of the state health secretary as the chairperson of the steering team. Such a structure helped build a collaborative model with the SMAs helping SACS in Kerala, Andhra Pradesh, Odisha, and Gujarat in the selection, training, and management of NGOs for TIs. This experience was then replicated into full-fledged TSUs for high-prevalence states to help them scale up the TI and related interventions. Many of the professionals working in the SMAs subsequently provided the leadership needed to scale up the TI/NGO component under the NACP III.

The TSUs' mandate was to implement all aspects of the TI strategy with SACS, concurrently building their capacity as also that of the implementing partner NGOs. While in most states, TSUs proved useful, in Odisha,[7] Chhattisgarh, and Madhya Pradesh, their efforts were stymied due to the choking institutionalized corruption. The TSUs could be effective only if allowed to function objectively. Instead, in these states we faced problems of pressure being mounted on the TSUs by the SACS officers to renew the contracts of NGOs or give favourable reports about their work. TSUs would, in turn, be threatened that if they did not cooperate, an adverse report would be sent against them to NACO.

Special Vehicles for Condom Marketing and Trucker Interventions

Two areas—condom marketing and implementation of the trucker's project—needed special focus and skills. These capacities were clearly beyond those available in SACS. Under the pilot Healthy Highways Project, the DFID had directly managed the truckers' intervention through its two RMUs that worked under the social sector and its own management professionals. This innovation was adapted and scaled up as a technical resource group. Professionals were selected and designated specifically for condom marketing and for the trucker's projects, with both directly reporting to NACO. Professional management agencies selected through open bidding in turn recruited experienced hands to work with SACS teams in the mapping of HRGs, identifying the NGOs and training them, and overseeing other aspects of implementation through frequent visits to the NGOs.

By the end of 2009, NACO had 18 Technical Resource Groups (TRGs). The TRGs consisted of domain experts, target group members, leading NGOs, state representatives, and experts from donor organizations and academicians working in this field (totalling about 300) with defined terms of reference and quarterly meetings. Most TRGs were chaired by the DG but some such as Research or Ethics were chaired by experts. TRGs helped NACO expand its field of experts advising and critiquing the programme and providing advice on how to improve and do better. All proceedings were minuted and action taken on decisions reviewed at the next meeting to ensure serious follow-up.

Other institutional innovations were the TSUs at NACO and SACS and eight state technical resource centres to help with the TI work. Ninety-five people in NACO were working on prevention programmes. The total staff at NACO was 152 as compared to 31 under the NACP II.

District AIDS Prevention and Control Unit (DAPCU)

As implementation assumed scale and speed, the need for further decentralization and integration with the health system emerged, be it in the siting of testing centres in primary health units located for every 30,000 population in high-prevalence districts or in establishing ART link centres for drug delivery in the block-level health facilities. The need to have a district-level presence to coordinate and link the various NACO activities gave rise to the DAPCU. By the end of 2011, a survey of 182 districts showed the presence of 44,753 people paid for by NACO in the form of salary or honorarium and working for the NACO programme in 9,120 delivery points—half working for the TIs and 10 per cent for treatment. Personnel included managers, doctors, microbiologists, epidemiologists, pharmacists, laboratory technicians, counsellors, nurses, link workers, outreach workers, PEs, janitors, cooks, cleaners, and a host of others.

Implementation of the Strategy

Standardization

Any effective well-designed scale-up normally follows the phase called 'proof of concept'. New interventions or policies are usually piloted, experimented with, and evaluated for their replicability and 'scaling up'. By the time the NACP III was launched, the proof-of-concept stage had been completed. It was time for expansion. However, the challenge was not replication in quantitative terms but ensuring quality and sustainability. In other words, it was important for every intervention to have a standard design and structure to ensure uniformity and reliability with inbuilt resilience to withstand temporary setbacks.

Operationally, this entailed four processes: designing the intervention, standardizing the implementation guidelines, disseminating them, and monitoring compliance.

The first is designing the content and substance with clarity, disseminating them to the front-line workers, and monitoring to ensure a uniform understanding irrespective of the geographical location of the intervention.

Second, scheme design led to the need for operational guidelines to be written in an easily understandable language. An operational guideline was conceived in the form of a document that laid down the statement of goals, objectives, and rationale; provided details of the activities, process features, unit costs, and monitoring formats with periodicity for report submissions. The guideline also indicated the qualifications, functions, responsibilities, and suggested band of remuneration of the human resources that are required to be deployed. To ensure ownership and accountability, the operational guidelines were developed in-house but in consultation with and the approval of the TRGs that were established for each intervention. The idea was to standardize and align budgets and outcomes with NACO's expectations with minimum loss in transmission of ideas and approaches. It was also to ensure that the residence of the beneficiary (patient) should not deny access or quality of service. By the end of 2009, about 40 *operational guidelines* were developed.

Third, ensuring compliance of the operational guidelines meant that they had to be read, understood, and internalized by the concerned staff in the SACS and the DAPCU through training and during visits and reviews. For example, Suresh Mohammad, in charge of the ICTC, personally interacted with and gave training to each of the 250 district supervisors on the operational guidelines developed for supportive supervision. All the other divisions did likewise and developed the appropriate training software.

As the requirements of the TI division were complex due to the varied educational backgrounds of the concerned, teaching aids including animation films and flip charts were developed. Given the large numbers involved, training was institutionalized and standardized to the extent possible. Eleven training institutions were identified and provided long-term support for recruiting staff and strengthening their capacity in TI work. Similarly, medical colleges, schools of social work, and other such institutions were identified for training doctors, counsellors, and so on.

Fourth is the tight monitoring of the scaling up of execution. For understanding the directional flow of the programme, it was critical to have good-quality and reliable data and to have it available on a regular basis. But NACO had no capacity for developing such an HMIS. An expert committee was constituted that developed 156 indicators, a dashboard, and a format. UNAIDS was made responsible for obtaining the reports from donors. It was a tough task as many such as the Gates Foundation and USAID were often not open to sharing their data.

Within NACO, a full-fledged HMIS unit with 12 professionals was established that directly reported to the DG. The SACS was also provided with staff, but the biggest challenge was finding epidemiologists. The HMIS unit developed guidelines and trained the state units, closely following up data submission, outliers, and discrepancies. This data was read with the surveillance data and also compared with the data received directly by the programme officers that, at times, was exaggerated. Calibration took both time and effort. Subsequently, in 2009, substantial efforts were made for triangulating all the rich data available to plot the trajectory of the epidemic and action points. Front-line workers were to be trained to furnish and analyse the data and get involved in preparing the district plans. But this was not followed up to the extent envisaged and continues to be a need. The only antidote to the fudging of data is that the primary worker understands the meaning and implication of the data being collected and feels her input is being valued.

Monitoring of the programme consisted of weekly reviews, bimonthly reviews, field visits, and state-level reviews. Once every quarter, a team of officers representing all the divisions undertook a five-day visit for indepth reviews of the key states. And once a quarter, indepth reviews of each division lasting half a day or more were undertaken by the DG. Records and minutes of every field visit and meeting were maintained and actions taken were reviewed until the problems were resolved. Besides, field visits entailed preparation with details of issues proposed to be addressed and follow-up of previous visits. Such systems are rigorously implemented in the private sector while public systems tend not to accord much importance to these aspects, explaining to a large part the reason for the hiatus between policy articulation and implementation.

Standardization and uniformity helped costing, budgeting, and the eventual scale-up. It is, however, entirely in the realm of possibility that it may have been at the cost of innovation and local initiative. In the initial stages, balancing such trade-offs was difficult. My experience shows that before innovation, it is more important to build in habits[8] and a culture of valuing evidence, monitoring, and evaluation for achieving the targets already agreed to. Once this sets in, innovation and the ability to use evidence to solve local problems in a constructive way follows.

Change is always resisted and has to be overcome by laying down clear guidelines on what has to be done, how, when, and by whom and diligently monitored, leaving no room for mistakes. Persuasion and constant repetition of the given instructions are also important. In other words, consistency, along with clarity, is critical. Over time, as the results begin to flow in, resistance reduces and confidence develops that the new way of doing things helps in getting better results within a shorter time. In the third year, resistance gives way to acceptance and the scale-up. Graphs of periods of reform and policy shifts show a dip in the first year, a slight increase in the second year, and a jump in the third year and onwards. Likewise, a leader starts with total centralization and as acceptance increases, new habits and systems get institutionalized, there is 'controlled delegation'. Total delegation kicks in when all systems are completely institutionalized. Then the leader becomes less important for the sustainability of the intervention. But a leader also must know when to centralize, when to let go, and also what should never be delegated to another and lost sight of.[9]

Thus, monitoring of implementation had three threads: operational guidelines, training, and enforcement through structured reviews for course correction. Flexibility is an essential component for such course corrections. Large impersonal organizations that have limited interactions with stakeholders forget this principle of management and develop rigidities.

Components of the Strategy

India's strategy was three-pronged and had three major pillars that had to be simultaneously strengthened with equal vigour and on scale for maximizing impact.

1. *Prevention* that had six distinct subcomponents and accounted for 55 per cent of the budget: a) expanding access to treatment of STDs, b) reducing HIV transmission from 1 per cent to less than 0.3 per cent by promoting blood safety, c) promotion of condom use, d) raising awareness and communication, e) increasing access to diagnosis through ICTCs, and f) mother-to-child transmission.
2. *Treatment, care, and support* of opportunistic infections (OIs), cross infections, and provisioning of free ART.
3. *Reducing discrimination and working with the marginalized HRG*—commercial sex workers (CSWs), men who have sex with men, injectable drug users, bridge population groups—who accounted for a disproportionately high incidence of the HIV infection. This aspect of the programme strategy called TIs accounted for a quarter of the budget and half of NACO's attention space.

Every intervention had its own design features and institutional structures that again had to be knitted together. Using data and evidence resulted in constantly innovating for addressing new challenges that kept emerging as we went deeper into the issues.

Prevention

Sexually Transmitted Infections (STI)

Against an estimated[10] 30 million STI/Reproductive Tract Infection (RTI) cases per year, hardly 2 million were being treated in the 845 STI clinics in public health facilities. The current strategy was clearly inadequate and co-opting the private sector to scale up access to STD treatment an imperative.

Avahan introduced two innovative approaches to STI treatment. The first approach was through static clinics within the HRG premises. In these clinics, HRGs were incentivized for early check-ups and meticulously tracked for the frequency and timeliness of seeking medical care. It was thereby possible to develop a cohort of the caseload that enabled tracking disease progression—the shifts from bacterial to viral and the drastic reduction and the gradual elimination of syphilis and other venereal diseases. A study conducted for the years 2000–8 showed that HIV and syphilis prevalence declined substantially among young pregnant women. Each additional STI treated (per 1,000 people) reduced the annual risk of HIV infection by −1.7 per cent (95 per cent, CI −3.3 to −0.1) and syphilis infection by −10.9 per cent (95 per cent, CI −15.9 to −5.8).[11]

The second approach was the introduction of a protocol-driven treatment consisting of pre-packaged colour-coded drugs—each colour representing a typical clinical condition and the drugs to be administered for treating that condition. Standardization and easy usage reduced the scope for error. At the same time such standardization ensured the appropriateness and effectiveness of the treatment.

The scaling up of this approach was then attempted nationwide. A strategy that consisted of centralized procurement and supply of colour-coded drugs, issuance of operational guidelines, standardization of training modules, and training of doctors working in public health facilities was implemented jointly by NACO and the NRHM to ensure uniformity.

STI facilities in public hospitals were improved with audio and visual privacy along with space and equipment for examination. Counsellors, doctors, and nurses were assigned and provided with computers to better enable them to record and report cases. Staff was trained on STI management and services scaled up to all the medical colleges, district hospitals, and sub-district health facilities. Another 330 facilities were added to the existing 845. But this conventional approach was found to be inadequate as was the concept of static clinics in the HRG sites.

In 2007, a mapping of private providers revealed that over 8,000 providers were treating STI but over three-quarters of them were located in cities/towns. Another round of mapping of preferred providers in consultation with the HRGs and NGOs implementing TIs revealed that over 3,700 'preferred' providers were the ones the key population groups went to and trusted. These people were then trained and supplied with the colour-coded drugs; the TIs provided an additional budget of Rs 50 for every case of referral to the clinic and encouraged the appointment of an ANM to undertake periodic examination and maintain health records.

The treatment access points were branded as 'Suraksha Clinics' to ensure that these appeared user-friendly and non-stigmatizing. An IEC strategy helped raise awareness and dispel common myths related to sexual health. It also helped generate demand for standardized services. This approach resulted in an uptake of services by sex workers—from less than 0.23 million in 2007–8 (per year) to over 3.55 million by 2014–15. Syphilis reduced to less than 1.2 per cent in STI attendees as against over 3.2 per cent, and among pregnant women it came down to 0.4 per cent from 1.8 per cent. The overall service utilization increased from the stagnant 2 million to over 7.4 million in 2014–15.

Blood Safety

In 1991, contaminated blood was responsible for 15 per cent of HIV infections with almost three-quarters of the blood procured from paid donors. This alarming data led to blood safety being shifted from the DGHS to NACO. However, as a systemic issue, it was a bad decision since blood safety is not only for HIV infection but also for general health. As a result of a PIL filed in 1992, the Supreme Court in its order of 4 January 1996 directed the constitution of an independent organization called the National Blood Transfusion Council (NBTC). With this, a further stimulus was accorded to the relatively neglected programme. The programme sought to shift focus towards promoting voluntary blood donation; establishing blood banks and blood component separation units; training personnel; providing equipment, testing kits, and so on. A national blood policy was released in 2002.

As a result of these developments, NACO strengthened 1,137 blood banks. HIV seroreactivity declined from 1.2 per cent to 0.2 per cent and availability of safe blood increased from 4.4 million units in 2007 to 9.8 million units (of which blood collected by NACO's blood banks was 5.7 million units) by 2013 against the total requirement of 12 million units per year. Seventeen training centres were identified to provide training to a range of personnel: blood bank medical officers, technicians, counsellors, nurses, clinicians, donor motivators, and programme officers of SACS. Quality assurance systems were put in place and voluntary blood donation boosted to reach a level of over 84 per cent of the total blood collected. Such statistics made professional donors history in some states like Tamil Nadu and West Bengal.

Blood transfusion services in India, however, are plagued by a multiplicity of controls rather than a centralized policy. For instance, licensing is under the drug controller general of India, policy under the national and state blood transfusion councils, and implementation with the states. Recently, a national blood cell has been created in the Department of Health and Family Welfare, with an identical mandate as the NBTC leading to further confusion.

Despite NACO's efforts for the reliable transportation of blood, access to safe blood continues to be limited, especially in rural areas of states such as Uttar Pradesh, Uttarakhand, Jharkhand, Bihar, and Chhattisgarh. Almost 48 districts have no facilities for blood transfusion. This issue requires resolution through policy reforms and strengthening linkages with the National Health Mission (NHM) and preferably the outright inclusion of this programme under its direct ambit. The inability of government systems to coordinate availability of blood to those in need is one of the reasons for the large number of deaths and rampant black marketing of blood. There is an overall absence of accountability[12] in the system on the one hand while this critical component of healthcare is neglected on the other.

Marketing Condoms

Promotion of condoms as a family-planning device started in the 1960s with the establishment of a public sector entity Hindustan

Latex Limited (HLL) to manufacture good-quality condoms at affordable prices. Global companies like Unilever and the Indian Tobacco Company (ITC) were the main social marketing agencies, replaced later by Population Service International (PSI), Drammen Kommunale Trikk (DKT), and others with funding from bilateral agencies and private foundations. In the meanwhile, several manufacturing companies also came up giving HLL tough competition in terms of price and quality and bringing down its market share to less than 40 per cent.

Programme administration of condom promotion was with the MOHFW. Over the decades, with no marketing skills, corruption, and poor governance, the government's role gradually reduced to that of a subsidy provider. The ministry had no understanding of forecasting market demand and also had inadequate programme funding for condom promotion. Social marketing programmes focused on areas of donor priority rather than need or on family planning. The overall lack of accountability of social marketing organizations and questionable practices by some of them were aggravated by weak oversight of the programmes. All this was a huge challenge for expanding the market in the states with high prevalence of HIV but low fertility.[13]

For NACO, condom was a lifeline. In the absence of any alternative protective devices such as vaccine or microbicides, condom was the only effective barrier to the transmission of HIV infection. The NACP III had an ambitious plan of marketing 3.5 billion pieces from the baseline of 2 billion, establishing 2.5 million sale points and expanding from the existing 7 or 8 social marketing agencies to 25. Aware that achieving these ambitious targets would require marketing professionals and an institutional mechanism, a rearrangement of roles was worked out between NACO and the concerned division—condom programming for HIV and family planning under NACO, while the ministry would continue with the procurement and subsidy management.

Funded by the Gates Foundation, the Hindustan Latex Family Planning Promotion Trust (HLFPPT), a subsidiary of the government-owned HLL, helped NACO set up a technical support group (TSG) consisting of marketing experts to drive the condom programme. Getting the TSG team to work was an uphill battle requiring careful navigation through a complex bureaucratic landscape that had a negative, stonewalling approach and a problem of inflated egos. Even a seemingly simple task such as changing the packaging of a brand needed approval from multiple levels with decisions guided more by the preferences of joint secretaries rather than evidence from market research. Changing this mindset was a big challenge and it was only in 2008—almost 20 years after the proposal had been initiated by HLL—that NACO was granted permission to redesign the condom pack to align with consumer preferences. The long wait for a simple package change is a pointer to the prevailing situation within which NACO had to work.

To estimate the funds required for condom marketing, the TSG analysed the geographies where the scale-up of social marketing programmes for family planning and HIV could be undertaken. The MOHFW was at that time operating on a limited 'mental' model of sales-linked subsidies that were useless while dealing with 'hard-to-crack' geographies and customer segments. The cost of promoting condoms in a red-light area among reluctant sex workers and their clients was significantly higher than that of promoting them in a city for the general population.

The price differential led to allegations of many social marketing organizations (SMOs) selling off the condoms in cities through traders and pocketing the subsidy meant for condom promotion. The need for programme-based funding in high-priority geographies and consumer segments was acutely felt. After a lot of back-and-forth discussions with the MOHFW, it was finally decided that the required funds for administering the social marketing programme would be released under the NRHM to the TSG.

Based on learnings from the donor-funded social marketing programmes implemented between 2000 and 2006, the TSG developed a programme management framework, undertook retail trader training in marketing, and put in place a performance-based funding model. These performance metrics were focused on sales offtake, retailer penetration, and indicators for behaviour change. An effective monitoring mechanism was institutionalized for reviewing the programmes on the ground and for making all funding contingent on performance. The social marketing programmes were launched in all high-priority districts. After years of stagnation, under the NACP III the condom offtake increased from 2 billion to 3.5 billion sold in 1.2 million retail units and by eight social marketing agencies. Condom sales were monitored through the Operations Research Group (ORG) market surveys that also showed a substantial increase in the proportion of commercial sales signalling behaviour change where people were willing to buy condoms and practise safe sex. Female condoms were also introduced in all sex-worker interventions as part of the NACP III with marginal success. Such concerted efforts helped reduce condom-access time from 30 to 19 minutes and increased awareness from 81.8 per cent to 98.4 per cent. There was also a growth in the rural commercial condom market by 81 per cent as against the 47 per cent increase in the socially marketed condoms from 287 million to 422 million during the same time period. Rural condom stocking outlets also increased from 0.44 million in 2007–8 to 0.58 million in 2010–11.[14]

Innovation in Communication

A major weakness of the public health policy has been the insufficient attention to IEC aspects. Barring the two successful campaigns launched to propagate Nirodh and the red triangle, and later the universal immunization programme, IEC has by and large been confined to posters, pamphlets, and a few intermittent TV campaigns by way of short-duration advertisement spots. Attempts in the ministry to integrate and converge the IEC requirements of all national health programmes under one budget head did not succeed. Thus every programme has its own IEC budget and campaign strategies resulting in waste and duplication of efforts. Besides, due to the procurement rules of awarding contracts to the lowest tender and the order of having to first and foremost utilize the services of government media, quality did become a casualty.

NACO was fortunate in this regard as donors provided funds for the IEC campaigns. The Gates Foundation seconded the BBC World (far more expensive than our local agencies but has good quality) to NACO. Besides, it also helped commission four short films on issues related to HIV/AIDS by top film producers like Mira Nair, Vishal Bhardwaj, Farhan Akhtar, and Santosh Sivan.

Likewise, the support of UNICEF in putting up innovative visual displays in the Red Ribbon Express (RRE) campaign made a major contribution to expanding awareness into the interiors in an effective way.

The RRE was a great innovation and the most visible mass communication campaign.[15] Over the years, it traversed 187 stations. Besides visuals, the train also had teams of dramatists fanning out on cycles into the rural hinterland performing skits and holding interactive sessions with the community. Government departments, local bodies, NGOs, and corporate and industrial houses participated in the campaign reaching an estimated 25 million people and about 250,000 district resource persons were exposed to the message.

The nature of the infection makes AIDS communication a complex process. Social stigma and the difficulties in reaching out to highly vulnerable populations are challenging as a mix of contradictory messages have to be related: abstinence with safe sex, fidelity to a single partner with condom use, promoting condoms without hurting the population policy, and so on. Besides condoms, communication efforts were also aimed at promoting a more caring society, reducing stigmatizing attitudes towards the HIV-infected, and also creating awareness about how the infection spreads. Donors helped mobilize media icons: Shabana Azmi embraced an AIDS-affected child in a television advertisement and assured that the 'disease does not spread this way but what spreads is love'. Amitabh Bachchan, Shilpa Shetty, Sharmila Tagore, Jackie Shroff, Sachin Tendulkar, Rahul Dravid, and others also helped with raising AIDS awareness, promoting condoms, and appealing to youth to stay safe and healthy.

Behaviour change communication (BCC) was critical. Animation films and communication materials were developed for use by outreach workers, counsellors, nurses, and so on under the programme activities.

NACO's attempt to expand access to young teenagers about life-skills education under the School AIDS Education Programme (SAEP) later renamed as Adolescence Education Programme (AEP) was a major problem area. This was a collaborative programme with the Ministry of Human Resource Development and UNICEF to impart life-skills education to schoolgoing adolescents. Life-skills education is about sensitizing young schoolgoing children to undesirable behaviour patterns and enabling them to recognize those that need to be avoided, cope with an unsafe environment, and so on. As per NACO's understanding, the parents were also keen for their children to be taught such life skills. However, this programme had to be suspended in a number of states due to opposition from the more conservative forces that felt that exposing children to matters of sexuality meant instilling unnecessary ideas in them, not realizing that these children were facing such issues every day—in the bus, on the street, in the classroom.[16] Later some states did resume the programme. A major effort was also made towards mainstreaming HIV/AIDS messages in other departments to promote understanding and reduce irrational behaviour against those infected. This may not have contributed to reducing HIV prevalence per se, but it did help develop a more concerned and less hostile social environment.

Testing and Counselling

In 2005, about 6 per cent of the total estimated HIV people were diagnosed and the stigma attached to the disease was very high. Demystification of HIV testing was essential. Voluntary testing centres were located in district hospitals that were too far to access and, not surprisingly, located in the most unlikely areas of sprawling hospital complexes, which even the savvy and educated found hard to access. HIV testing consisted of pre-test and post-test counselling, which was a time-consuming, slow, and cumbersome protocol.

Taking the example of decentralizing testing centres to primary healthcare centres from Tamil Nadu, the first step towards scaling up testing and counselling services was by decentralizing their location to the facilities as per the ABCD categorization based on the gravity of the infection—CHCs in the C and D districts and PHCs in the A and B districts. This was a mammoth task as it not only required trained laboratory technicians but also recruiting a new category of personnel called counsellors. But very soon it was realized that such a conventional approach to scaling up was inadequate.

Clearly, a paradigm shift was required in two ways: one, decentralizing patient motivation to undergo HIV testing directly with the providers; and two, the introduction of whole blood finger-prick test kits for HIV testing. In the first instance, such provider-initiated counselling and testing was particularly emphasized for target groups such as pregnant women, TB patients, and others at risk. In the second instance, it was felt that the test kits would reduce dependence on laboratory technicians besides helping labour-room nurses to undertake HIV testing of pregnant women in labour, who are often rushed in for delivery at night when the laboratories are closed. By having a simple, user-friendly test kit available, an HIV-positive woman could be tested and administered timely treatment that could save the unborn baby from being infected by HIV.

The availability of easy-to-use technology and counselling services helped to better integrate HIV testing in routine antenatal care through a systematic convergence between the NRHM and the NACP. Such convergence was first achieved in the high-prevalence state of Karnataka as a result of the personal initiative of the PD of the NRHM. The stigma and reluctance of the Reproductive and Child Health (RCH) programme officers was so high that it took the PD (who was also the commissioner of health) eight rounds of meetings with the RCH division to persuade them to integrate HIV as a part of ANC. Besides, since a large number of facility-integrated ICTCs were established as part of this convergence in 24×7 PHCs, further integration became easier with HIV counselling and testing services being provided by the existing staff nurses and lab technicians. ICTCs were also established through PPPs in large maternity homes and missionary/charitable hospitals.

All these sets of measures enormously improved HIV counselling and testing. The number of ICTCs increased from 982 in 2004–5 to 7,548 in 2011–12 while testing increased from 1 million to 19.47 million per year in the corresponding period, covering almost 75 per cent of the total target of 22 million tests per year.

Scaling up meant expanding centres, ensuring their proper location, a patient-friendly atmosphere, and appointing trained laboratory technicians and counsellors. For example, it was observed that persons recruited from schools of social work as counsellors had a fairly low skill base as their teaching and curriculum was didactic and classroom-oriented. Massive investments in terms of time and energy had to be made to make these counsellors effective. Under Round 9 of the Global Fund, NACO identified TISS as the primary implementer for a USD 30 million grant to network the 45-odd schools of social work on a uniform curriculum, training, mentoring, and faculty development on counselling skills for HIV and thereon for chronic disease conditions.

Counsellors were the real lifeline of the HIV strategy and therefore dominated our attention space. They were trained and graded for their increments. Annual tests were prescribed for the continuation of their contract. This raised a mountain of protests and a certain amount of unionization in Maharashtra and Andhra Pradesh. The issue was regarding the 'fairness' and 'legality' of setting performance standards and competency measurement tools for one category of employees that did not apply to others in the health system, resulting in a feeling of 'harassment'. In terms of perception, this was partly true but the compulsions of having well-trained counsellors to help the 'infected' cope with the trauma did not allow the luxury of waiting for the whole health system to improve.

Since all ICTCs were located within public hospitals and health facilities, insulating NACO services from the rest in terms of quality and professionalism was a challenge. And speed and ambition were often curtailed by the weaknesses of the general health system. For example, Odisha was emerging to be a concern as it had serious problems of availability of certified lab technicians, severely hampering expansion.

Closely related to ICTCs and testing were issues of quality of reagents and their procurement. HIV is a laboratory-based disease as only blood tests can reveal not just the HIV status but also the progression of the disease once inside the human body. Laboratories and the quality of testing, standard of reagents along with the equipment and competencies of technicians were therefore critical and required focus and attention.

The External Quality Assurance Scheme (EQAS) was developed to strengthen laboratories involved in HIV testing. A three-tiered structure was set up with the NARI as the apex laboratory, 13 national reference laboratories, and 117 state-level reference laboratories. By developing standard operating procedures, capacity-building programmes, and technical support from Elizabeth Dax, an international expert from Australia and the CDC, laboratory practices were strengthened to ensure the quality of HIV testing at all ICTCs. Proficiency panels, periodic reviews, and training activities enabled most of the national and state reference laboratories to obtain the tough accreditation from the National Accreditation Board for Testing and Calibration Laboratories (NABL). Currently, more than 55 laboratories are accredited. This led to the strengthening of the health system. In fact, public sector laboratories applied for accreditation by the NABL only after NACO had initiated the process. It was a landmark achievement of NACO.

Issues of quality assurance need not have been of any concern to NACO if the health system was functioning well. If, for example, the drug regulatory authority was not such a corrupt, incompetent, or understaffed body, NACO would have moved towards standardization and making quality products available rather than having to get into several of the manufacturing and licensing issues. Likewise, if the health system had paid adequate attention to laboratories and functioned according to the protocols and quality standards, NACO would not have had to spend so much time in training, supervision, drilling down quality standards, and the rest.[17] These issues got no traction in the health ministry, yet they could not be ignored by NACO as they were central to the treatment and survival of HIV-infected people.

Prevention of Parent-to-Child Transmission (PPTCT): Use of Nevirapine

An interesting issue that arose in the ART programme is the time lag between discovery of good science and its adoption in policy. In other words, science may be sound but this may not imply an automatic acceptance as policy is often a compromise of the possible. For example, the combination of ART drugs administered at the end of the last week of the last trimester and continued for three months thereafter for pregnant women was better than administering the single dose nevirapine. Yet its adoption took time due to cost and programmatic implications. In an environment where antenatal care continues to be provided to less than 50 per cent, it was problematic to identify HIV-infected pregnant women and follow up with medication after delivery. This called for training and monitoring ANMs. For, this intervention implied identifying about 60,000 HIV-infected pregnant women out of a denominator of 23 million, which is like finding a needle in a haystack. Besides, though this intervention had no impact on the goal of reduced transmission, its implementation was pursued vigorously on ethical grounds. This was yet another instance that demonstrated the limitations of a vertical programme in expanding and scaling up when the basic health system itself is deeply flawed.

Things have changed now. With clinical trials, better knowledge, and effective drugs, it has become possible to scale up the programme to provide lifelong drugs to five categories of people irrespective of their CD count: pregnant women, breastfeeding and lactating women, TB patients, children under five years of age, and those with Hepatitis B and C having severe liver problems.

Treatment, Care, and Support

Prior to 1 December 2003, when Sushma Swaraj made the dramatic announcement of the government's intention to provide free treatment to people living with AIDS, there were heated debates about the implications of including treatment in the national programme. India's understanding and the core strategy for stopping transmission was the successful implementation of targeted interventions among HRGs and launching information campaigns to calm down the irrational fears and stigma surrounding this infection. It was apprehended that by introducing treatment when the prevention strategy itself was in a nascent stage, attention and resources may get diverted. This apprehension was because of the high cost of treatment at over Rs 30,000 per patient per month—a great deterrent given the small resource base.

Whatever it be, the die had been cast and the juggernaut of ART slowly rolled out on 1 April 2004 in eight hospitals. In 2005, NACO obtained a grant of USD 122 million from the Global Fund under Round 4 project. Under this project, there was a target of establishing 188 ART centres and reaching 0.3 million patients by 2012. Against this target, India established 313 ART centres, 641 link ART centres (LAC) as drug delivery points, and had over 0.5 million people living with HIV (PLHIV) on ART.

Globally, since the mid-1990s, the questions of treatment for HIV-infected people and price of drugs were acrimoniously discussed and debated in every international conference since the lack of treatment had resulted in the loss of lives on a scale and at a speed never witnessed before. The IPR regulations of 1995 had given monopoly control to patented drugs and medicines manufactured by large multinational pharmaceutical companies. The price at USD 12,000 per patient per year made them clearly unaffordable. Negotiations brought the price down at first by 10 per cent and later by 90 per cent. Yet even the USD 1,000 per patient per year was too high for a people living on incomes of a dollar a day (Brazil, South Africa, and India). The game changer was when in 2000, Cipla, an Indian generic company, offered to supply combination drugs for AIDS patients for USD 300. The sheer audacity of it stunned the world grabbing media headlines. This changed the tide in favour of AIDS patients and at once opened up a floodgate of possibilities and hope.

Emboldened with the sharp fall in prices and the easy availability of drugs, UNAIDS and the WHO launched the '3 by 5' initiative in 2003, under which three million PLHA in low- and middle-income countries were to be provided life-prolonging ART by the end of 2005. In the previous year, the Global Fund came into existence providing financial support and the US set up the President's Emergency Plan for AIDS Relief (PEPFAR) with a generous budget of USD 40 billion essentially for scaling up access to treatment. This, then, was the context in which India was holding out the introduction of treatment in the national programme. It was but a matter of time before it gave in to the demands of the infected people for treatment. From the government's viewpoint, the choices were a question of optimizing resource use. For the infected, it was quite simply a question of survival.

The infirmity in understanding and interconnecting the several aspects of the epidemic led to complications. With no treatment, HIV was a death sentence and with minimal nutrition and no treatment for OIs, patients acquired full-blown AIDS status within a short span of time and faced premature death. The absence of any hope of life and the certainty of death were at the root of the fear and stigma that were so closely associated with HIV. Shunned and abandoned, HIV-infected patients suffered immense isolation and pain. Human suffering apart, another critical aspect was that AIDS patients were also the most effective transmitters of the infection and since ART reduced the viral load, the risk of transmission also reduced significantly, making treatment an effective option.

The conundrum was the balance between finances and approach. In arguing that treatment stopped transmission, most countries gave up efforts to prevent the spread of HIV in the first place. India believed that in view of the large and growing sexually active population base and the major mode of transmission being heterosexual relations, a treatment-led strategy alone would be risky. Not only was the base of sex workers and clients expanding, nebulous, and ever-shifting but accessing it was also a constant challenge in itself. In such a situation, focusing on treatment would not only have been disastrous financially but would also have meant losing control over the epidemic.

With reduced prices and funding by the Global Fund under rounds 4 and 6 projects, the scenario changed dramatically providing the possibilities of building a two-pronged strategy that simultaneously scaled up both prevention and treatment. The technical complexities of the diagnostic tests, treatment consisting of highly potent drugs, and the poor condition of district hospitals made it imperative to locate the ART centres in medical colleges despite their overall inaccessibility to the patients. By definition, the ART centres were to be located in the departments of medicine that in all hospitals were typically understaffed and overcrowded. With no assistance, these departments refused to take the responsibility of providing treatment to AIDS patients, seeing it as an additional burden on their already scarce resources. On the other hand, in NACO it was argued that HIV was a new infection and should be treated in the department like any other instead of verticalizing it since that would only deepen the stigma.

In reality, the medical colleges were poorly financed and understaffed with weak infrastructural support and poor infection control processes. And in this context, we were introducing a highly infectious disease that also demanded intensive attention. This led to

NACO providing financial support for a whole package: physical infrastructure in terms of renovation and refurbishment, furniture, computers, and toilets; additional staff consisting of doctors, laboratory technicians, nurses, pharmacists, counsellors, record keepers; and all drugs and diagnostic equipment and even nutritional support in some places—in other words, a full-fledged, self-contained unit. Concerned that it may not be 'owned' by the department, the funding was channelized through the superintendent of the hospital with the head of the department held accountable for the proper functioning of the centre. The story did not end here. One of the most trying and difficult challenges was coordinating patient care that spread across departments—paediatrics, gynaecology, medicine, blood transfusion, and the rest—once again exposing the limitations of verticalized programme implementation.

As a large number of cases of lost to follow-up came up in the reviews, the PLHA organizations were requested to help find the missing patients and bring them back into the programme. This then gave rise to the appointment of a PLHA as the core coordinator in all ART centres. This was found to be very fruitful as PLHAs helped keep watch on the availability of drugs; ensured that they were not siphoned off; observed instances of denial of care, rude or stigmatizing behaviour; and followed up with patients who did not report on the scheduled day. They also helped in tracing the lost to follow-up cases that accounted for about 8.5 per cent of patients on treatment. Additionally, in order to improve the levels of adherence to ART, special initiatives were also undertaken such as dispensing antiretroviral drugs for two months to reduce the number of visits to the ART centre and liaising with concerned ministries to provide concessions in rail and bus travel.

The treatment, care, and support programme had other components: LACs, centres of excellence, treatment for pregnant women (PPTCT), HIV–TB patients, and community care centres. These are detailed further.

Link ART Centres (LACs)

By 2008, the number of ART centres had expanded coverage but also entailed a high number of dropouts because of the difficulties and expenses involved in coming all the way to the ART centres located in medical colleges to collect the monthly quota of drugs. Taking a cue from Thailand's example of demystifying ART, NACO decentralized ART drug distribution to the block-level health facilities—each catering to a population of 100,000—thus innovating the LACs. This greatly benefited the HIV patients who now got their monthly drugs close to their residence, saving on travel and the day's wages. As per protocol, they were required to visit the mother ART centre once in six months for their CD4 count checks.

Another idea that unfortunately did not take root despite concerted efforts by NACO was the electronic linking of patient records from the point of diagnosis in the ICTCs to registration and treatment in ART centres. Such a system based on biometric cards would have alleviated the portability aspect. Regular treatment on a long-term basis is required for chronic patients and more so for migrant labour. The electronic records would have helped in terms of identification and immediate access to medical reports. Though money and technology were available and computerization of the records and uploading were also done in substantial measure, the proposal languished for want of follow-up.

Quick expansion can affect quality. In 2007–8, regional coordinators (RCs) were appointed to closely monitor, mentor, and supervise ART centres under their charge through frequent visits. Periodic meetings of RCs were held at NACO to review the various issues pointed out by them. Additionally, NACO officials, particularly Dr Rewari, frequently visited ART centres to sort out problems on the spot. However, in hindsight, more could have been done with regard to treatment, education, and adherence.

An evidence-based approach was adopted from the very beginning to scale up the ART services network in order to improve access to care without compromising quality. Site selection for setting up ART centres was based on an analysis of district-wise ICTC data of seropositive people to map catchment areas and ensure distance does not become a barrier to access.

Centres of Excellence (CoE)

As time passed, the complexities of the programme and the extra-medical factors that affected the treatment outcomes necessitated

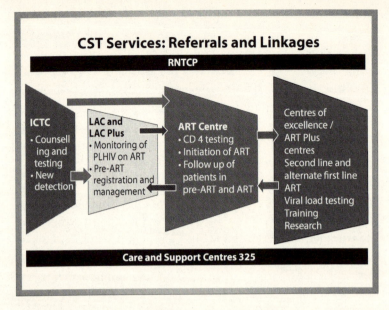

Figure 4.1 Scaling up ART
Source: NACO.

operational research, effective health delivery systems, and a trained workforce. There was a need for medical institutions that would deliver high-quality care, treatment, and support to PLHIV. Consequently, 10 CoE in HIV care were established (Figure 4.1). Alongside, seven regional paediatric centres were also established to cater to the needs of children infected with HIV. India, in association with the Indian Academy of Pediatrics (IAP) and UNICEF, became the first country to develop paediatric ART and paediatric dosages.

Integrating HIV with TB

Coordination, convergence, and integration are words most often used and least realized. In the roll-out of the HIV programme, evidence clearly showed that most HIV-infected people developed TB necessitating a close coordination with the programme. The TB division in the ministry was unwilling to cooperate and join forces with NACO. They were apprehensive that the stigma against TB, which was in decline, may get revived by its being associated with HIV/AIDS. Finally, the programme coordination was

TABLE 4.3 Comparison of HIV Testing for TB Patients and Treatment for HIV-Positive TB Patients: Global versus Indian Averages

Country/Region	% of Notified TB Patients with Known HIV Status	% of TB Patients with an HIV Test Result Who Were HIV-Positive	% of Notified HIV Positive TB Patients Started on CPT	% of Notified HIV-Positive TB Patients Started on ART
Global	48	18	85	70
India	63	5	95	88

Source: TB Division, MOHFW, GOI, 2015.

facilitated at the WHO's insistence under the National Framework for Joint HIV/TB Collaborative Activities developed in 2007 that extended basic TB–HIV activities nationwide. An intensified TB/HIV package of services was developed to offer additional services in states with higher burden of HIV–TB. Coordination mechanisms such as the coordination committee and National Technical Working Groups (NTWGs) were established at the national and state levels. This programme was important as approximately 120,000 HIV-associated TB cases occurred in India annually,[18] out of which an estimated 42,000 died each year, making India the second-highest burden country for people living with these co-morbidities. Case fatality rate among the notified HIV-positive TB patients in India is about 13 per cent, four times higher than that among HIV-negative TB patients.

The global TB report of 2014 stated that 63 per cent of TB patients knew their HIV status and 95 per cent of HIV-positive TB patients received the cotrimoxazole preventive therapy, while 88 per cent received ART. As shown in Table 4.3, HIV–TB collaborative activities were performing relatively better in India as compared to the global averages. However, TB-related outcomes have remained poor among PLHIV with a treatment success rate of less than 80 per cent.

Second-line Treatment

The role of the private sector was a significant issue that called for serious attention. Reports of PLHAs being fleeced, provided wrong dosages, wrong treatment and second-line drugs when the patient could be on first-line therapy were routinely surfacing. In 2003, the Human Rights Law Network filed a PIL in the Supreme Court to direct the government to extend treatment. This PIL came up for a decision in 2008. Since NACO had already rolled out first-line treatment, the PIL focused on providing second-line treatment alongside other non-medical facilities such as free bus fares while travelling for treatment and a higher quota of subsidized rations, pensions, and so on. NACO decided not to confront or contest this petition as is generally the case with government-related litigation. A negotiated outcome was hoped for. Vasu Murthy from the solicitor general's office and Dr Rewari from NACO helped negotiate a fair agreement. The main bone of contention was the introduction of second-line treatment that NACO did not have the institutional capacity to provide at that stage. Several rounds of discussions were held. Finally, a consensus was reached. As a result of this agreement, the Supreme Court ordered that HIV patients be provided with ration cards with additional rations, free bus passes for travelling to the treatment centres, and pensions. The SC also ordered the constitution of grievances and redressal committees under the chairmanship of the health secretary with PLHAs as members who were to meet quarterly and review the functioning of every ART centre. All the states were made party to ensure compliance—a matter of great importance as the actual provisioning of the relief as ordered by the court was in the domain of states. Besides, on seeing the huge evidence that NACO placed before the court to show the extent of poor-quality treatment by the private sector, the SC also directed the private sector to follow NACO guidelines while providing treatment. This was one of the rare instances of litigation where both parties were on the same side!

NACO was not against offering second-line treatment per se but two issues had to be considered: one was NACO's technical and institutional capacity to handle this. Given its limitations, it was felt that in the first instance the available resources should be used to ensure a rapid expansion of coverage to the first line. This seemed ethical too. It was argued that timely medication and good case management could delay drug resistance. This was compelling as it was believed that the toxicity of the second-line drugs resulted in a speedier resistance. In other words, the strategy was to prolong life by conservative and well-managed treatment—the focus being on patient management and not merely on more potent drugs. This line of thinking also led NACO to provide ART to those with a CD4 count under 250, except for pregnant women and TB patients who were initiated at 350 counts. Under pressure from the WHO, the line kept going up to reach 500 CD4 counts as many experts felt the cut-off line for introducing treatment is erroneous. But now there is better evidence and decisions are being taken on those parameters.

The second was NACO's limited capacity to monitor and treat second-line patients. The institutional capacity had to be developed: better diagnostics such as polymerase chain reaction's (PCR) for viral load testing, specialists to head ART centres for managing the complex side effects that more toxic drugs inevitably entail, patient management for other OIs that were a consequence, and so on.

In 2008, the second line was introduced after a survey was conducted that also included visits to the houses of PLHAs on first-line treatment. Straightaway, the State AIDS Clinical Expert Panel (SACEP) was constituted to screen patients eligible for the second line. A condition was incorporated that the second line would be provided free only to those who took treatment for the first line from government hospitals. This was plain competition and to ensure that the private sector did not exploit patients' vulnerability, mismanage their treatment, and dump them for the second-line on the government hospitals. This was also an incentive for the PLHAs to come to government ART centres that were providing free-of-cost high-quality treatment. It was argued that those wealthy enough to afford private care for the first line could afford second-line care too. And so, in the first round, free-of-cost second-line treatment was made available for all those below the poverty line, widows, children, and those taking treatment in a government facility since at least two years. In 2010, as NACO gained experience, this condition was waived.

There are now 510 ART centres and 1,060 LACs. In 200 of these LACs, CD4 count tests are carried out. Over 9.7 lakh HIV-infected are being treated. What is, however, worrying is that while

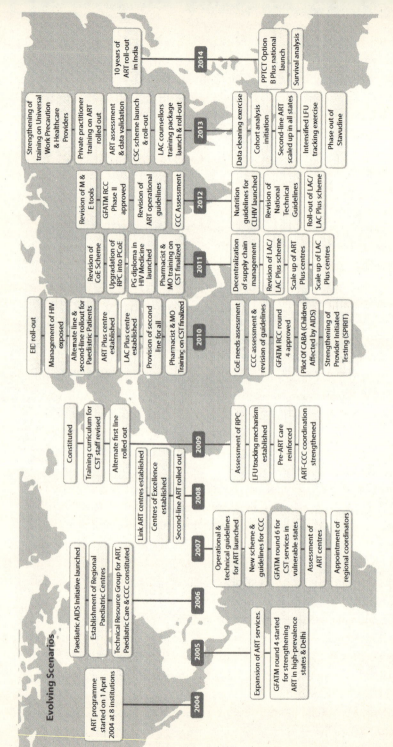

Figure 4.2 Scaling up of the ART Programme Guidelines
Source: NACO.

the number of patients has increased, the supervisory cadre has not with just six RCs (appointed when the patients were one-third of the number today) and two programme officers at NACO. This is likely to impact quality. Lack of budgets during the last two years resulting in stock-outs of drugs and consumables might have also contributed to increasing drug resistance.

Community Care Centres (CCCs)

The establishment of CCCs by NGOs—mainly faith-based organizations were judiciously incorporated into NACO's care and support scheme—was an institutional innovation to provide treatment for all OIs and board and lodging for HIV patients coming from rural areas until their pre-treatment workups were completed. This was a low-cost intervention with the twin benefits of quick, hassle-free treatment for OIs and reduction of patient load from the already overcrowded public hospitals. Around 2009, NACO undertook a survey of the 250 CCCs and categorized those that were doing well, those needing improvement, and those that needed to be shut down. A lot of effort went into building capacities of these care centres. NACO's financial support also motivated many faith-based NGOs to improve their facilities and infrastructure.

In April 2013 when NACO unilaterally shut down CCCs being run by several highly committed and motivated institutions, there was outrage, particularly since a credible alternative was not put in place. As social activist Sanghamitra Iyengar of Samraksha noted:

> One of the reasons for this is also the timing of the closure of the CCCs. There were some non-performing CCCs. Instead of improving those, all the 250 CCCs were closed down in April 2013. These were actually helping to manage acute drug reactions, respite, and family psycho-education on treatment adherence and palliative care support, which allowed people often to get over an acute stage of reactions from drop out on multiple OIs or resistance to first line. Not having this has led to enormous number of deaths last year. With CD4 cut-off for ART raised to 550, we will not need the CCCs in three-to-five years. But we need them now.[19]

Closing CCCs was an unfortunate decision since many NGOs had developed good infrastructures and directly helped the poor.

The effective implementation of the TI strategy was the key to reversing the epidemic. However, 'effective implementation' required going beyond implementing rules and procedures and entering the realm of social activism to fight prejudices and discriminatory attitudes that inhibited access to these groups which was required for initiating interventions.

'TI' is a term used by the NACP III to indicate programme activities among hidden and outlawed groups of people: CSWs and their clients, men having sex with men (MSM), and injectable drug users. The focus was to identify among them those prone to high-risk behaviour. Stopping the transmission of the infection required behaviour change that could, however, not be forced by diktat. In other words, earlier strategies to promote abstinence or condom use that had clearly been ineffective necessitated NACO to get more proactively involved with the issues, debates, and controversies that were of concern to these groups. It became important to understand the contradictions between established laws and social norms, with NACO having to take a position on the rights of the marginalized sexual minorities. As these issues generated much controversy and were also of critical importance in the context of NACO's strategies, a digression to explain the rationale and understand the significance of NACO's work and contribution is necessary.

The Judiciary

On 15 April 2014, the Supreme Court recognized transgenders as a third gender to be listed under the other backward classes (OBCs) and eligible for all benefits and entitlements: quotas, right to education, ration cards, loans, housing, employment, property rights, and, above all, the right to vote. Two years on, in pursuance of the Supreme Court order of 2014, the Ministry of Social Justice and Empowerment has come up with the Transgender Persons (Protection of Rights) Bill, 2016. At a meeting held on 22 August 2016, prominent civil society groups of transgenders criticized it as inadequate and against the spirit of the court judgment. They found faults with the definition of 'transgender' and the processes followed for identifying them. They felt that their rights and entitlements had been diluted and no mechanism or amendment in the IPC was proposed for addressing the problem of abuse or violence against them. Besides, they found the draft act inadequate with regard to proposing mechanisms for ensuring effective coordination with the reltated departments for enabling transgenders access their rights as granted by the Supreme Court. They called upon the ministry to hold widespread consultations and review the draft.

The 2014 judgment was significant as it reiterated the rights and entitlements of transgenders. But in doing so, it also exposed the limitations of the Constitution and the deep-seated social intolerance towards sexual minorities. Though fundamental rights are a cardinal principle of the Constitution, yet at every level, denial and discrimination against such stigmatized social groups are routinely practised. We are forced to confront the fact that issues of intolerance and discrimination fall into a grey area where social norms, beliefs, and cultural traditions seem bigger than the law of the land. Is it the job of judicial pronouncements to modify social behaviour and attitudes to align with the Constitution's Directive Principles or social standards?

Sociopolitical systems ordain what is good and bad behaviour, and what kinds of behaviour can be condoned and who is to be punished.[20] Thus, two homosexual adults having sex in private can be incarcerated for 10 years and denied bail, but a serial rapist could, until recently, be granted bail with his citizenship rights intact. While the homosexual is seen as a threat to our cultural traditions, the rapist is not.

Definitions of morality, social values, or ethical standards and norms have evolved over time influenced by external factors and discourses, social conditioning and cultural history. India's literature is replete with the social acceptability of transgenders, homosexuals, and prostitutes as a part of our social–sexual behavioural diversity. In the nineteenth century, however, the British rejected this aspect of our history as symptomatic of a debased morality. Homosexuality was declared to be 'against the order of nature' and in 1860, the draconian section 377 of the IPC was instituted. The UK itself decriminalized gay behaviour between the years 1965 and 1982. India has not only continued with this section in its statute but soon after Independence, with the colonial mindset bent upon 'being like the British', the country even banned the devadasis, who were repositories of music and fine arts. The withdrawal of zamindari patronage followed by a legal ban reduced most of these devadasis to poverty and prostitution.

Patriarchal mindsets and social prejudices are often concealed in religious verbiage. This kind of mindset often stems from an ahistorical understanding of cultural traditions and misplaced definitions of modernity. Electoral politics and populism have, maybe inadvertently, sustained and advanced social intolerance. In fact, over the years electoral politics has resulted in greater bigotry and led to compromising values of equality and individual freedoms be it the Shah Bano[21] case or the recent Supreme Court judgment overruling a landmark Delhi High Court order legalizing homosexuality on grounds of the inviolability of an individual's right to choose his/her sexuality. Thus, the Indian state continues to enforce unconstitutional moral codes through its institutions: Parliament, courts, and the police. And against this formidable state power and the loud protests from multiple layers of 'respectability' is pitted a motley crowd of 2.2 million people who are denied their fundamental rights as citizens for living in accordance with their sexual choices, natural inclinations, and circumstances.

Even as late as 2000 when a new millennium dawned, subalterns like CSWs, MSM, transgenders, and drug addicts (injecting drug users [IDUs]) were shunned, harassed, and ridiculed with their very existence declared illegitimate. They lived hidden lives in fear of social disapproval and police beatings. They lived amidst us, near our homes, on our streets, and were yet invisible.[22] The fear of HIV compelled the very same repressive society and government agencies to seek out prostitutes, transgenders, and homosexuals, and acknowledge their presence and condescend to negotiate with them. Such concern arose from disturbing data and disquieting media reports. In 1998,[23] Peter Piot, the executive director of UNAIDS, had warned:

> HIV is now firmly embedded in the general Indian population and is fast spreading into rural areas that were previously thought to be relatively spared.... In five years, the infection rate among

prostitutes has increased from 1 per cent to 51 per cent in Mumbai. Among injecting drug users in Manipur, the infection rate has risen from 1 per cent to 55.8 per cent. And among attendees of sexually transmitted diseases clinics, the infection rate has shot up from 23 per cent to 36 per cent in one year in Mumbai.

Alarmed and afraid, NACO was accorded an implicit social sanction to work with criminalized groups. Explicitly though, these groups would continue to be denied social recognition and their constitutional rights. Ironically, the HIV epidemic compelled societal engagement with these 'invisible' and stigmatized groups, kindling hope that one day they might be included in mainstream society. Well, at least partly.

Values and Ideologies: Empowerment and Dependence—Commercial Sex Workers

Debates and discussions around the HIV clearly opened up a can of worms, exposing social hypocrisy and raising uncomfortable questions related to sexual morality. But the issue confronting NACO was not about upholding morality but how to address matters of sex and drugs. In other words, the issue was not 'should we' but 'how should we'. For a nascent NACO, reaching out to or working with sex workers was unthinkable. So the strategy focused on educating the clients through campaigns about the dangers of unprotected sex with prostitutes and the regular use of condoms.

In 1992, the WHO sanctioned small grants to experiment with two different strategic approaches: one promoting the use of condoms through information campaigns and the other promoting treatment for STDs. Two specific areas were selected as the most apt sites for testing the approaches: one in Mumbai's Kamathipura and the other in Kolkata's Sonagachi—the two largest brothels in India.

Kamathipura

Partnering with the local NGOs of Mumbai, NACO's strategy focused on educating sex workers, clients, the police, and others about the risks and dangers of HIV in the tightly closed network of the sex industry. I.S. Gilada, a gutsy young doctor from Mumbai, promoted health education and condoms. Convinced of the growing risk of HIV, Gilada had, prior to 1990, started the condom

> **Box 4.3** Kamathipura, Mumbai, 1992[24]
>
> The Population Services International (PSI)—a leading international NGO for social marketing of condoms and ORS—had been working in Kamathipura as part of their IEC and social marketing strategy, painting up teashops located opposite the brothel in bright colours, providing TV sets, promotional films, and condoms. Elegant booklets earnestly advocating abstinence, use of condoms 'always' for not transmitting HIV, and the importance of good nutrition were diligently prepared by the WHO consultants and provided free to the sex workers. A sex worker I met asked me for one good reason why she should use a condom. HIV and death clearly did not frighten her. 'I don't care if I die—that is better than this wretched life and it serves those b****s right if they get HIV and die too,' she said, her eyes full of contempt and bitterness. 'Then why don't you run away to your home?' I asked. 'Because I will be caught and beaten ... and ... besides, I can't go home as my family will not accept me.' Her parents had sold her to sex work for money to pay off a debt. By the end of 1995, an estimated 30,000 sex workers had been infected and large numbers succumbed to the disease.
>
> *Source*: Author.

promotion movement through his NGO, the Indian Health Organisation (IHO). Along with his volunteers, Gilada would perch himself atop a vehicle, mike in hand, and go up and down the busy street of Kamathipura explaining to the bewildered sex workers and their clients the dire consequences of unprotected sex. He distributed condoms to them, even as the sex workers, quite unmindful of his exhortations, continued to recruit new clients. Given the conservative social environment, Gilada's style was innovative and attracted media headlines. But as a strategy, it had limited impact. What Gilada and Thai activists had in common was their passionate advocacy of the condom as the only barrier for stopping the transmission of HIV. An important difference was that while Gilada had to convince and persuade, Thailand legalized prostitution and strictly enforced the 100 per cent condom use by prostitutes (CUP) policy by making the non-use of condom a punishable offence, resulting in a drastic reduction in HIV.

Sonagachi

An intervention of the AIIHPH, Kolkata, supported by the WHO was to establish STD clinics for the sex workers in Sonagachi, a brothel with about 40,000 of them. Dr S. Jana, a young epidemiologist working in the AIIHPH was made the project-in-charge of the Sexual Health Intervention Project (SHIP). The objective was threefold: to bring about behavioural change among sex workers, to promote the regular use of condoms, and to reduce STD infections. A baseline study of 450 prostitutes revealed that STD infections were 80 per cent and HIV prevalence and condom use was about 1.1 per cent.[25]

It was not long before Jana and his team of professionals realized that talking about condoms and STDs was not making any impact. The sex workers had different priorities and concerns. Reducing syphilis or HIV/AIDS prevalence implied reduction in the number of sexual contacts and ensuring the regular use of condoms. But such behavioural changes were dependent on the power dynamics that underscored behaviour—the unequal power relations between the more powerful client and the vulnerable prostitute. It was argued that in a competitive market, the prostitute has no power over a client who puts pleasure above the use of condom. The prostitutes were women lacking in self-confidence and self-esteem, socially alienated, and used to brutal violence and being routinely beaten up by the police and local goons. It was a milieu where even the murder of a sister by a client was not to be reported.[26] 'Stigma, discrimination, violence, harassment and social equity issues are critical concerns of FSWs [female sex workers].'[27] In such circumstances, refusing sex without condoms would mean losing customers and having to choose between hunger now and disease later. Safe sex was clearly not a priority.

It was becoming increasingly evident that to make the bio-behavioural intervention work, it was most important to first gain the trust of this disparate group of sex workers and educate them to realize why they should use condoms and refuse sex without it, why condoms were important for themselves and the future of their children, as well as to understand the pathology of power. Thus, the 'initial period of the project was spent in listening to the voices of the sex workers and being empathetic, not judging but understanding in an environment of informality and equality'.[28]

It was also realized that an 'insider' or a member of the group could communicate messages with greater conviction and also access other sex workers more effectively. This gave rise to the concept of PEs, introduced for the first time in community development dialogues. As PEs, they were given training on HIV-specific issues and also 'formally attended training on legal and human rights, civil and criminal laws related to their lives, gender issues, sex and sexuality, sociopolitical processes and a host of other issues'.[29] More important was the perception part. Being associated with a respectable government institute, having the title of PE instead of the reviled term 'prostitute', and using words spoken by English-speaking professionals were hugely empowering and gave them a certain status.[30]

Redefining themselves as sex workers and not prostitutes—a term that was derogatory and associated with shame and immorality—was the first step. And being able to articulate their exploitative relationships and marginalization at the hands of powerful 'madams', goons, boyfriends, pimps, and the police through a process of understanding gave them confidence. In a book on Sonagachi titled *Community Led Structural Intervention*,[31] Evans, Jana, and O'Reily trace the process of knowledge and understanding followed here to Paulo Freire's theory of praxis—a theory centred around 'power, how to grasp it and utilize it effectively for social change' expounding that 'for those who are most disadvantaged in society, the Freirian model of reflection, consciousness raising and political action is the only coherent theory to have been explicitly applied in community participation and development with clearly measurable success'.

Within three years of project implementation, the gradual awakening wrought by an ideological framework of respect, reliance, and recognition revealed to the sex workers that their struggles went beyond mere condom use. In fact, sustaining even the limited goal of regular condom use was inexorably connected to their fundamental desire to work in a safe environment that would allow them to carry on their profession with dignity. But achieving this freedom to choose their own lifestyle while continuing to live as a part of mainstream society was fraught with challenges. The major test was to defy the political system and the rules of social morality, both of which worked in tandem and reinforced each other. A space had to be negotiated through dialogue and a well-calibrated strategy because it was apparent that society would be unwilling to grant those freedoms without 'a fight and pressures from below'. As Freire had noted four decades ago, 'freedom is acquired by conquest ... not by gift. [It] has to be pursued constantly and responsibly.'[32]

In 1995, praxis led to a structural instrumentality in the form of a collective.[33] The collective was an innovation and a contribution of Sonagachi. It arose as a means of neutralizing the vulnerability of a single individual and raising her bargaining power as a member of a group. Thus was born Durbar, the first large collective of sex workers. They set to work with great energy and enthusiasm building solidarity and trust, a common vision, and an ability to articulate and demand their rights by forming strategic partnerships and having a flexible strategic position to issues as they evolved.[34]

The collectivization concept had three components: agency, resources, and the creation of an enabling environment. Agency was the means of providing them the necessary capabilities and skills required to assert themselves, while resources consisted of acquiring soft skills needed to build the necessary social capital. The term 'enabling environment' is liberally used in HIV/AIDS discourse. It implies the creation of a supportive or facilitative environment to enable sex workers to live in dignity in three spaces: as individual sex workers, as a part of the larger sex industry, and as members of the wider society. Over time, such collectivization led to Durbar being visualized as a political construct that sought 'sex workers' social recognition, participation at policy level, and access to resources [alongside] challenging discrimination, oppression and injustice against sex workers ...'[35]

These ideas took the mission far beyond what the small WHO project had envisioned in 1993. By 1999, Durbar had evolved into an ideologically driven self-governing entity. Its ambition was to heighten political activism to scale by a strategy of social activism and by working across with other sex workers as well as other exploited groups on a common platform of action. They needed to gain strength to face the political and social power system that exploited them. What was difficult was that the established social norms that excluded them or the laws that criminalized them had to be challenged by living within those very social and democratic constructs as law-abiding citizens.[36]

By forming alliances with the local power structures and the CPI(M) leadership, Durbar was able to get the West Bengal legislative assembly to amend the Cooperative Act—dropping the clause that only persons of moral character be allowed to establish a cooperative. With this amendment, a credit society was formed, followed by a school for their children, a cultural society, their own health clinics, and developed networks for taking up the social marketing of condoms. The credit society was also one of the many efforts to get mainstreamed into middle-class society. Durbar became a model for HIV efforts and by 2000, regular condom use went up by 90 per cent and HIV plateaued at less than 2 per cent.

Sangli

Meena Seshu, a graduate from TISS, a feminist, and a lawyer inspired the third model of sex-worker empowerment. Thakur of IHO, Mumbai, introduced Meena to the world of sex workers. In 1992, Meena set up a rights-based NGO called Sangram and in 1995, she set up the Veshya Anyay Mukti Parishad (VAMP)[37]—a mock acronym for a sex workers collective. It had similar beliefs of empowering sex workers as a collective as in the case of Sonagachi but provided a narrower room for accommodation and negotiation. It marked a shift from the strategy of pleading for understanding to demanding as a matter of right. Such an understanding had implications for the programme as it meant, for example, that the government was duty-bound to provide services. And equally, the sex workers as citizens also had the fundamental right to demand them. Therefore, be it condoms or STD treatment, the sex workers would not run any separate clinics or social marketing networks. VAMP, unlike Durbar, did not have an expansionist political vision. Instead, it focused on stimulating a transformative self-development among the sex workers in the collective through a process of thinking and developing an identity, a sense of self-worth, and assertiveness. These features were then seen as attributes to, and critical preconditions of, behavioural change—from a psychology of helpless victimhood to one of being empowered, independent, and confident.

By the time the NACP II was to be formulated, India had solid experience of what works and how. In the meanwhile, the World Bank researchers like Prabhat Jha, Martha Ainsworth, David Wilson and others also built up theoretical arguments demonstrating the irrefutable correlations between unprotected, multipartner heterosexual behaviour—practised by female sex workers, truck drivers, and MSM—and HIV transmission. This research provided the justification for implementing interventions targeted at HRGs using the World Bank funding. TI was thus designed as a structural approach aimed at HRGs, moving away from blaming and shaming to working with them as active partners—an approach that the Indian experience had conclusively and successfully demonstrated on scale.

Given this background, it was reasonable to expect that the collectivization approach as implemented in Sonagachi and Sangli would be scaled up, particularly because there were very few NGOs willing and able to work among the socially ostracized sex workers and the goons that surrounded them. Instead, NACO decided to adopt the usual approach of NGOs and granted 'projects' to implement TIs. In hindsight, this raised several questions.

Jana, who had turned Sonagachi STD project into a sex worker collective, hypothesized that there could have been three possible reasons for such a decision: a) the policymakers in general were apprehensive to use radical terminology and strategies related to empowerment and rights as that could be viewed as 'promoting sex work', b) the absence of an understanding of the concepts of social medicine and public health approaches among the rank and file in NACO, and c) the lack of commitment to address structural barriers that made sex workers vulnerable since it was more comfortable to follow traditional approaches even though they were inadequate to create a significant impact.[38]

Jana was not entirely wrong. In fact, he was profoundly correct on all the three counts. There was mounting criticism from the conservative middle class against the rights-based approach, alleging that the socially condemned classes were disturbing the status quo. The opposition of the middle classes to NACO's work with sex workers was resented as they feared that supporting sex workers may be construed as promoting and condoning promiscuity, a fear that has not been substantiated with data. As Freire notes, 'Any restriction on their way of life in the name of rights of the community, appears ... as a profound violation of their individual rights.'[39] Secondly, the instrument to bring about transformative change as envisioned by Sonagachi was a bureaucratic set up that was by its very nature conservative and 'status quoist'. In other words, NACO lacked the institutional capacity at the national and state levels to catalyse this change, even if it desired to do so.

Whatever be the reason, a replication of collectivization models was not easy. It was a leadership-dependent model that made it inherently limiting. Scaling up required inspiring leaders like Jana, Sushena, Sanghamitra, or Meena who were not available in the numbers required. As for NACO of the 2000, just the task of building capacity even among NGOs was considered a 'revolutionary' task. Besides, it was also easier to work and communicate with NGOs as they came from the same middle-class background as the policymakers in NACO and spoke the same language. In other words, NACO had little capacity to directly deal with sex workers or transgenders.

By the end of 2005, there were nearly 1,100 TIs, though not all focused on HRGs. Over 700 were called 'composite' TIs that consisted of a few sex workers, many street children and ragpickers. Mixing up target population groups was a deliberate strategy to provide the NGO a veneer of social respectability, as during those days working with sex workers was considered indecent. Most NGOs at this time were focused on expanding access to condom use. Though some guidelines were framed, there was no systematic mapping, hardly any monitoring, evaluation, field visits, or guidance, leaving the states to struggle with the 'how to' questions. The emphasis during this period was IEC, STI awareness, and condom use.

Some argue that not learning from Sonagachi and Sangli and instead resorting to a 'projectized' NGO approach was a strategic mistake. But in hindsight, broadening the involvement of the middle-class NGOs to work with the subalterns was useful for NACO as it helped in building up a constituency of support from within the same class. After all, morality apart, social equality for sex workers is also always a class issue. Tactically, therefore, having articulate middle-class (largely) women fighting for sex workers helped strengthen the latter's voices.

Ashodaya (Mysore)

Unlike Sonagachi, Mysore had no brothels. The sex workers were either street- or home-based. A majority of the Ashodaya members came from villages. They were a part of society but lived dual lives—lovers in the mornings and mothers and wives in the evenings. Their families and communities thought they were factory workers or worked in a telephone company and so they were respected as breadwinners.

Mentored by Jana, Swarup Sarkar,[40] and Sundar, the young epidemiologist Sushena started her work by walking through 60 per cent of the villages of Bijapur and Mysore districts and got a firsthand understanding of the way in which sexual networks were organized and operated. She got into the network through Asha Kiran, a poor vegetable seller, who told her that she supplemented her income by doing sex work at night. Asha Kiran then told her about others and the others told her of yet more sex workers till she met Akram, a transgender, who became her mainstay in helping set up Ashodaya. The BMGF funded Ashodaya through the University of Manitoba's Indian NGO called the Karnataka Health Promotion Trust (KHPT). Sushena then organized an STD clinic, from where she began making a list of women whose major source of income was sex work. When she approached sex workers, a scattered lot whose main concern was maximizing their earnings for the day and to not miss the evening bus back home, she was met with suspicion and silence. As in Sonagachi, daily contact promoted trust and faith in the strength of their own unity. As sex workers began to respond, the need for a place to talk and bond was felt. Thus came into existence the drop-in-centre (DIC) that also had an STD clinic. A caring ambience became a critical component of the CBO funding package.

Ashodaya is not a brothel-based collective. It consists of rural women who lead 'respectable lives' in society as opposed to Sonagachi where women had left their homes to live in an urban brothel. Physical concentration need not be a prerequisite for forming collectives. Ethnographic studies show that only about

> **Box 4.4** Ashodaya, 2006
>
> My first interaction with sex workers was during a visit to Ashodaya in 2006, a few weeks after I took over as DG. It was an eye-opener. I was interacting with sex workers who were not embarrassed of their profession. Clearly, this reflected my middle-class upbringing and bias where subconsciously I viewed sex work as something to be ashamed of. Instead, here I witnessed a lucid and sophisticated PowerPoint presentation on mapping and tracking techniques given by a relatively illiterate male sex worker.
>
> Ashodaya had a DIC located in rented premises. The sex workers had painted the hall depicting rich, brightly coloured scenes of the sea with boats and palm trees, vivid blue skies with happy birds, and so on—scenes that reflected peace and tranquility, a sharp contrast to their traumatized lives. The centre provided beds where tired women could come and rest, a dressing room and a kitchen to supply hot meals at very low cost, a TV and a clinic for medical care. The DIC gave them a safe space to meet, talk, rest, and share their problems with others who were in similar situations. It was a haven that they could escape to and hide from the pressures of living dual lives with multiple identities. Bonding of these disparate groups was made possible and enabled by the DIC.
>
> *Source*: Author.

10 per cent of all sex workers were brothel-based, while the rest were street- or home-based. The precursor for this kind of an understanding of rural sex work was Samraksha. In 2003, Sanghamitra established a collective called Samraksha in the little-known district of Kuppole in Karnataka. Samraksha focused on the mobilization of hidden sex workers and was unique in demonstrating the principle of collectivization among non-brothel based and geographically scattered women.

Ashodaya has now come a long way with a microfinance programme, a restaurant, a training academy, a home called Ashraya for those infected with HIV, and other facilities. On the day of my visit in 2006, sex workers complained of how they were made to wait for long hours and make multiple visits to get treatment. Today there appears to be a better bonding between the health staff and sex workers. Working as volunteers with the HIV-infected patients, the sex workers earned respect. There is no stigma and no sex worker is frightened of the AIDS disease or the doctors. Most importantly, collectivization backed by substantial sensitization of the police force reduced violence against them by 80 per cent.[41] And finally, the difference between Ashodaya and other groups lay in the attempt to 'deconstruct science'. Such deconstruction meant that sex workers were made to demystify myths and perceptions, to think through their own reality critically, and to articulate and present their views based on self-understanding and not because someone asked or said so.[42]

The common thread that bound all these experiences cutting across the country was that social inequities hurt the female sex workers: illiterate, lonely, vulnerable, struggling to survive, and at risk. 'Clients often offer more money for unprotected sex, and, in the context of extreme poverty, negotiating condom use as well as taking time to access sexual health services can be less important than the immediate need for sex workers to provide for themselves and their families.'[43] Therefore, the strategy was clear. They had to be empowered and supported in order to give them the confidence to change their risky behaviour. It was also clear that collectivization was the only way even though government benefits including free housing, food, and schooling are available.

> [S]tructural barriers often prohibit FSW access to these schemes. The application procedure requires levels of literacy beyond that of many FSWs, and discrimination of FSWs by government officials often lead to the explicit denial of those FSWs who do apply. The requirement of a residential address to access food ration cards (providing 10 kg of rice per month), and the requirement of a child's father to be present to access free schooling, present additional structural barriers.[44]

NACO's Approach to the CSW Issues

Inspired by the models of Sonagachi, Sangli, and Ashodaya detailed earlier, the NACP III aimed at scaling up TIs to cover all HRGs and proposed that at least 50 per cent of them should be collectives.[45] By the end of 2012,[46] there were 1,873 TIs covering 0.78 million sex workers, 0.26 million MSMs, and 0.13 million IDUs accounting for about 80 per cent of the estimated numbers, including the bridge population groups namely migrants and truckers. There were, however, only 140 collectives and most were of MSMs. Two factors inhibited NACO's ability to achieve the target for establishing sex workers' collectives: a dearth of visionary leadership and time for building the social capital. India seriously lacked a critical mass of such leaders and NACO lacked the time to wait for the social capital to train them. Besides, a careful review of both Sonagachi and Ashodaya showed a substantial investment of both financial and human resources and a large supply of high-quality, non-community techno-managerial expertise that were available to them during the formative years. According to Manilal, a NACO project officer, 'Involvement of non-community experts to guide the community/CBO is one of the important factors for the success/establishment of these organizations … These CBOs also had resources that took care of the various socio-economic needs of the community members'—something that a government-funded agency like NACO operating with tight budgets could ill afford.

Yet the learnings from these examples were not lost. Sanghamitra of Samraksha reflected that the 'collective spirit is deeply entrenched … the rights and entitlement issues have been mainstreamed and communities have taken it up squarely'. In other words, the rights-based empowerment approach in an enabling environment influenced all TI work even when implemented by NGOs. In fact, as recently as 2010, in Kuppole NGOs such as the South India Action AIDS Programme (SIAAP), Samraksha, and Women's Initiatives (WINS) have collaborated to constitute a collective of 10,000 sex workers that is federated and is functioning without the support of NGOs, the BMGF, the KHPT, or other funders.

While the NGOs used the language of empowerment such as 'the right to make choices, participatory decision-making' that are now the hallmarks of a collective, they held on to their power as well as their control over the sex workers, who operated as project beneficiaries and not as self-actualized individuals.

The sex workers were objects and passive recipients of services and were perpetually dependent on the NGOs. Yet in some places like Ahmedabad,[47] Bangalore, Hyderabad, Mumbai, Bagalkot in Karnataka, Kannur in Kerala, Kolkata, Chennai, and a few other small cities like Tirupati and Bhiwandi, NGOs did try to capacitate the community regarding their health and other issues within a framework of collectivization.

Ironically then, sometimes the main barriers to sex workers' empowerment were often the NGOs themselves. As a sex worker of Ashodaya explained to me, 'For them [NGOs], the project is the bread and butter and they do not want to hand over to community.' This was a predictable contradiction but one that was not easy to resolve. After all, NGOs were yet another facet of the same class and social structure that sought to retain control over subaltern movements.

The NACP III had a methodical approach. Mapping enabled fixing the geographic jurisdiction and number of sex workers to be covered. Sites were tendered out to NGOs in a two-step process. Detailed guidelines of how to conduct participatory site assessments were drawn up and the prospective NGOs were provided training. The second step consisted of developing their capacities to use the operational tools to prepare project reports. Upon submission of project reports, SACS would give final approvals, enter into contracts, and release funds. The monetary amounts per NGO were trebled as compared to the NACP II. TIs were also structured into three tiers: the project officer, outreach workers, and PEs. In the PEs' category, sex workers were selected from among the active, mobile, and more vulnerable with a maximum of two years of standing in the profession.[48]

With the focus on HIV, NACO adopted approaches that helped it to change behaviour and attitudes among sex workers. NACO deliberately adopted a non-judgemental policy on the issues of morality, though it was aware that the two issues could not be separated beyond a point. This position was the outcome of umpteen debates around the question of choice and the co-option of sex workers as active partners in the struggle to reverse the HIV epidemic.

Hollywoodizing[49] or Being Humane?

The NACO approach did not go unchallenged. Several activists condemned collectivization and according recognition to sex workers. Allegations of 'Hollywoodizing' India, abetting the trafficking of women and children into sex work, and promoting sexual slavery were made against NACO. NACO was also under scrutiny of the media and Parliament. Part of the problem was exacerbated with Sweden legislating a law that punished clients. According to our reports, sex work in Sweden had not only gone underground but had also been pushed across the borders. The US, under Bush, was anti-abortion, anti-sex work, anti-condom, anti-clean needles and persistently pushed the anti-trafficking bill.[50]

Under this pressure, the Department of Women and Child Development (DWCD) produced a draft law on the lines of the Swedish law that criminalized the clients and demanded 50 per cent of the TI budget to be spent on alternative livelihood options for sex workers. Sex workers were perceived as 'fallen women', victims of poverty and circumstance who needed empathy and state support against 'male exploitation'—an approach that reeked of a sanctimonious, self-pitying victimhood against the very principles of rights-based approach. The flattening and simplification of a complex problem was astonishing. It was unclear how imprisoning male clients who numbered millions would help, besides being unfeasible. Additionally, the assumption that all sex workers were trafficked was not evidence-based. A study carried out of over 130,000 sex workers by Swasthi, a Bangalore-based NGO, shows that not more than 5 per cent of the sex workers are trafficked. The DWCD had no independent sources of information and relied on NACO's data. An analysis of over 5,498 sex workers across 22 districts between 2007 and 2008 for reasons of entering sex work indicated poor or deprived economic conditions, negative social circumstances in life, own choice, force by an external person, and family tradition.[51] But the data was twisted to suit its argument that all sex workers were slaves and trafficked.

It was distressing to see the Left parties having negative perceptions of issues related to sex work, charging NACO with commodifying women, and disagreeing that women be given any choice[52] regarding lifestyle. However, while the party leaders in West Bengal did not agree with the 'freedom-of-choice' concept as demanded by sex workers, they were nevertheless sympathetic to the latter's demands for ration cards, pensions, and other amenities. None of the indignant voices, however, raised the issue of state inaction and complicity in trafficking, though they knew fully well that powerful mafias connected to, and abetted by, powerful politicians were behind the trafficking industry. The police knew who controlled the trafficking rackets and where exactly the hotspots were. They could differentiate between trafficking and routine sex worker addas. But no one ever challenged this larger context as that would mean questioning the sociopolitical set up. Instead they focused their energies to fight an already beleaguered NACO that was struggling to contain an infectious disease and that, too, in a humanitarian manner. Some of the self-righteous NGOs also had no idea about how to 'rehabilitate' the sex workers. Their suggestions of sewing or petty vending for the illiterate and unskilled sex workers were not as lucrative or even seen as viable substitutes by the sex workers themselves.[53] It was clear that some NGOs were playing up to the US-funded global movements. NACO was unwilling to take these NGOs seriously. From the start, NACO felt that often the NGO attitudes were hypocritical and glib.

The issue of sex work was not just one of poverty but of structural infirmities. It was also about aspirations in a rapidly changing society and state. The tilt towards neo-liberalism demonstrated that only money was valued and what it could buy in terms of upward mobility and fine living. The tilt reiterated that patriarchal attitudes, the state's failure to create safety in workplaces, low wages, absence of the enforcement of labour laws, and the appalling conditions in which most men and women work have enhanced vulnerability to sexual abuse. At another level, with employment opportunities shifting to urban centres and the sharp declines in farm incomes, in many villages women-headed households have increased and so has their vulnerability. With the breaking down of family and social cohesion, the social security of women is getting tenuous even as predators scour the villages for helpless women to traffic them. All this was further exacerbated by a poor redressal and legal system; lack of access to social security, credit, health care; and an ungendered environment for single women. Such situations cannot be redressed by blaming, shaming, and hurting the worst victims of this situation.

In India, gender violence is a structural issue and sex work is perhaps an extreme manifestation of it. In fact, surveys showed that in terms of sexual abuse and violence, sex workers were probably a shade better-off compared to married women within the so called 'safe space' of their homes. Many women run away to sex work for the 'freedom' it provides from oppressive domestic environments. The activists simply did not understand the broader issues of gender violence that plague our society. Some feminist movements, too, stood exposed as often elite women were unable to cross class boundaries and join the rights-based movement of sex workers and transgenders. If class differences were one factor, the other that compounded the attitudinal differences was their failure to understand the nature of the state. The state was ready to grant rights to food, education, and information but not to sexuality. The ideological bias persists even in developed countries like the US where the most contentious arguments even today revolve around sexuality and reproductive rights.

Sex workers were agitated at this combined assault on their rights and aspirations. Once some frustrated and angry sex workers stormed into my office and told me, 'We sell our bodies, and you sell your mind. It's the same!' One sex worker argued that while the women activists called them 'dirty', it was they (the sex workers) who sacrificed their lives so girls could be safe and not raped! Were male clients the lesser evil who exploited the vulnerability of sex workers, or the latter who were only responding to a demand? 'Who has brought the virus?' They demanded to know.

Around 2007, sex workers from all over India were mobilized for a march in Delhi to protest against the anti-trafficking bill. NACO's decision to stand solidly behind the rights of sex workers and sexual minorities drew the line where no ambivalence on the question was permitted. But this was easier said than done. The bureaucracy does not like to let go of power and did not really believe in the rights-based approaches. It was a matter of time before NACO reverted in part to the NGO-projectivized approach, though in an improved manner.

MSM: Fighting Section 377

The problem of MSMs was more acute than that of sex workers due in large part to societal conditioning. While thieves, murderers, rapists, and goons walk away many a time unpunished, those who exercise their choice of sexual behaviour in private are punished. The illegality of homosexual behaviour and the social disapproval that accompanies it means that MSMs lead dual lives—respectably married but having a parallel relationship in secret with a male partner and living in dread of being found out. In addition to the law under Section 377 of the IPC, they have to live with shame and the pain that their families would undergo if they knew. Handling the problem of MSM was also compounded by the fact that 'coming out' could mean breaking up family structures due to the deeply entrenched social ostracism and disapproval.

Ashok Rao Kavi, a Mumbai-based journalist, was among the first few gay men to come out in the 1980s. He was a great help in sensitizing NACO staff on issues related to gays, the various categorizations among the homosexual community—the double deckers, the *koti*s, the transgenders, the cross dressers—and their specific problems, fears, and loneliness due to social exclusion. Discussions revealed that many MSMs were from middle- and upper-middle-class echelons, so it was not as if MSM behaviour was the result of poverty, or material deprivation, or compelling social circumstances. Rather, it was a matter of an intensely individual sexual preference. In other words, gays can not help their sexual orientation. They are not making a choice. Neither they nor society has any option but to accept them as they are and give them the required social space.

The question of determining the number of MSMs at high risk and getting access to them was tricky and not easily amenable to the tools and techniques of snowballing or contact-tracing. Some wild estimates were made and cleverly clothed in respectful jargon called 'epidemiological modelling'. After trying several different methodologies, it was surmised that 10 per cent among the 'homosexual population group' were highly promiscuous and tended to change partners frequently. The focus was on identifying them, but how? Given the nature of the behaviour pattern, NGOs could not be effective entry points to do so. The high risk MSMs had to be tracked through their own networks.

A majority of homosexuals were virtually compelled into bisexuality due to fear of family disapproval and social approbation.

Marriage was imposed as was the pressure to raise a family and lead a 'normal' life. Data from Mexico, a conservative catholic country, clearly showed the spread of HIV was attributable to bisexual men who had several partners and who passed on the infection to their wives due to the prohibition of using condoms. NACO also had to keep in mind the trauma that families may go through on realizing that their father, brother, or husband is bisexual. Therefore, bringing gay or bisexual men to clinics for counselling in full public view was clearly out of the question. It was for these reasons that NACO's work among MSMs prior to 2006 remained relatively ineffective. Avahan's pioneering work among this community led NACO to replicate that model and scale up under the NACP III.

NACO gained the trust of MSMs when it filed an affidavit as a respondent in a PIL case by Naz, a Delhi-based NGO, in the Delhi High Court. Naz sought the repeal of Section 377 of the IPC[54] on grounds of it being inconsistent with the Constitution that guaranteed several freedoms including sexual freedom. Based on the interactions with Sankalp in Bangalore and subsequently others, NACO took a stand in support of the petitioner. The affidavit was approved as a routine matter and filed in the high court. As the first respondent, the Department of Home Affairs squarely opposed the removal of Section 377 of the IPC arguing that homosexuality corrupted society and promoted a debased value system.

The high court commented adversely on how a government, namely the Ministry of Home Affairs and the health ministry (through NACO) could take two contrary stands and directed the government to file one affidavit. A meeting to reconcile the two viewpoints was called. The home secretary agreed with NACO's standpoint and the formulation that sought the repeal of those portions of Section 377 that made consensual sex in private punishable. But the then home minister Shivraj Patil was livid. In a meeting with some donor organizations and UNAIDS, he asked for data on the number of cases that had been filed under Section 377. It was impossible to explain that cases were not filed and registered because of police corruption—the police took bribes in return or demanded free sexual favours.

One afternoon, the minister of home affairs called the health minister A. Ramadoss to his house for a discussion to reconcile their respective positions. Naresh Dayal, the secretary of health, and I accompanied the minister. Heated arguments followed with Shivraj Patil vehemently arguing against the position. But Ramadoss did not give in. If today the NACO affidavit stays unchanged and if it helped the favourable outcome in the high court in any way, a lot is owed to the outright support that Ramadoss gave to the issues of MSM and transgenders.

Three other factors enhanced an environment of support for the gay community: a supportive media, mobilization of MSMs and transgenders in Tamil Nadu under the Avahan-funded project, and the advocacy work of UNAIDS among the judiciary. The Lawyers Collective of Anand Grover was at the forefront organizing workshops and talks with the higher echelons of the judiciary by Supreme Court judges from South Africa and Australia who were sympathetic to the plight of people infected with HIV and issues of homosexuality. Such sensitization efforts helped break down barriers and reduce societal prejudices.

In 2009, the Delhi High Court presented a well-argued judgment favouring the repeal of Article 377. The extreme Right groups among Christians, Hindus, and Muslims appealed to the Supreme Court against the judgment. Given the political fallout that would result by opposing religious fundamentalism, the government took an ambivalent view. The cabinet was itself divided over this issue. Such vacillation was not taken note of as all were sure that the Supreme Court would most definitely endorse the lower court's verdict. This was a grave error. In hindsight, if only NACO had got the amendment pushed through Parliament! It was the right moment as there were powerful politicians who were supportive of NACO's stand. NACO and the gay community lost a historic opportunity.

In December 2013, the Supreme Court pronounced a most unexpected judgment that stunned every liberal-thinking individual. While the Supreme Court was procedurally correct in stating that amending laws was the business of Parliament, yet it was felt that scrapping Section 377 would have been consistent with its role of safeguarding individual rights and liberties as laid down in the Constitution.

In February 2016, the Supreme Court heard a batch of curative petitions and agreed to hear the case by a five-judge bench to go to the root of the matter afresh. There is palpable anxiety as to the outcome since the current government is conservative in its approach to matters related to sexual freedoms. However, while the issue of decriminalizing homosexuality is back to square one, the situation is vastly different from what it was even a decade ago. There is a much higher level of social acceptability and conscientization. Media attention gave many homosexuals the courage to come out. Standing up for MSMs also won NACO their trust and support which was seen as vital for the organization's work. A TRG for MSMs was constituted, surveillance sites sanctioned, TIs approved, and a USD 30 million grant from the Global Fund was obtained to build capacity, train PEs, and support their collectives.

In fact, Avahan's work among transgenders in Tamil Nadu was significant as it resulted in the state government providing a quota for transgenders in all educational institutions. This victory was decidedly a precursor to the Supreme Court judgment of 2014 which ordered that another category of 'third gender' be created and included under backward classes for the purpose of extending all government benefits. Strong reactions to NACO efforts to create social spaces for sex workers and MSMs either through legal means, or raising awareness by way of information campaigns clearly demonstrated that work being done was making a difference.

Giving Hope to Injecting Drug Users (IDUs)

The ICMR bulletin in 1990 recognized the use of injectable drugs as a risk factor but limited the geographic focus to the three north-eastern states of Manipur, Nagaland, and Mizoram. These states form part of what is called 'the golden triangle' between Pakistan and Myanmar. From the estimated 70,000 addicts in India, a majority were from the North East. There was hardly any evidence of IDUs in the rest of the country except in metropolitan cities, and of them Kolkata had significant numbers.

NACO was not involved with the issue of drug abuse per se. It was concerned only to the extent that addicts shared needles, thereby spreading infection among themselves and to others. The focus of NACO's rather limited harm-reduction strategy

> **Box 4.5** Society for Community Intervention and Rehabilitation (SCIR), Kolkata, 2006
>
> Supported by the West Bengal SACS initiative, the SCIR, an NGO run by Soumen Mitra (an IPS officer), functioned from a building located along the sidings of railway tracks. The building was in desperate need of repairs—peeling walls and broken windows gave it an air of desolate shabbiness. The corridors were lined with addicts sitting listlessly, their arms raw with abcesses and their hollow eyes staring with expressions of hopelessness. Makeshift shacks of the poorest of the poor abutted the facility. There they lived amidst filth and unimaginable squalor—an environment totally degrading for humans. The location of the SCIR was perfect as most drug addicts lived around these parts. Besides treatment, the NGO also attempted to provide skill development with a view to gradually build confidence and wean the youth away from drug dependence.
>
> *Source*: Author.

consisted of giving new, sterilized disposable needles to the IDUs in lieu of old ones. It was called a safe behaviour practice and like the condom for heterosexual behaviour, it pivoted around the Needle–Syringe Exchange Programme (NSEP). There were some 90 TIs working with IDUs—70 or so in the North East. There was little data available. For example, there was no information as to whether the needles being provided were adequate or if there was any differentiation or categorization of heavy shooters and casual ones. And there was no monitoring as NACO had no expertise, skill, or knowledge about this technical matter.

While the harm-reduction strategy undoubtedly helped bring down the numbers of the infected in states like Manipur, India had no interventions for those who were willing to stop injecting but were unable to do so. In fact, there was not even an understanding of such options.

In 2007, NACO was approached to not stop the Opioid Substitution Therapy (OST) programme. It transpired that under a DFID assisted programme (that NACO was unaware of), the OST had been piloted in the two states of Manipur and Nagaland.

Since their funding was ending, they set up beneficiaries to ask NACO to foot the bill. Sometimes when donors find bureaucracies unsupportive, they tend to go directly to the implementation level and initiate pilots. It was the same in this case as not only did NACO lack the capacity to introduce the OST but it could also not afford to. However, now NACO was stuck with a fait accompli as a beneficial programme could not be suddenly shut down.

Globally, the OST has gained some recognition as an effective strategy to wean off addicts. It implies administering small doses of the opioid to be taken orally and every single day without interruption, gradually reducing the quantum until the addict is completely weaned off. India's official policy, however, had not recognized it as it involved administering a contraband drug that was listed under the Narcotic Drugs and Psychotropic Substances (NDPS) Act. Administering it or even seen to be administering it without prior approval was against the law, as was the distribution of needles.

The OST was a complex programme that had the scope of being misused if improperly implemented and this deterred NACO. While the NGOs lacked the knowledge necessary for treatment of such disorders, there were very few medical institutions in the country that dealt with addictive disorders and administering the OST. The second challenge was that there was no platform where medical institutes and NGOs could talk to each other and harness each other's strengths to serve IDUs.

More complex were the entangled institutional arrangements in the government to deal with IDUs: the finance ministry (Department of Revenue) along with the home ministry (Narcotics Control Bureau [NCB]) were responsible for enforcing the ban on availability of, and access to, contraband drugs. They were opposed to any action that would tantamount to 'encouraging' drug consumption. Demand reduction was handled by the Ministry of Social Justice and Empowerment (MSJE) through their de-addiction programme while the MOHFW also ran some drug de-addiction programmes. There was no institutional mechanism to enable the four departments to even talk to each other. So while the MSJE believed in total abstinence irrespective of what the drug user wanted/was capable of, NACO's approach focused on harm reduction, that is, on reducing immediate harms first than insisting on abstinence. This approach was in direct conflict with the MSJE and the supply-control departments.

Involving drug users, talking to them as equal stakeholders in the designing and delivery of programmes were alien concepts for most of the other departments. This ideological divide between the ministries as well as the individuals/NGOs associated with these ministries was also reflected in the United Nations Office on Drugs and Crime (UNODC), which was also split down the middle—between the lobby advocating for the OST as an effective means of weaning away the addicts and the promotion of abstinence. Since the US, not unsurprisingly, was for abstinence, the UNODC could not be too strident in their support of NACO since their funding depended on the US. In these circumstances, even as NACO tried to engage with the various ministries, it received a lukewarm response—they reluctantly endorsed NACO's strategy, but they did not want to have anything to do with its programmes. It was a 'to each his own' stance by various ministries.

NACO lacked sufficient knowledge about drugs in general and the OST in particular which gave rise to fears and doubts: what if the OST does end up legitimizing drug consumption and facilitating further expansion of drug availability? What if the OST is black-marketed or siphoned off to corrupt more youth? Thailand and China had decided to implement the OST. China's ability to turn an idea into reality was awe-inspiring: within six months of taking the decision, over 300 methadone sites had been established. Most sites were well located in the midst of busy bazaars and easily accessible. The family of the drug addict was also co-opted, actively involved, and made responsible for providing moral support and an enabling environment to help the process of weaning off.

In January and March 2008, Dr Robert Newman from the USA and Dr Nick Crofts from Australia visited NACO and intervention sites and provided some insights into fine-tuning the IDU strategy. The challenge in implementing the OST strategy was to develop a system where this drug could be administered every day without a break and secure the commitment of the addict's family that was seen as a vital and an integral component in the transformative process of this intervention. But there was no approval for introducing the OST since it was not a part of the NACP III strategy. NACO needed a technically sound plan to withstand critical scrutiny and obtain concurrence from the related departments, namely the MSJE, the NCB, and the Department of Revenue, before submitting it to the Expenditure Finance Committee (EFC). It managed to do this in January 2008 and got all approvals in the June of that year.

To make a further headway, it was crucial to build technical capacity within NACO. In August 2007, Dr Ravindra Rao from AIIMS was seconded to NACO as a consultant. He was a huge asset who single-handedly managed to bring in some order. A TRG was formed for IDU interventions to deliberate issues as well as inform/guide on how to go about addressing this challenge.

To implement and scale up the OST programme, the first step was to transfer all the pilot project sites to NACO. To ensure uniformity in the functioning and assure consistency in quality and approach, the 'Clinical Practice Guidelines and Standard Operating Procedures on Implementation of OST' were brought out in 2008. At the same time, before starting OST centres, all the 30-odd centres were inspected by the NABH. Only those centres that were in accordance with NACO guidelines were permitted to provide the OST. This therapy was the first NACO intervention to have been accredited by the NABH. The entire supply chain of OST delivery was planned and implemented to ensure the regular flow of medication as even a single day without medication could jeopardize the impact of the intervention.

In the meanwhile, other challenges emerged. In January 2008, UNAIDS report on size estimation of IDUs in Punjab and Haryana showed that there were an estimated 25,000 IDUs in these two states alone. Also, HRG mapping revealed a number of other states that showed IDU presence in thousands. States that hitherto had no IDU problems started reporting them: Madhya Pradesh, Chhattisgarh, Odisha, Bihar, Uttar Pradesh, and even southern states such as Karnataka and Andhra Pradesh. Building capacity became imperative. Guidelines/training manuals on IDU intervention were developed.

It was clear that if the OST was to be sustained in India, it had to be integrated within government hospitals. A plan to implement the OST in government-hospital settings in active collaboration with TIs was prepared. An innovative GO–NGO model of OST delivery was conceived. To test the feasibility of this model, a pilot was initiated in the five districts of Punjab in 2010.

By 2009, we made steady progress on the intervention's side. The number of harm-reduction TI sites in the country increased to about 200 or so and much of the expansion took place in states other than those in the North East. By 2012, 57 OST intervention sites had been established providing therapy to 5,350 people. Systems were in place for a further scale-up including technical documents, supply-chain mechanisms, capacity-building, and dedicated teams at national and state levels to deal with the IDU problems in the country.

It was a long and, at times, hopeless struggle. All said and done, drugs were dangerous stuff and it was difficult to detect and control their availability. This was brought home to me when I met the chief minister of Nagaland. He clearly expressed his helplessness as he pointed out that the borders with Myanmar were so porous that in the border villages, drugs are used as barter for other goods like toothpaste! Besides, the North East had nothing—cinemas or pubs were not allowed by the church (though they were allowed in Kerala), sports were not developed, and in the villages educational institutions hardly functioned. The youth had no outlets except drugs to overcome their boredom. They had to be brought back through careful nurturing. The government's response was de-addiction centres. As per NACO's assessment, many of them were reported to be functioning on paper. Besides, a habitual drug addict cannot be weaned away within 15 days at a centre! It is a far more complex issue that needs a multi-pronged approach.[55]

Similar methodologies of mapping, tracking, and identifying high-risk behaviours among other vulnerable population groups such as truckers and single male migrants—referred to as bridge populations—were followed. The Transport Corporation of India was contracted to map the hubs and trucker routes, develop strategies in consultation with trucker organizations, and implement the initiatives. Lack of clarity regarding the behaviour aspects of the highly mobile and invisible groups like migrants was a major hindrance. Visits to worksites of migrants, say, in Bhiwandi or Surat revealed the abysmal and inhuman living conditions, focusing the spotlight on the hollowness of the implementation of labour laws. Therefore, the Ministry of Labour was persuaded to engage with NACO and funding for undertaking advocacy work in construction, manufacturing, and textile industries was obtained from the Global Fund. The funding came but the Ministry of Labour was excluded subsequently by NACO that feared loss of authority and power. Based on some scanty evidence, a strategy to cover the source (point of origin of labour) and the point of destination (where migrants work) was developed. Its effective implementation was, and continues to be, a problem.

Role of Avahan

In 2003, the BMGF, a US-based philanthropy, established Avahan as its Indian vehicle to implement TI strategies in 85 districts of India. It was provided USD 250 million for five years—the same amount that NACO had for all its activities under the NACP II. In a majority of the 85 districts that constituted the epicentre of the epidemic, NACO had already set up TI interventions. These were handed over to Avahan to further expand and improve while NACO focused on opening up new areas.

Avahan's entry provided momentum and undoubtedly raised the profile of the battle against HIV/AIDS generally and more importantly for the marginalized population groups. The annual trips of the world's richest 'father-son duo'—Gates Sr. and Bill Gates—to India, their visiting and talking with sex workers not only captured media headlines but also gave the programme 'respectability' and 'legitimacy'.

Avahan was quick to incorporate the learnings of DFID experiments with sex workers and truck drivers under the Healthy Highway project. In states like Andhra Pradesh and Tamil Nadu, Avahan built on the impetus created with TIs supported by SACS and bilateral agencies (USAID in Tamil Nadu and the DFID in Andhra Pradesh). For leveraging the on-the-ground implementation capability, Avahan appointed the same management agencies of SACS as its State Lead Partners (VHS in Tamil Nadu and HLFPPT in Andhra Pradesh) and speeded the scale-up in Karnataka and Maharashtra, where the state-level responses were tardy. It engaged seasoned and experienced civil society leaders like Jana, Sundar, Meena, Swarup Sarkar, Senthil, Nandinee, and Amit, among others, to advise them. Avahan also contracted the University of Manitoba's KHPT to replicate the Sonagachi model in Mysore. This copycat version was called Ashodaya. With a work culture very different to that of the government—based on competition and performance and tightly monitored for results—Avahan scaled up rapidly.

The Avahan project was for a fixed five-year period—2003–8. As their term ended in 2008, it raised several important implications. Explaining this will require a small digression.

Process of Transition from Avahan to Government

Donor-assisted projects generally do not incorporate an exit strategy at the time of entering into an MoU with the government. So when the KHPT exited from their projects on migrant labour in Rajasthan, NACO could not take them over for want of a budget. As NACO alerted Avahan of a similar danger at the cessation of their project in 2008, the project was extended for another five years with an inbuilt exit strategy that included handing over of the TIs to NACO in a phased manner: 10 per cent in 2010, 20 per cent in 2011, and 70 per cent in 2012. Such phasing was necessary as the NACP III budget had not earlier incorporated the contingency of taking over Avahan projects. However, NACO laid down four conditions: one, it would take over only after a third-party evaluation and an agreed baseline. Such evaluation was essential as NACO wanted to sustain the good work and not be blamed if there was a discrepancy between claims and reality on ground. Two, only those found to be performing well; and three, only those that were found to be functioning as per the financial norms followed by NACO. The fourth condition was that the transition should be in phases to enable the absorption of costs.

Accordingly, the exercise for the scheduled transition was taken up in 2009. The process of transition consisted of two steps: a) an independent assessment of all the 182 TIs implemented by

Avahan, and (b) categorization of the TIs into good, satisfactory, and poor. So those that were fully qualified for immediate transition were taken over by NACO, those that were partially qualified had to be extended support and hand-holding and made ready for transitioning, and the poor ones had to be replaced with new management.

The process adopted for transition was exhaustive. During the first phase of the transition, NACO developed quantitative and qualitative tools and a manual for the assessment of the shortlisted TIs at the field level. Assessment teams were constituted for each state with external experts, donor representatives, and SACS representatives. A detailed protocol of the team's visit to the TIs was prepared and a comprehensive briefing on the content, aims, and objectives of the review was provided. The reports of the assessment teams were then shared with all concerned and the SACS directed to take over those TIs that were ready for transitioning and aligned with NACO costings and guidelines. Each such transitioned TI had a baseline that became the basis for monitoring by NACO. The project director of SACS and his team were provided detailed briefing on the transition and post-transition plans.

Such a detailed process was necessary as until then Avahan had functioned largely autonomously and NACO was not necessarily aware of the actual work being done, relying only on the reports submitted by Avahan.

The reports and feedback received were a mixed bag—good work in some while room for improvement in others. In several cases, the teams found data discrepancies. The problem appeared to be in Avahan's implementation processes. Under this structure, NGOs to run TIs were contracted by a state-level partner (SLP), and SLPs were accountable to the Avahan management team that consisted of highly qualified people with degrees in business management or work experience in management. With SLPs as the 'custodians' of data collection, processing and reporting to Avahan, the onus was squarely on the former. NACO teams found this to be an obstacle as in some cases, they either found the project beneficiaries and workers unaware of the data or unwilling to provide data for fear of it being found inconsistent with that furnished by the SLP. Overall, out of the 182 TIs assessed, 41 were found to be fully qualified for transition, 130 were recommended for further hand-holding, and 11 were rated as poor.

Avahan was unhappy and its partners upset. The internal contradictions of Avahan's implementation structures created problems that needed to be resolved. Besides, the partners and NGOs did not want to come under the government fold and for good reasons: funding was lower, untimely, and often released only after some harassment. Avahan had to then put in a lot of effort to harmonize interventions and costs to get aligned with NACO and come up with proper data sets—this had to be, therefore, done only in collaboration with NACO teams at state and district levels.

Avahan has continued to hand-hold the TIs it funded by providing the NGO Swasthi a USD 10-million grant for three years. Under this support, the members of the 84 CBOs in five states have been listed. The listing showed a shortfall of 30,000 members. The focus has been on strengthening the CBOs by not merely talking about condoms and violence but expanding the agenda to include access to government programmes such as ration cards, pensions, credit from banks, scholarships for their children, and so on. Each member is being computerized and tracked to address her special needs. About 86 per cent of the members have an ID card and applications worth Rs 3.6 billion have been processed to banks and life insurance policies worth Rs 0.24 billion have been taken. Sex workers have indeed come a long way. This is possibly the first example of an exit strategy being incorporated at the early stages of project implementation and phasing out gradually.

Often it is believed that the problems of transition are attributable to the poor capacity of governments. Such a situation can be resolved with training and aligning modules and monitoring formats. But in reality the situation is more complex, depending on the extent of the autonomy in which the donor operates. There are trade-offs in these kinds of situations. Autonomy provides scope for innovation, and often innovation is what takes the agenda forward. But then at the time of transition, converting innovative practices into public policy and implementation frameworks is fraught with problems. For example, a key pioneer in the success of India's battle with HIV was the DFID. It was the DFID that did the proof of concept in establishing workable models of community-based organizations, management structures, and contracts with CBOs, or the monitoring tools, or TSUs, and so on. These lessons were available, yet they were not adopted by NACO automatically. It was Avahan that had the funds to operationalize them on scale and establish their viability before NACO could incorporate them under the NACP III.

The important issue in transitioning is not just the physical takeover of project costs into domestic budgets. Equally critical are the quality aspects. For example, the identification of elements central to empowerment and most vulnerable to be attacked in case of regime change. Under the NACP III strategy, behaviour change was to be achieved through a process of empowerment, which then resulted in the provisioning of budgets for processes that facilitate collectivization of the workers. A PE in such a process is expected to be in close touch with her peer group to effect changes in behaviour. On the other hand, the NACP IV approach is using key population organizations for service delivery. In operational terms, this has meant a budget cut on all activities related to mobilization and experience-sharing, and one where the PE is reduced to a low-paid worker filling 16 forms—a shift from a public health approach to a techno-managerial one.

In hindsight, it is in this context that the process of transition from Avahan could have been better. Today NACO does not have the evidence to justify investment in collectivization to counter the current government policy that is against community-based organizations and the importance of empowerment as a means of effecting change. In other words, the 'thinking' did not get transitioned. Very often such soft but critical concerns do get overlooked and fade out particularly in situations when the donor has also moved on, as seen in this case where the BMGF shifted focus to other agendas. In other words, issues related to the poor and their empowerment that could be disruptive in the short run often get off the policy agenda in political environments that are volatile and unstable.

Avahan was an important partner. Its distinct contribution in five specific aspects substantially influenced NACO and the trajectory of the epidemic:

a) It revived and reiterated the importance of instilling ownership in the community and focused on community mobilization, particularly the MSMs. Some of the best practices in community mobilization like Participatory Site Assessment (PSA),[56] community-owned clinics, peer education, and others were mapped and scaled up with consistency across TIs in all the Avahan programme states.
b) A platform for sharing good practices among partners was also created.
c) It created a strong management and process-orientated approach that enabled standardization of interventions and professional management practices such as supervision and very tight monitoring and reporting systems including data analysis.
d) It focused on quality.
e) It created space for innovation and flexibility.

While their contributions to, and legacy in, India's fight against HIV/AIDS cannot be minimized, there were three negative and unintended fallouts. One was the distortions Avahan created upon entry into the narrow NGO market. The salary scales and bias towards promoting international non-governmental organizations (INGOs)[57] such as the FHI, CARE, Pathfinders, HIV Alliance, and Futures drew away many of the best and most experienced people from local NGOs, decapacitating an already weak and fragmented civil society. Besides, other equally qualified people, too, demanded similar pay scales and work conditions. In fact, one of the problems in the transition was NACO's inability to pay such huge salaries to staff in the SLPs and implementing NGOs, making them reluctant to work with the government.[58] The situation was similar in the case of salaries of the experienced personnel seconded to NACO, who were paid for by donors. To this extent, Avahan did adversely impact the building of internal capacity.

The second was the inability of the Avahan management to 'discipline/control the SLP, losing the plot half way' as commented by an activist. Avahan had funded and supported the replication of the Sonagachi model, but such a rights-based approach was not in the interest of the SLPs/NGOs who leaned towards fostering a dependency syndrome. Avahan's praise of Ashodaya only generated jealousies and insecurities among the SLPs. Actually,

Ashodaya's attempts to expand its learnings to other sex worker interventions were viewed by the KHPT and even by Avahan as 'disruptive', making many feel that the concerns of the INGOs mattered more for Avahan. Many activists who were interviewed were unhappy with Avahan,[59] accusing it of inadequate commitment to the rights-based approach—of being only interested in data and results than in the real welfare of sex workers. In fact, it was alleged that there were people within the Avahan senior management itself who had no faith in the 'mumbo jumbo' of collectivization and the rights of sex workers and had a deductionist approach of a clinic and standardized treatment. Since empowerment and collectivization were process-driven and time-intensive, support from such people was weak largely due to 'the fear of not being able to meet their project targets'.[60]

Jana and other activists feel that the major barrier to empowering sex workers is ideological. Deep-rooted prejudices cannot agree to a rights-based strategy and so capacity-building or mobilization of financial resources can only go so far. So while the Avahan management team did, in principle, agree to, and were supportive of, the approach to form CBOs, in reality they did not necessarily follow it up with the SLPs. 'Avahan leaders ignored its avowed policy to hand over interventions to its natural stakeholders, that is, the CBOs.... There was inherent resistance from within the implementing agencies and individuals who ran these HIV interventions which was overlooked by the Avahan leaders ...'[61]

Many in NACO and Avahan believed that sex workers could be mobilized around an HIV agenda as opposed to their own agenda, namely police raids, violence, social stigma, marginalization, and so on, which led to the adoption of a narrow focus on community mobilization. In this narrow focus, the role of NGOs was also left vague and community mobilization was seen as capacity-building and not a structural agency to bring change. The dialectical process that had been envisioned was clearly not understood, partly because of the result-oriented, 'projectized' approach that was adopted. But frankly, such projectized, results-oriented approaches suit bureaucracies well, be they of the government or of private foundations like Avahan, as they are more amenable to measuring successes and outcomes within predetermined time frames.

Unfortunately, this narrow understanding continues to pervade NACO even today. It fails to see the importance of enabling the marginalized so that they could be freed from the hold of NGOs. NACO, in its anxiety to arrest HIV transmission, has consciously opted to go with the project approach. Giving up the two principles of collectivization and value of cross learnings that Avahan taught and NACO replicated will impact the latter's ability to control the epidemic at times when the sex worker's industry itself is undergoing considerable transformations, calling for new approaches and strategies but founded on principles that go beyond the HIV agenda. It would be useful for NACO to bring back to the centre stage the application of public health principles and learn from India's negative experience with population stabilization when it was designed around the narrow focus of contraception.

The third fallout was Avahan's tendency to take all credit for the success of India's model that was, in fact, the result of combined efforts. While all partners worked as a team, Avahan was perceived as standing out alone, narrowly focused on its own project, its own SLPs, and its own results. They had the money and resources to dominate the press and media and to also stake a large presence in multiple sessions at international AIDS conferences. It felt as though Avahan, and not India, was being showcased. The Avahan experiences were written about and commissioned to reputed universities like Harvard and John Hopkins and journals like the *Lancet*. So while the world knew about Avahan, little was known about NACO and the dedicated work done by other partners.

Such skewed publicity riled many as Avahan's success was contingent on NACO giving away successful and already 'worked upon' project areas with very few virgin areas where they had to start the intervention from scratch, so much so that some alleged it was a NACO 'sell out'. It was after all NACO and its partners (DFID, USAID, AIIHPH, HLFPPT, and others) who had put in the pioneering work in the early and difficult times before Avahan stepped in. Besides, Avahan borrowed and adapted ideas, concepts, and successes—a fact it never acknowledged. Finally, what is often overlooked is that NACO's TIs, at half the cost, had comparable high-quality outcomes as compared to those implemented by Avahan, giving rise to the comment that Avahan 'brought the money, not the thinking'. Avahan also benefited from the unconditional support it got from all partners, NACO, and all other levels of bureaucracy. This support enabled it in the effective implementation of policies that led it to achieve its goals. Avahan's reluctance to acknowledge the role of partners made it a poor team player.

Linking TIs with Services

An important aspect of the NACP III strategy was linking TIs with health services and not staying engaged with empowerment and condoms only. Caught up with the dual tracks of rights and empowerment in the initial stages, NACO had lost sight of the fact that empowerment also meant gaining access to life-giving services, namely testing for HIV and ART treatment. Providing such services, however, entailed individualized monitoring, which in turn implied listing and naming the beneficiaries. The civil society cried foul as it felt that such listing was a form of coercion. Undoubtedly, government employees could be insensitive,[62] yet they did need a denominator to evaluate their efforts. This gap in understanding had to be corrected without once again raising the debate over whether NACO's mandate was to only enable the empowerment process of the marginalized or to have the larger responsibility of arresting the epidemic on the one hand and ensuring on the other hand that every HIV-infected person, irrespective of his/her profession, got access to treatment and other entitlements. Full access to clinical services—medical check-ups, STD and ART treatment, and testing services—were accordingly included in the reviews along with the supply and utilization of condoms. In other words, NACO interpreted true empowerment of the marginalized to mean that they had full, hassle-free access to all government programmes. Today NACO has over 31 indicators for the TI programmes it monitors. But the danger of such an approach is that over time the aim to achieve the measurable targets takes over the process issues that are actually much more important. That is what happened here too. An illiterate PE—whose actual strength lay in talking with and keeping in touch with her group and ensuring that new recruits are sensitized on prevention—has been reduced to becoming a health worker who has to fill 16 forms. The programme has rapidly slipped to a target-driven techno-managerial approach rather than the social–humane approach and will undoubtedly plateau like the TB programme.

Stigma and Confidentiality

A contested issue in the treatment of HIV has been the confidentiality of an individual's HIV status. Globally, there was strong censure of any attempt at either mandatory testing or disclosure of HIV status on grounds of human rights as the disease conjured irrational fears, shame, and stigma. There was so much fear built around this infection that NACO had to unleash a series of campaigns just on how it does and does not spread—not through mosquito bites, shaking hands, hugging or touching, or sharing lavatories. The most irrational instances of fear were demonstrated in the removal from employment or schools as if the mere presence of an HIV-infected person in the room would infect others. A UNDP survey showed that 90 per cent of women who got the infection from their husbands were thrown out of their marital homes, denied property, and reduced to destitution.

Dealing with such deeply entrenched perceptions and fear psychosis required constant public demonstrations of state authority to lend assurance. Sushma Swaraj or A. Ramadoss were seen hugging HIV children, or the chief minister of Karnataka staying overnight at the home of an HIV-infected person. These were all meant to reassure the public. With time, the virulence of the stigma did begin to reduce but many feel that it is still latent, not far beneath the surface.

A memorable incident helps illustrate the fear psychosis. In 2008, two eight-year-olds were diagnosed as HIV positive in the 100 per cent literate district of Kottayam in Kerala. The news was inadvertently printed in a newspaper that led to loud protests from other parents demanding the immediate removal of the children from the school. Senior officials of the education department visited households and explained to them the irrationality of the demand. But the parent community was adamant and threatened to withdraw their children. It was a dicey moment. It could unnecessarily become political and adversely affect the government's efforts to destigmatize the infection. The government, to its credit, announced that the school would continue to function for the two children and the parents could withdraw their children if they so wished. That was a strong response and a mark of statesmanship. After some amount of squirming, all the children quietly trooped back to school and normalcy was restored.

Likewise, village visits amply showed how the HIV-affected families received social support in several cases. Essentially, discrimination and stigma did reduce with the introduction of treatment. Public hospitals did deliver HIV-positive women. However, overall such attitudes do persist, though with much lower intensity.

While the protagonists of the confidentiality policy had some merit, there were many who were not convinced. In response to public demand, the Andhra Pradesh legislative assembly passed a resolution making HIV testing mandatory before marriage; this was subsequently dropped under pressure from NACO. But the issue did not necessarily go away. As seen in the case of Kerala, a greater gain lay in social acceptance. Society needs to be educated, made aware, and helped to confront realities sensibly and rationally. And state power must strongly handle attempts to discriminate and compel, if required, society to be tolerant, caring, and sensitive. This is true for all forms of discrimination, be it against MSMs or women, or on the basis of caste or religious denominations. NACO did moot the idea of proposing an anti-discriminatory law. Since it was a wider issue, NACO supported a bill that Lawyers Collective helped to draft for protecting those vulnerable to, and infected by, HIV/AIDS. Non-discrimination was included.

Financing NACP III

India's HIV/AIDS control programme was largely donor-funded for the first three phases. From USD 85 million for the NACP I to USD 500 million for the NACP II, the amount increased to USD 2.5 billion under the NACP III. Of this sum, almost USD 1.7 billion came from donors like the World Bank, the Global Fund, other UN bodies, and international foundations like the BMGF.

Given the increased quantum of money, interventions, and partners, finance had to be strengthened. Establishing a full-fledged division with almost 10–12 accounts officers drawn from the government was an uphill task. For the six high-prevalent states that received more than Rs 1 billion, NACO insisted on a joint director-level officer to be deputed to SACS. Straightening discrepancies and shortcomings in financial-record maintenance, computerization of financial and physical performance, building up records voucher by voucher, developing financial manuals, and training finance staff on aspects of public finance and accounting procedures meant hard and meticulous work as every rupee under various heads had to be reconciled and accounted for. Such work was crucial for increasing the scope for absorbing funds. The pipelines have to be unclogged before flows can be assured.

For the NACP IV, an amount of Rs 134.15 billion was approved in the Twelfth Five Year Plan. During the current Plan period

TABLE 4.4 Releases for HIV/AIDS during the Twelfth Plan: 2012–17 (Rs Crores)

Year	Budget Estimate (BE)	Revised Estimate (RE)	Actual Expenditure
2012–13	1,700	1,759	1,316
2013–14	1,785	1,500	1,473
2014–15	1,785	1,300	1,287
2015–16	1,397	1,615	1,605
2016–17	1,719		
Total	8,386	6,174	5,681
Percentage to total allocation in Twelfth Plan of Rs 13,415 crore	62.5	73 (BE)	92 of RE and 42.3 per cent of Twelfth Plan allocation
Amounts released under the NACP III, 2007–12, against Plan allocation of Rs 11,585 crore*			8,910 † (77 per cent of total Plan allocation)

Source: NACO (figures rounded off).
Notes: 100 crores equal to 1 billion.
* Includes the domestic budget of Rs 8,023 crore and the rest is extra budgetary.
† Total spent (includes donor and budget expenditures).

(2012–17), an amount of Rs 55.76 billion has been spent during the last four years. Despite including the amount allocated for this year—2016–17—it still falls short of what was spent under the NACP III. Besides, under the NACP VI, the coverage for ART has doubled. Lesser resources and more treatment explain the massive cutbacks on prevention activities particularly related to the key population groups, not without having long-term adverse consequences.

Unpredictability in releases and sudden cuts in budgets have had an adverse impact on programme activities. Media reports of stock-outs of drugs, testing kits, consumables; non-payment of dues to NGOs; and closing down of TIs are coming out with regular frequency.

Back to Square One

Early 2014, the NACP IV was released to the public, though consultations had begun in 2011 itself. Until then, it was a top-secret document that no one had any access to. Preparation of the NACP IV was initiated with 16 working groups. Several 'think pieces' provided insights into the changing nature of the epidemic, calling for re-strategizing the approach. Receiving no response to these inputs, the civil society caucus and members of the working group on AIDS for the Twelfth Five Year Plan submitted in March 2011 a note to Rangarajan, the economic advisor to the PM, wherein they emphasized:

> [I]f we want to strengthen the continuum from prevention to treatment, then we need to move away from the present dependence on highly resourced techno-managerial system of managing the epidemic and instead invest in more economically viable and result-oriented community systems that can make the programme work on the ground. This implies scaling up and further mandating the already evolved and highly experienced community systems to manage the epidemic as the latter will not only help us to reach out to the most vulnerable individual but also enable us to build a more organic, sustainable and uninterrupted response.

They received no response.

On 12 May 2011, 100 civil society members, many of whom had dedicated a good part of their life to this struggle against HIV/AIDS, gathered in Delhi to appeal collectively for a more inclusive process for preparing the NACP IV. They passed a resolution: 'Expressing deep concern at the ad hoc and top-down non-consultative process used by NACO to draft the NACP IV program plan, the civil society organizations hereby urge NACO to ground the process on principles of inclusion and transparency, particularly with regard to information and knowledge sharing.'

They suggested that a rigorous review of the NACP III be undertaken by an independent body and widespread consultations be facilitated across the length and breadth of the country. They urged for making 'the process of evolving the NACP IV meaningful, participatory and transparent. And it must be taken far beyond the design and consultative standards established by the NACP III.' Across the regions five consultations were held and all organizations representing populations affected by the epidemic participated. The report prepared by civil society and community organizations was given a quiet burial and erased from all official records.

The civil society members wanted that documents be shared with them and also expressed 'concern that international agencies were taking over much of the consultative process'. They also stressed to the DG the 'strong sense amongst civil society that there is a lack of respect from NACO' and a direct contrast to a measure of openness that characterized the NACP III.

Finally, when the NACP IV was released, they found to their dismay that it was no different from the earlier plan—a 'document of intent totally lacking in strategy as none of the rapid changes in the epidemiology of the epidemic were taken note of and was essentially a weak update of the NACP III'.

Basically, the NACP IV was a wasted opportunity. The objective conditions have changed. Brothel-based sex work has gone down and there are rapid changes in the organizational structure of sex work. With the cell-phone technology, sex work is increasingly becoming home-based, making access difficult and a challenge calling for innovative approaches. Besides, there is a need to undertake the remapping of sexual networks as most have shifted with the lapse of time. Other unfinished agendas pertained to issues related to transgenders, expanding the IDU programme in the northern states where drug addiction was increasing rapidly, and finally the issue of programme integration with the NRHM, particularly in the northern states that were vulnerable but did not have adequate case load to justify verticality. These issues found inadequate attention in the NACP IV.

Besides, NACO has erred in giving up the CBO approach. It no longer provides funds for institutional development, the time lag for getting funds is almost 10 months, there are no more DICs that could be an invaluable way of accessing the hidden sex workers, and so on. And more importantly, when sex workers are empowered, they talk and raise issues. PEs selected from among the community were not valued so much for mobilizing sex workers for getting their tests done but for being in touch, building contacts, and bringing behaviour change through bonding. CBOs talk and their voices can be heard, but in NGO-run projects, one only hears the NGO that says only what the NACO bosses would like to hear. CBOs have no incentive to inflate figures as funds are not based on membership, while NGOs fudge figures as their funding depends on the number of sex workers in their project. Finally, there is enough data to show that CBOs' response to the HIV epidemic in terms of behaviour change, reduction in STIs, availing of treatment, and so on has been far better than that of NGO-run TIs.

The CBO strategy conformed to the classical public health approach of bringing the affected people centre stage. Yet NACO reversed the policy demonstrating once again that bureaucracies dislike true empowerment of people and prefer dependence and being 'in control'. Unlike in the earlier decades, public health professionals within the government are losing touch with their science and becoming obsessed with governmentalism or allowing personal biases to dictate strategy. These attitudes explain why India is unable to overcome its burden of infectious diseases. It is important that the government provides in-service training and establishes a well-trained public health cadre.

It had taken over a decade of dedicated work to build NACO. It took less than three years to bring it down to the level where the very people for whom NACO was working expressed a lack of confidence in it. Their troubles were not over. The new NDA government brought no cheer. In 2014, the health minister visited NACO for a briefing; he disapproved of the strategy and asked for abstinence to be promoted. In September 2014, the department status of NACO was withdrawn and the status quo ante restored with the AS and DG becoming part of the Department of Health. Though not an issue, civil society interpreted this move as yet another demonstration of the falling priority of HIV/AIDS in the eyes of the new government, though it is the Planning Commission that had suggested the merger in 2012.

Due to a lack of attention NACO has fallen silent. Almost all the well-trained people have left. TRG meetings are held but not with the same passion or rigour; dialogue with and among the stakeholders has collapsed and civil society kept at an arm's-length. There are lesser number of review and tours. Monitoring has declined and inter-ministerial partnerships have also been dropped. NACO seems to stand alone, a position worsened with the budget cuts resulting in stock-outs of diagnostics or drugs.

NACO was built brick-by-brick by several individuals who, for years, stood committed to the HIV/AIDS programme. They now see their efforts flattened and NACO once again standing at the crossroads. Funds are not reaching the intended and there is dismay that if this indifference continues, there may be a backlash and HIV may rise again. A new dynamism and a new flush of energy are urgently called for to address the demoralization and fatigue that has crept into NACO. But there is hope. Past efforts have not been in vain. This year, due to media editorials and pressure from the PLHIV whose very survival seemed to be on hold, the budget cuts imposed were restored—the only programme to be so fortunate!

The story of NACO and its struggle to contain an infectious disease provides a salutary lesson for policymakers and public health practitioners. Understanding the way India fought the HIV infection in a sexually conservative and traditional society, the processes followed, and the approaches adopted to implement strategies have important lessons for those interested in understanding implementation science.

Designing strategies and processes based on evidence, prevailing realities, and the social and behavioural contexts of the stakeholders; synchronizing inputs to achieve the desired outcomes; strengthening the managerial capacity to implement the interventions at the field level and the capacity to closely guide, monitor, and facilitate at the apex level; valuing inclusion and active engagement of all stakeholders; respecting knowledge, debates, thinking, and innovations; and finally, accepting the limitations of the top-down bureaucratic approaches with limited engagement of all stakeholders are some key lessons that need to be adopted in policymaking. India's success was the result of the commitment and direct involvement of those who had the most at stake, a factor that is often overlooked, especially in circumstances where there is an increasing perception that technology can replace human interactions. The NACO experience aptly illustrates the importance and value of the classical public health approaches that are premised on the need to contextualize the medical with the social and moral. This holistic understanding is rapidly being replaced by techno-managerial approaches that tend to substitute human behaviour, perceptions, and environmental changes with technology.

The focus during the NACP III was on building systems that have enabled most initiatives to continue despite attrition and change in leadership styles at the top rungs of management. But then, systems need leaders as much as leaders need systems to get transformative results. The truism of this statement is amply evident in the experience of the NRHM that was unfolding at the same time as the NACP III.

HIV is no ordinary disease. Unlike any other, it challenged the social order and value systems, and in the process helped enhance a measure of social acceptability of different sexual orientations and behaviour. That India with its multiple problems was able to develop a strategy and achieve the highest reductions in incidence in the world, averting disease and saving millions of lives is a tribute to the political leadership as much as to the selfless work of the thousands of individuals who worked on the programme for over two decades. Contact with the HIV/AIDS programme transformed the lives of those who worked in this area, making them humbler and less judgemental.

TABLE 4.5 Achievements under the NACP (End Phases I, II, and III)

S. No.	Indicator	Achievement		
		End NACP I	End NACP II	End NACP III
1.	No. of TIs established	199	721	1,821
2.	Coverage of HRGs (%)			
	FSW	55	80	
	MSM	06	64	
	IDU	53	80	
3.	STI clinics set up (cumulative)	494	974	1,112
4.	STD Coverage %	NA	17.98	91.25
5.	No. of ICTCs set up	109	4,027	12,897
6.	No. of people diagnosed	10,583 (in 1998–9)	202,485 (in 2006–7)	245,830 (in 2011–12)
7.	No. of blood units collected (in lakh per year)	NA	46.5	81.8
8.	Blood collected through VBD (%)	26	58.9	83.1
	No. of ART centres	NIL	107	355
	No. of PLHIV on ART	NIL	65,907	516,412
9.	No. of HSS sites set up	180	1,130	1,359
10.	Modes of HIV transmission (%)			
	Sexual transmission	74.15	85.8	89.7
	Blood and blood products	7.05	2.0	1.0
	IDUs	7.3	2.2	1.7
	Mother-to-child	NIL	3.8	5.0
	Others	10.92	6.2	2.7
10.	Awareness levels (%)	76.1%	84.6	>90
11.	Consistent condom use	51.9	61.7	74.0
12.	Funds allocated (in crores)	267.88	2,064.65	7,717.18
13.	Expenditure incurred Rs crores (%)	274.26	1,965.92 (95.2)	6,237.48 (80.8)

Source: NACO.

Note: 100 crores equal to 1 billion.

Notes and References

1. The National Institute of Health, Fogarty International Center, available at https://www.fic.nih.gov/researchtopics/pages/implementationscience.aspx (accessed on 21 December 2015).
2. According to the WHO, surveillance is defined as 'the ongoing systematic collection, collation, analysis and interpretation of data … in order that action may be taken'. See http://www.who.int/countries/eth/areas/surveillance/en/ (accessed on 17 July 2016).
3. 'State HIV Epidemic Fact Sheets', 2014, Department of AIDS Control, MOHFW, GOI.
4. HIV Sentinel Surveillance, 2012–13, 'India's Voice against AIDS', A Technical Brief, Department of AIDS Control, MOHFW, GOI, available at http://www.naco.gov.in/upload/NACP%20-%20IV/HSS%20TECHNICAL%20BRIEF/HIV%20Sentinel%20Surveillance%20Technical%20Brief.pdf (accessed on 25 August 2016).
5. Today NACO is conducting a national IBBA in 350 districts with a target of 160,000 respondents using standardized methodologies and operational aspects showing the maturing of NACO capacity.
6. My experience in the health ministry helped me to identify Dr Bachani, Dr Sokhey, Dr Venkatesh, and Dr Khera from the ministry and entrust them with ART, STD, epidemiology, and HMIS programmes respectively, while Dr Shaukat managed the blood-safety programme. Suresh Mohammad, a doctor-turned-police officer-turned public health expert, looked after the ICTC and PPTCT. Mayank Agarwal from the Information Service was in charge of IEC, and Suresh Kumar, a young IAS officer from the West Bengal cadre, who had worked as PD, State AIDS Prevention and Control Society of West Bengal, was appointed as director for administration and finance.
7. I recall an instance when the Odisha SACS, on one plea or another, delayed payments to NGOs adversely affecting work. Payment was finally made when I went to the state and insisted on the cheques being issued in my presence!
8. Otherwise, the process of adaptation to a new way of doing things also, in the immediate sense, creates a sense of loss—loss of control (Professor Heifetz of Harvard University, class notes, 2012).
9. Even after many other senior division heads and I left between 2010 and 2011, the programme implementation continued and expanded, at least for a while.
10. Survey conducted by the ICMR in 2002–3.
11. P. Arora, N.J.D. Nagelkerke, R. Moineddin, Madhulekha Bhattacharya, and Prabhat Jha, 2013, 'Female Sex Work Interventions

and Changes in HIV and Syphilis Infection Risks from 2003 to 2008 in India: A Repeated Cross-sectional Study', *BMJ Open*, DOI:10.1136/bmjopen-2013- 002724.

12. In 2009, cabinet approvals were obtained for establishing four state-of-the-art blood banks in the metro cities with a capacity of 100,000 units and two fractionation plants with a capacity of 150,000 litres. Land was identified and building plans drawn up. However, six years later, nothing has happened.
13. As a joint secretary handling this division, I was only too aware of its inadequacies.
14. Strategic Document of NACP IV (2012-17), 20 October 2011, NACO, GOI, p. 107.
15. This idea mooted by my predecessor in 2005 took form and shape in 2008 after several visits to the railway ministry, letters from the health minister to the minister of railways, from the PMO to the railways ministry, and so on.
16. The Petition Committee of Parliament under the chairpersonship of Venkaiah Naidu was very critical of this programme resulting in a revamp of the teaching materials, disassociation of the NCERT from the effort, and greater consultations with states. Overall, the state response was positive.
17. In fact, E. Dax, the Australian expert who we took to advise us, told me that our laboratories would take more than 10 years to reach the standards of Thailand and 15 years to reach global standards.
18. *Global Tuberculosis Report* (Geneva: WHO, 2014)
19. Sanghamitra Iyengar of Samraksha, in an interview (2014).
20. 'Violence is a symptom of power and linked intimately to the social conditions that so often determine who will suffer abuse and who protected.' See Paul Farmer in *Pathologies of Power: Health, Human Rights, and the New War on the Poor* (Berkeley: University of California, 2003).
21. Mohd. Ahmed Khan v. Shah Bano Begum, (1985) SCR (3) 844.
22. Though we are with all, yet we feel alone. If only we had that little identity that we are human beings like others … our pain is that though we are living in society … we are outsiders—does anyone understand this? This suppressed pain is always looking for a way out. And nothing else do we want—just an identity, a social recognition—is that so difficult? (Das quoted in Catrin Evans, Kevin O'Reily, and Smarajit Jana, *Community Led Structural Intervention* (Saarbrücken: Lambert Academic Publishing, 2013).
23. The second thematic meeting of UNAIDS Programme Coordinating Board, 9–11 December 1998, New Delhi.

24. My first visit to Kamathipura was as director in the MOHFW in charge of international health. The place was a cause for concern as HIV prevalence had sharply increased from 1 per cent in 1988 to over 30 per cent in 1991 and to 51 per cent in 1998 against an increase from 1 per cent to 5 per cent in Sonagachi during the same period.
25. Evans et al., *Community Led Structural Intervention*.
26. As informed by Meena Seshu of VAMP.
27. Vandana Gurnani, Tara S. Beattie, Parinita Bhattacharjee et al., 2011, 'An Integrated Structural Intervention to Reduce Vulnerability to HIV and Sexually Transmitted Infections among Female Sex Workers in Karnataka State, South India', *BMC Public Health*, 11: 755.
28. Evans et al. *Community Led Structural Intervention*.
29. Evans et al. *Community Led Structural Intervention*.
30. 'None in my family knows I am a sex worker.... I can tell them I am working for the Hygiene Institute. I have not told them I am working in Sonagachi.... If they question me, I show them my green coat and my identity card and this makes them silent. This work lends a sort of respectability to us' (a PE quoted in Evans et al., *Community Led Structural Intervention*).
31. Besides the rich discussion in the book *Community Led Structural Intervention* by Evans et al., I learnt a great deal about these issues from Jana himself in an endless round of meetings when he was advisor at NACO, 2007–8.
32. Paulo Freire, *Pedagogy of the Oppressed* (New York: Herder and Herder, 1972).
33. This was later called Community-led Structural Intervention or CLSI. It essentially meant that the community organizes itself to fight the barriers that are systemic and integral in the social structure in which they are situated.
34. Evans et al. *Community Led Structural Intervention*.
35. Evans et al. *Community Led Structural Intervention*.
36. Bandyopadhyay and Gooptu quoted in Evans et al., *Community Led Structural Intervention*.
37. There were others along with VAMP: a sex worker collective called Sangram, an MSM collective called Muskan, a research foundation called CASAM, and so on.
38. This information was gathered from an interview with Jana (April 2014).
39. Friere, *Pedagogy of the Oppressed*.
40. Sarkar is an epidemiologist by training and is currently working as director in the WHO South East Asia Regional Office (SEARO).

41. Reza Paul Sushena et al., 2012, 'Sex Worker-led Structural Interventions in India: A Case Study on Addressing Violence in HIV Prevention through the Ashodaya Samithi Collective in Mysore', *The Indian Journal of Medical Research*, 135 (1): 98–106.
42. Paramita, a prostitute, was homeless and a drunk. In 2007, she was infected with HIV. After she joined Ashodaya, she gained self-confidence and her self-esteem was revived. She began to value life. This is the transformation that can take place when 'deconstructing science' is practised. Within three years she not only learnt English and Hindi but was also sent to South Korea in 2011 for an AIDS conference to give a PowerPoint presentation. She is currently the treasurer of Ashodaya.
43. Vandana Gurnani, Tara S. Beattie, Parinita Bhattacharjee et al., 2011, 'An Integrated Structural Intervention to Reduce Vulnerability to HIV and Sexually Transmitted Infections among Female Sex Workers in Karnataka State, South India', *BMC Public Health*, (11): 755.
44. Gurnani et al., 'An Integrated Structural Intervention'.
45. There is substantial research and evidence available to show the utility of such community-based interventions as opposed to the traditional approaches where the key stakeholders are treated as recipients of government grants. Sonagachi's success in registering low infection rates of STD, HIV, alongside increased condom use, is evidence of the efficacy of strategies that are centred around ideas of inclusion, participation, and collectivization. The Sonagachi model based on such principles gave the sex workers a sense of empowerment that then brought about behaviour change.
46. HIV Sentinel Surveillance, 'India's Voice against AIDS'.
47. Ahmedabad is a salutary story of what bureaucratic mindlessness can do. The city had an established 400-year-old brothel located near the port. An enthusiastic superintendent of police wanted to 'clean' up the place and thus conducted raids that scattered all the sex workers all over the city. Due to the loss of steady income and incapability to pursue any other means of livelihood, sex work increased, and so did HIV. It became very difficult to reach out to them with information or services.
48. This rule emerged from an analysis of the PEs who were found to be elderly. They also tended to double up as procurers of new sex workers to keep the trade going and were also found to be not in touch with the rapid shifts in the nature of sex work from static to mobile.

49. Rami Chabbra, former additional secretary in the MOHFW and an activist, often used this word to describe NACO's work among sex workers. She was very opposed to the NACO strategy and felt that it was spreading licentious behaviour. Her charge, however, was never proved by any evidence.
50. NACO was also completely against trafficking. Its point of difference with the DWCD was that NACO did not believe that every sex worker was trafficked. Besides, the solution to stop trafficking was to penalize the gangs and big interests that were behind human trafficking and not the sex workers.
51. N. Saggurti, R.K. Verma, S.S. Halli et al., 2011, 'Motivations for Entry into Sex Work and HIV Risk among Mobile Female Sex Workers in India', *Journal of Biosocial Science*, 43(5): 1–20, DOI:10.1017/S002193201100002
52. Basically, I saw this debate of choice being tautological as women resorted to sex work to fight poverty. They were merely a symptom of a development model gone wrong. Not one sex worker I met aspired to be a sex worker—it was always the circumstances. But once in, most found it difficult to opt out.
53. In Maharashtra, sex workers were provided with buffaloes. After six months, the BDO visited them and found that all buffaloes had been sold off. The sex workers admitted that they had indeed sold off the animals and repaid their bank loans as they found that feeding the buffaloes, taking care of them, and repaying loan instalments meant that they had to undertake extra sex work! (as related by Meena Seshu).
54. Section 377 of the IPC reads as: 'Unnatural offences: Whoever voluntarily has carnal intercourse against the order of nature with any man, woman or animal shall be punished with imprisonment for life, or with imprisonment of either description for a term which may extend to ten years, and shall also be liable to fine.'
55. I had met some NGOs from Pakistan who informed me of their efforts to develop wastelands into the richest grape-growing vineyards that are today exporting grapes—all done by drug addicts. Trained, skilled, and put to work, the drug addicts were weaned away from drugs even as their own self-worth got enhanced. I was convinced that it was a worthy model to emulate.
56. PSA meant mapping of the spread of the target group by the NGO in consultation with the key stakeholders and the community.
57. Even in the current projects being implemented in Bihar and Uttar Pradesh, it is CARE and the KHPT that are the TSUs. The people

working there are, however, all Indians getting remuneration far beyond that prevailing in the Indian markets.
58. There were other reasons too, of course, and I suspect the main one was having to pay bribes and the untimely release of funds. In the Avahan project, neither were any bribes paid nor were there any uncertainties or delays in the release of funds.
59. According to Sanghamitra of Samraksha, '[H]alf the problem was the unwillingness to seek accountability from their State Lead Partners who ruled the roost in different states and were more interested in collecting data for their own papers and research than looking at tying in with the national programme objectives …'
60. Personal communication with Jana (2014).
61. Personal communication with Jana (2014).
62. 'SACS officials went to a village (in Karnataka) presumably for line listing high-risk persons. As all the women assembled, they announced that only sex workers may stay and the rest could leave. All women got up and left' (interview with Sanghamitra of Samraksha).

CHAPTER FIVE

Revitalizing Rural Primary Healthcare: The National Rural Health Mission

An Overview

By the end of 2004, the public health system, particularly in rural areas, was in serious need of repair and reconstruction. On the other hand, the technologically driven private sector had medicalized healthcare and was skewing demand towards treatment rather than prevention. India's task was complex as it was faced with multiple problems—a huge burden of communicable and non-communicable diseases and an increasing load of injuries, a spiralling cost in healthcare impoverishing people in the absence of social security, and a lack of clarity in policy and direction required for setting priorities and making appropriate investments. As a first step, revitalizing primary care and resuscitating a failing public health system was of critical importance.

In April 2005, the newly elected UPA government launched the NRHM with a threefold increase in the budget. The increased budget helped to make substantial inroads in addressing some of the most basic issues facing the sector. Since 2005 institutional deliveries have increased from 47 per cent to 68 per cent, doubling the rate of decline in maternal and infant mortality compared to the period prior to the NRHM. Polio has been eliminated, bringing closure to a 25-year struggle; immunization coverage has increased from 48 per cent to 68 per cent; nearly a million CHWs have been recruited in rural villages; a country-wide emergency transportation system has been launched with over 1,200 ambulances ferrying patients to hospitals; and adequate drugs, personnel, and equipment have been ensured in health facilities, increasing footfalls dramatically, particularly in the states of Bihar, Madhya Pradesh, and Rajasthan. With over 0.15 million personnel recruited to work in the health facilities, the government developed enough confidence to declare the provision of free maternal and child health services in government facilities. The NRHM triggered institutional innovation; smoothened, in part, a dysfunctional public health system; established processes for people's participation; widened access to basic healthcare; and restored a measure of confidence and trust. Most significantly, in its early years, the NRHM initiated the process of dismantling centrist approaches and encouraging state participation and ownership. These are no mean achievements.

Yet the perception that these shifts and changes were not transformative enough persisted. It was felt that despite a supportive environment and enhanced funding, the NRHM's achievements were limited, though the yardstick on which these achievements were being measured was not always clear. By the end of the Eleventh Plan period, questions were raised about whether the NRHM was the right strategy to have been adopted at all. And furthermore, whether the shortcomings could be attributed to a flawed policy and strategy or faulty implementation? Did the problem lie in the lack of leadership and diffused centres of power, or simply in the lack of institutional capacity to bring change at the centre and state levels? Such doubts even resulted in a concerted attempt to abandon the NRHM during the Twelfth Plan. The issue is whether these questions were justified and how do we measure success.

Some of the answers to the questions are embedded in the way the NRHM policy evolved. This chapter seeks to trace the events as they unfolded during the period from 2005 to 2013. It explores the impact of the ideas, issues, and challenges that dominated the discussions in the early days, including the power struggles between individuals and institutions that together impacted the NRHM policy and its implementation. An understanding of the evolution of the NRHM policy can enable one to clearly see what needs to be done now and how. The chapter concludes with a short overview comparing management principles that were adopted by NACO and the NRHM that may have influenced the course of both these public health programmes—the largest since India's independence.

The Political Context of 2005: UPA I

In May 2004, the Congress rode back to power with a fractured mandate. Though the single-largest party with 145 seats, the Congress had to cobble up alliances with other parties to reach the magical figure of 272 required for forming the government under the banner of the United Progressive Alliance (UPA). Some parties like the Communist Party of India (Marxist) [CPI(M)] provided outside support, while others like the Dravida Munnetra Kazhagam (DMK) and the Pattali Makkal Katchi (PMK) joined the government.

The UPA had agreed upon a National Common Minimum Programme (NCMP) that laid down its vision and policies. Eager to shed its association with the 1992 reforms that were believed to have dented welfare and their pro-poor image, the Congress set out to re-establish itself as a left-of-centre party—a task made simpler because of the unqualified support extended by the CPI(M).

Sonia Gandhi was expected to become the prime minister. Instead Manmohan Singh was nominated after a dramatic sequence of events. This was the first time that India had a prime minister neither elected by the people nor the party. Nevertheless, the decision was welcomed as Manmohan Singh was respected as an honest and good professional and a progressive leader.

To stay engaged with policy issues, Sonia Gandhi established the NAC with the mandate to look at public policy issues and review the functioning of the government. She was the chair of the council that consisted of relatively prominent civil society activists, retired bureaucrats, and some of Delhi's elite selected partly on professional merit. The idea to bring together expertise and diverse opinions and dispassionately deliberate upon key issues facing the country was an inspired idea. In its early years, the NAC ushered in some fresh air with progressive policies such as the Right to Information (RTI) and the Right to Work[1] (RTW), but soon it fell short. There was no stamina or intellectual muscle to usher in the much-needed structural shifts and social transformations. Instead, the NAC unfolded as a pressure group and, before long, began to function like what a former member called 'a super cabinet' with no accountability to any institution, party, the government, or the Constitution. In other words, though the NAC's advice was not binding on the government and it was not accountable for its recommendations' immediate or future repercussions on the economy, it was expected that its instructions were to be implemented.[2] Or so was the public perception.

Coalition politics made the Congress dependent on the support of every small party. The PMK, a little-known party of Tamil Nadu with six MPs, became a crucial partner in this fragile coalition. It made its support to the Congress conditional on making Ambumani Ramadoss, the son of its founding leader, the cabinet minister of the health ministry. Thus, for the third time, the health ministry had a PMK party member as its minister. Ramadoss lasted his full term of five years. During the decade from 1998–2008, the PMK governed the health ministry for eight years in all. Unlike the previous times, this time around, the selection of Ramadoss was fortuitous as he emerged to be one of the more capable health ministers India has had since Independence.

Health policy had to be formulated in this maze of layered power centres—diffused political power, multiple interest groups, and contending with an array of decision- and opinion-makers along with the formal systems of governance that consisted of the ministry hierarchies, the PMO, and the cabinet. Added to all this were the institutional trappings of democracy: Parliament, the CAG, the judiciary, the media, and informal wielders of political power—the UPA and the NAC—all at the same time.

National Common Minimum Programme (NCMP)

A confluence of several unconnected factors during the period from 2000–4 led to declaring health a priority sector. The

Millennium Development Goals (MDGs) launched in 2000 set out a global resolve to achieve a set of outcomes by 2015. In the same year, the report of the Commission on Macroeconomics and Health (CMH) chaired by Professor Jeffrey Sachs was released. Both Prime Minister Manmohan Singh and Isher Ahluwalia[3] were members of the commission and their association with it certainly helped in prioritizing health in India. In 2001, the Indian Council for Research on International Economic Relations (ICRIER), a research institute headed by Isher Ahluwalia, facilitated the publication of *India Health Report*, the first comprehensive assessment of India's health system and the challenges it faced, authored by three government health officials.[4] At the same time, the release of the second National Health Policy in 2002; the constitution of the NCMH co-chaired by the ministers of health and finance in 2004; and finally as a run-up to the general elections in 2004, the strong lobbying by the civil society with political parties to commit themselves to the strengthening of the public health system created the ideal situation for bringing health to the fore.

The sensitization of influential leaders and powerful economists on the centrality of health in development and economic growth was a key component of the development dialogue. The NCMP of the UPA I made seven clear commitments as listed below. Their implementation was to be reviewed by the coordination committee of the UPA at regular intervals.

> The UPA will raise public spending on health to at least 2–3% of GDP over the next five years with focus on primary health care. A national scheme for health insurance for poor families will be introduced. The UPA will step up public investment in programmes to control all communicable diseases and also provide leadership to the national AIDS control effort.
>
> The UPA government will take all steps to ensure availability of lifesaving drugs at reasonable prices. Special attention will be paid to the poorer sections in the matter of health care. The feasibility of reviving public sector units set up for the manufacture of critical bulk drugs will be re-examined so as to bring down and keep a check on prices of drugs.
>
> The UPA government is committed to replicating all over the country the success that some southern and other states have had in family planning. A sharply targeted population control programme

will be launched in the 150-odd high-fertility districts. The UPA government recognizes that states that achieve success in family planning cannot be penalized.⁵

This was the first time that health had been put at the centre stage in any political manifesto. There was relief, hope, and high expectations that this sector had finally come out of cold neglect. Though limited, the NCMP's agenda offered possibilities for reviving the state's decrepit public health system and for widening access to privately provisioned health services through insurance.

By the end of 2012, the promised 'architectural correction' and 'community engagement' had been partly realized with the health system continuing to be fragmented, dysfunctional, and unregulated. Infectious diseases had not abated leaving India gasping with a dual burden of disease, calling for a more sophisticated policy and greater resources. Progress under some of the more specific commitments made in the NCMP were tardy. The health insurance policy was ad hoc and had a minimal impact in reducing out-of-pocket expenses or catastrophic expenditures, particularly among the poor. Essential life-saving drugs continued to be inaccessible—neither affordable nor available. The revival of bulk drug production did not take off. Instead, under pressure from the WHO, the three public sector vaccine-producing institutions—Kasauli, Conoor, and Chennai—were peremptorily shut down under what was termed a 'slash and burn policy'.⁶ And finally, public investment in health increased only marginally from 0.9 per cent of the GDP to 1.1 per cent against the 2–3 per cent of the GDP that was promised in the party manifesto.

As the following paragraphs will show, in this story, five issues clearly stand out. One, the role of NGOs and the enormous policy space they occupied in the initial years but could not sustain.

Two, the ahistorical approach of policy formulation. Even as new players came in, their enthusiasm was stymied due to an inadequate understanding of how the system works—the set-up, incentive structures, and the pulls and pressures. Changing the established ways requires basing policy on evidence and an understanding of the policy environment and past history—features that were absent in the initial years.

Three, the non-engagement and absence of platforms for a continuous dialogue with the key stakeholders—the people and the frontline workers—through intensive interactions and visits to villages, inspiring leadership among them and implementing the vision at that level.

Four, the varied levels of interest and commitment of state governments coupled with an inadequate understanding of the implications of the principles on which the NRHM was postulated.

And five, institutional weaknesses that made scaling up with the desired speed problematic. All these issues together created a peculiar dialectic of centralizing the decentralization process. By 2013, the NRHM had become yet another vertical programme. In other words, as a researcher opined, 'the NRHM was strong on the macro aspects but weak in its micro'.

The Birth of the NRHM (2005): Unfolding of the Policy

The initial correspondence in September 2004 between the prime minister and the health minister laid down the broad policy contours within which the NRHM was to be formulated. The focus had to be on improving service delivery in the rural areas of the laggard states and implementation was to be within the framework of the Panchayati Raj Institutions (PRIs) in order to facilitate the convergence of sectors that directly impact health, such as safe drinking water, sanitation, and nutrition. For scaling up the population-stabilization programmes in the 150 high-fertility districts, partnerships with private providers were to be forged and a cadre of community-level health workers be instituted.

The focus on the poorly performing states was, in reality, in line with the ongoing policy of the health ministry. In 2000, the five states of Bihar, Madhya Pradesh, Rajasthan, Uttar Pradesh, and Odisha—states with high population growth and poor health indicators—had already been identified as Empowered Action Group (EAG) states, enabling preferential attention to addressing their special needs, particularly under the family-planning rubric. In view of this, the health minister sought the inclusion of other 'backward' states, increasing the number to 17 states and 210 districts for fast-track attention under the mission. Population stabilization was to be considered within the framework of overall primary healthcare and delivery of RCH services, co-opting private providers 'as it is not feasible for the public health system in these states to make rapid progress [since they are] beset with governance and manpower issues'.[7] However, the two issues of decentralization and inclusion of the PRIs for inter-sectoral convergence as envisaged by the prime minister were not mentioned.

The NCMP resolution and these letters, when read together, reflect either a limited vision and political understanding of the issues plaguing the health sector or an unwillingness to look beyond the incremental for want of resources or capacity. But even within such a limited perspective, the inherent tension between the PMO and the ministry was palpable. While the PMO focused on changing the fundamentals of governance—differential planning, decentralization, inter-sectoral convergence—the ministry saw this renewed focus on health as an opportunity to intensify the implementation of several initiatives such as institutional deliveries and family planning without necessarily tinkering with the existing structure.

It was only after several rounds of discussions that the ministry[8] included in its outline of the strategy inter-sectoral convergence, integration of vertical programmes under the mission, strengthening of public health infrastructure by involving PR institutions, constitution of hospital committees with powers to levy user fees, creation of a cadre of CHWs, and involvement of private sector in health delivery and the rest. 'RHM [NRHM] was an effort to change the very structure and the methodology of functioning of the health sector in the near future.' Such a transformation was to be achieved by states taking full ownership of the mission.

Prasanna Hota, the secretary of family welfare, became central to this initiative by default. Rural primary healthcare fell under the ambit of the family welfare department, while the health department was responsible for disease-control programmes, hospital services, medical and nursing education, drugs and international health, among others. This dichotomy was the outcome of the decision in 1989 to constitute the family welfare department as a full-fledged department.

Verticalization into two departments created an institutional mess. While at the national level, the Department of Family Welfare was responsible for rural primary healthcare,[9] at the state level it was the director of health services who controlled the system in terms of siting facilities, HR recruitment, deployment, and disciplinary powers and was aligned to the health department at the centre due to the disease-control programmes. Such a split isolated family welfare as a department with no teeth and a mismatch between responsibility and authority.

Contextually, making the Department of Family Welfare as the main instrument of change for revamping the rural primary health system was flawed and not unexpectedly, the initial response was narrow, tentative, and disappointing. Caught in the traditional departmental mindsets, the political mandate to set right a deteriorating rural healthcare system was interpreted as a revved-up version of the RCH II that had been prepared for World Bank funding and was readily available.[10]

But the idea was not to implement the RCH II. Civil society would not be appeased by a World Bank project and approached Gopalakrishnan, the joint secretary in the PMO, to broaden the agenda from a narrow donor-led RCH and family-planning scheme to a broader mandate of revamping the rural health delivery system. Dr Antia, Dr Imrana, Abhay Shukla, and Mira Shiva[11] were among those who expressed reservations against the 'donor control' of the ministry, exercised through its funding of the various vertical programmes. Dr Antia was the most vocal among the civil society members in his assertions for a primary healthcare system that was accountable to the people it was meant to serve. He argued for a system where women would be empowered to take care of their own health by 'demystifying' and 'simplifying' healthcare in a language they understood.

Gopalakrishnan, as secretary to the chief minister of Madhya Pradesh, had earlier invited Dr Antia to design a community health worker programme called Jana Swasthya Rakshak (JSR) for Madhya Pradesh.[12] Both firmly believed in decentralizing and empowering PRIs to play their constitutional role in providing healthcare to people. They believed in the power of community-based initiatives and were against a large central government and private sector.

Several rounds of meetings of civil society members were held.[13] From this followed the push for creating operational mechanisms for community participation in decision-making and a decentralized approach based on public health system. Dr Antia also had a one-to-one meeting with the prime minister on these issues.[14]

Firm on its resolve, the civil society wanted nothing short of an overhauled, comprehensive primary healthcare system as defined in the Alma-Ata Declaration of 1978. Driven by the fire of 'Health for All', decentralization and community activism were to be the foundational principles to guide the NRHM process. In this power struggle, Gopalakrishnan emerged as the focal point for Dr Antia and his group to pressurize the ministry to back these initiatives. In this process, the idea of a whole new policy mix called the NRHM[15] was born.

Defining the NRHM

In January 2005, the cabinet accorded its 'in-principle' approval for a set of broad ideas. Further deliberations were required to give form and shape to what was a hazy vision. No one actually knew what to make of the mandate, but all were aware of the significance of the moment. On 10 February 2005, a formal consultation was called for at the Ashok Hotel in New Delhi. By the same evening, nine task forces were constituted to come up with a concrete framework.

The task forces provided scope for a wider debate on what the NRHM should include. In addition to the formal consultations, individuals and scattered groups of people continued to engage on a one-to-one basis with the ministry officials. The JSA[16] emerged as a key player in influencing and defining the contours of the future policy.

The prime minister formally launched the NRHM on 20 April 2005. In the meanwhile, the process of regional consultations had already begun. And in this flurry of activity, the health secretary who dealt with disease-control programmes was kept out, reflecting the acute problem of departmentalism, the conditioning of policymakers equating the RCH with primary healthcare, and the implication such exclusion during the early years had on the ability to integrate the programmes that were being implemented in vertical silos.

While the beleaguered ministry, with no time to study, deliberate, or analyse, sought to take full advantage of the already available strategies and systems, the NRHM document continued to be commented upon at diverse fora.

Only Advise

The Planning Commission and the Department of Finance dismissed the NRHM document as half-baked, with no goals or objectives linked to inputs, no timelines for implementation plans and outputs, and no delineation of anticipated impacts at the end of the Tenth Plan.

In the meanwhile, the NAC was given a presentation by the health ministry on 30 September 2005. The comments of the NAC members were wide and sweeping: '... architecture be more realistically and clearly defined particularly under Universal Health Care, infrastructure improvements, risk pooling, integrated and locally accountable service delivery mechanisms....'[17] Some members felt that the NRHM needed a proper 'management structure to deliver on goals with implementation strategies leading to definite outcomes arrived at in a realistic manner'.[18] Jairam Ramesh, a Congress leader and later a cabinet minister, wanted to know what would actually be achieved on the ground that a common man could see. 'What new services will be available and what changes will be introduced? Will the timings of the PHC be changed?' he asked. The NAC demanded nothing short of a 'specific road map, time-bound and with quantifiable targets and a concrete action plan to strengthen community-based public health system to go towards NHS of acceptable standards and universal coverage'. They wanted the NRHM to consider

> the need to create a political and a public climate for NRHM; making ASHA accountable to the Gram Sabha and training a number of women, so selection can be from among them; and a greater clarity on how the convergence between drinking water, sanitation, nutrition and HIV would be realized on the ground and modalities for formulating district and village plans with local bodies.

On 3 January 2006, a task force under the chairmanship of the prime minister was constituted to monitor and review every quarter the implementation of the NRHM programmes. Three non-officials were nominated to this task force: Jayaprakash Narayan, a former civil servant who is now leading an NGO and was a member of the NAC; Imrana Qadeer, professor of community health from JNU; and Dr Arole, a renowned public health activist from Maharashtra. Dr Arole was nominated to represent civil society.

The first meeting of the task force was held on 4 April 2006. In this meeting, members raised several pertinent issues and questions. For example, Montek Singh Ahluwalia, the then deputy chairman of the Planning Commission, asked about the role of ASHAs and whether they were facilitators or providers and also whether paramedicalization was being proposed to tackle neonatal mortality. Narayan called for wide-ranging institutional reforms such as constituting a district health authority to attend to the issues pertaining to infrastructure and manpower and ensure convergence, appointing an ombudsman, introducing risk pooling for service-based financing, accreditation and training of registered medical practitioners (RMPs), and so on—in other words, a structural reconstruction of the health system rather than incremental changes. Both Dr Arole and Dr Imrana suggested paramedicalizing primary care to ensure access to vulnerable groups.[19]

Thus, while the discussions were animated and rich in content, disappointingly enough, only three decisions were minuted: a) preparation of plans by states for their respective districts within the next six months, b) providing a time frame of activities that would be visible by 2009 (that is, before the next election), and c) putting in place a health insurance programme in consultation with the Department of Insurance and Financial Services. These were no doubt important process issues but did not reflect any action points emerging from the discussions that had called for a process of reforming the financing and delivery of healthcare in rural areas.

All these perspectives were profoundly important but fraught with huge policy implications cutting across sectors, with choices and decisions on resource allocations falling within the realm of political economy over which the ministry had little control. For example, the concept of decentralization and Panchayati Raj that the PMO and the NAC kept mentioning, was a complex political issue that had to be resolved through consensus-building by the political system as both Panchayati Raj and the delivery of health services were constitutionally within the purview of the state governments. Chief ministers of most states resisted any delegation of functions, functionaries, or funds to the elected members at the district and village levels. Several states complained that the panchayat members were only interested in the money rather than health outcomes, often distorting priorities. There were also fundamental contradictions between a Panchayati Raj system that consolidates the existing power structures and status quo in the villages and the civil society and women's groups that questioned their authority and demanded equality. This single issue merited a high-level engagement. Instead they were papered over without looking into how a minister or secretary in Delhi can engineer consensus on this sensitive matter of sharing power.

The expansion of the health agenda was going far beyond the scope of the NCMP, the original understanding between the prime minister and the health minister, and what the harassed ministry with its limited capacities was being asked to deliver, that too within an unrealistic time frame of five years. No one at any level paid attention to the ministry's institutional abilities to implement the ideas. Reinventing and cleaning up a system that was full of cobwebs due to decades of neglect was not easy, particularly when, constitutionally, issues like primary care, inter-sectoral coordination, and decentralization to PR bodies, among other things, were squarely within the state domain. The officials in the ministry were at the end of their tether as grand ideas and rhetoric were no substitutes for a sound policy based on a thorough understanding of evidence, institutional capacity, and the political implications thereof. But there was little support from any quarter. Instead, every day the officials were made to feel inadequate and incompetent. There was no effort by the PMO, the NAC, the Planning Commission, or the prime minister's task force to leverage their power to mobilize the funds the sector desperately needed. Nor did the political management at the national and state levels try to push the implementation of the NRHM initiatives. Vital issues were not discussed and doubts could not be raised, since any such attempt would immediately invite condemnation as bureaucratic resistance and an unwillingness to change.

Framework of Action

The immediate task of the NRHM team was to come up with the draft framework of action, laying down the objectives, mission goals, and the action plan for the next five years. Hectic backroom discussions with civil society and academics set in motion a series of consultations of a span and intensity the ministry had never witnessed before. Consequently, different agendas and formulations cropped up and the framework went through several iterations. Notwithstanding the scissoring approach of cut-and-paste, the framework document laid down a progressive agenda of reform.

Never discussed formally with the actual stakeholders like the state- and district-level officials, researchers and academicians, professional organizations, or village communities, the document was one big mass of ideas that often ran contrary to each other. It appeared more as one called it: an 'eclectic document running all over the place'.[20] The clear structuring of concept, aims, objectives, implementation design, and architecture, as we know them now, took time and further deliberations at Delhi. A few civil society representatives who had access to ministry officials actively participated in incorporating their ideas. The revised framework was also critiqued and seen as an amalgamation of inputs extraordinarily idealistic and simplistic which Sundararaman felt had 'no order, no consistency, absurd targets, idealistic/romanticized stuff'.

Such criticism was considered 'unfair' since the framework was not expected to be any more than a charter because the NRHM was not visualized as a project. The timelines and targets were inserted in the framework only to 'appease the rigidly reductionist thought process in the Planning Commission ... that wanted to see a return on investment....'[21]

The framework document sought to articulate the vision and strategies centred around decentralization, communitization, flexible funding, capacity-building, and skill augmentation.

It reworked the exclusive focus on RCH to rebuilding primary healthcare and obtained the cabinet's approval in July 2006. As Sundararaman said, 'Basically everyone was exhausted and so no one really read the framework document ... resulting in all kinds of things being included in.'[22] Two days before demitting office, Hota signed off on scaled-up JSY and ASHA initiatives. With this the first tumultuous phase of the NRHM came to a close, but not without generating heat.

The release of the framework document invited critical reviews in a spate of articles published by several academicians.[23] The harshest critic of the proposed strategy was the public health expert Debabir Banerjee who simply dismissed the entire effort recalling Romesh Thapar's famous phrase '*babu log* playing government government'.[24] He was scathing in his criticism of the NRHM for being ahistorical and simplifying complex matters. Other civil society members were clearly dismayed at the manner in which the ASHA model had been designed and what they considered to be 'stealthy attempts' at privatization.

Role of Civil Society

The civil society played a profound role in setting the tone and direction of the NRHM. They helped contextualize the NRHM within the broader socio-economic framework and move towards socialized medicine—a clear departure from the 'donor-supported' approach that tended to underplay the social aspects of health and accord a disproportionate reliance to technological fixes. Yet despite the repeated mention[25] of the fact that no country had ever achieved health transition without fixing the fundamentals such as access to water, sanitation, and nutrition, these issues were not given any importance. Instead, the NRHM took a departmental approach, reducing the role of social determinants to a schematic line of 'inter-sectoral convergence' without ensuring commensurate investments in the related departments—human, institutional, or financial. Convergence requires detailed attention to align vertically structured institutional arrangements that are typically fraught with power dynamics of control and patronage. In other words, convergence is politics, and perhaps that is why the ministry overlooked it, since it lacked the convening power and the institutional capacity to negotiate with the other departments.

In expanding the boundaries of the debate, civil society also sought to define the role of the modern state as the guarantor of certain entitlements to all its citizens. The state's role was critical, especially in the context of an assertive neo-liberal ideology that tended to minimize it and promote privatization directly or through PPP. The PPP route was increasingly being seen as a euphemism for strengthening private space in the public arena paid for and supported by the state.

In a series of emails addressed to the ministry officials during November 2005 to February 2006, Abhay Shukla of the Centre for Enquiry into Health and Allied Themes (CEHAT)—a Mumbai-based NGO—who is also an active member of the JSA drew attention to the dangers of the two 'models of restructuring' being attempted together. One model promoted market principles of governance through PPPs and making public hospitals autonomous entities in order to empower them to levy user fees, contract out services, and share resources with the private sector.

The second model consisted of strengthening the public health system that is anchored in the community and accountable to it within a framework of health rights, devolution of powers, and decentralization of decision-making. Shukla argued that the current public health system is essentially status quoist with a tendency to control and not innovate or improve. Therefore, any restructuring outwards to the private sector or downwards to the community would imply shifting power to a new set of forces 'with different interests and goals and methods of functioning'.[26] He warned that an eclectic mix may favour semi-privatization, as it is in line with the prevailing ideology of 'market fundamentalism as the solution for all problems but if unthinkingly combined ... it will be the privatization portion (that) will be implemented rather than the community one'. This was prophetic as with budget cuts from 2014 onwards, it is the communitization aspects of the NRHM programme that have been effected.

These were important concerns that deserved consultations with experts and meetings at the highest political and administrative levels. The two-legged policy of the government as envisioned in the framework was simply unfeasible and opportunistic. Unable or unwilling to take on the private sector and afraid to let go of the public sector, a policy of allowing both to flourish in the same space without defining the roles and demarcating the boundaries was bound to fail. The framers of the NRHM seemed unconcerned that an unregulated and unaccountable private sector and a 'strengthened' public sector cannot coexist within the present ecosystem.[27] The insinuations of the trend towards the commodification of medical and nursing education by corrupt regulatory bodies was never raised either. This was largely on account of a poor understanding of the dynamics of the health system rather than any preconceived ideological moorings.

Unable or unwilling to understand the import and centrality of these issues,[28] Shukla's concerns never crossed the desk of the joint secretary. Civil society, too, did not pursue these concerns. It was perhaps unwilling to acknowledge the existence of a private sector, however small, for fear that it may compromise their ideology of the public sector being the only provider of health services. Ignoring the evidence of the growing presence of the private sector in the NCMH report, the refusal to deal with the issue was a serious policy omission as it amounted to the implicit acceptance of the default position of the private sector. The issue of the private sector was never raised again until the Twelfth Five Year Plan.

By lumping the whole spectrum of the private sector that ranged from solo practitioners, missionary and not-for-profit hospitals, to for-profit and corporate hospitals as 'greedy', an opportunity was lost in not harnessing and protecting the not-for-profit sector, faith-based organizations, and other charity hospitals that were serving the poor in remote areas at a very low cost while providing good-quality care. In a way, the government mortgaged its policy to the dominant views of the civil society representatives who had access to its corridors.

However, it was also not as if the JSA knew how to resolve all the contradictions that plagued the health sector at every level—be they between the private and public sectors, community and Panchayati Raj, or maintaining the balance between integrated primary care while not losing focus on the disease-control programmes, and so on. It raised important issues but rarely provided solutions. It charged that the NRHM was displaying notions of privatization and alleged that while the need for a comprehensive public health system had been recognized, the 'response is fragmented and lacks an integrated, health systems approach'. Its impact seemed to have been limited even though its members 'were located in all the core committees and participated in all the politics'.[29]

By the end of 2006, having failed to get an unambiguous policy statement on the primacy of the public health sector, civil society got embroiled in intense internal debates regarding its position vis-à-vis the government. These debates proved to be divisive and broke up civil society into three groups: a) one consisting of people who felt that the government was insincere about improving the health and well-being of people, b) the other that saw no harm in collaborating with the government to achieve a pro-people agenda, and c) the third that sought to maintain its neutrality and watchdog role while recognizing the value of engaging with the government and 'influencing' policy so as to 'make it work in a pro-people direction'. Accordingly, the JSA directed its constituent organizations to critically 'engage with the Mission to influence it at local, State and National levels to shape and influence the Mission activities'. It was interested in being involved with a wide scope of issues ranging from ensuring additional domestic funding, better design and implementation, universal access to free healthcare to strengthening comprehensive primary healthcare, developing structural mechanisms for the involvement of community members, beneficiaries, and local organizations in the planning and monitoring of health activities, and so on.

Glossing over key policy issues related to the role of the private and the NGO sectors in the design of the health delivery system was a serious omission. Reversing the current trend towards privatization needed strong political leadership as in the unregulated environment, the tentacles of private sector had grown strong and deep. Civil society alone had the ability to make the political system accountable. Instead, it got embroiled in the schematic approach of programme formulation at the joint-secretary level. Frustrated, many thought leaders withdrew and, sadly enough, fell silent.

Civil society's commitment to the notion of no one being denied healthcare for want of means is laudable. But its lack of preparedness and incapacity to provide leadership became evident. Instead of staying firm as a pressure group to force the government to stay the course on the agenda charted out, civil society representatives were co-opted and reduced to becoming members of the various policy advisory committees that the government established from time to time—NAC, MSG, Empowered Programme Committee (EPC), ASHA Mentoring Group (AMG), NHSRC, Advisory Group on Community Action (AGCA), CCHFW, and so on. The government's failure to broadbase participation meant that many of the same people were nominated to several of these committees. The government was thus able to provide a veneer of inclusivity but it resulted in the accompanying loss of diverse opinions and leadership driving policy towards greater participation and activism. This lacuna was felt acutely since political support for pro-poor policies for health was strong but the health bureaucracy at the implementation levels lacked both confidence and the technical ability to translate the political vision to implementable policies. By 2009, civil society had lost the plot. Several articles critiquing the NRHM were published.[30] A historic opportunity to change policy was allowed to go by but the high-level involvement of civil society did shape the NRHM in those early years, particularly on issues related to communitization.

Institutional Innovation

Within a year of the launch in 2005, the ministry established the mission office to design, implement, and monitor the NRHM framework document. The governance structure consisted of the MSG chaired by the health minister, ministers of other departments that impacted health, the member of the Planning Commission in charge of health, and some civil society representatives. In 2007, the MSG was empowered and provided with flexibility and autonomy for speedier decision-making and quicker implementation. An economic steering committee (ESC) headed by the health secretary was constituted to screen the proposals before they were submitted to the MSG. Similar structures were also to be established in all the states—with the chief ministers chairing the state missions.

A critical omission at this stage was to not give the mission an institutional structure like NACO's. Instead, it was kept within the ministry hierarchy by adding an additional secretary, a joint secretary, and some youngsters taken as consultants. Unlike NACO, no attempt was made to build internal capacity within the ministry, particularly for nontraditional areas like communitization or district-level planning.

The first additional secretary and mission director (2005–6) was Jalaja Sinha who was there for a year and worked under the shadow of the secretary who was the man at the wheel. As Jalaja noted, '[I]t was Hota who thought of the JSY and PMU [Programme Management Unit] and his leadership was solid over the concepts of creating a society mechanism, providing for flexi funds etc. and drove the system .... He did the work of the Mission Director as well....'[31]

In early 2007, Girish Chaturvedi took over as the MD of the NRHM. Chaturvedi had earlier worked as the health secretary in Uttar Pradesh and was sympathetic to the idea of providing states the liberty to develop plans as per their needs. Thus the dominant focus was on decentralization in both priority-setting and implementation. Plans were to be formulated by the states and PIPs were only to be notionally screened and approved by the centre, 'more for the purpose of fixing the budget and releasing funds', according to Chaturvedi.

Such freedom to states to set their own priorities gave rise to a diversity of options and a measure of innovation. Kerala from the beginning focused on issues related to old age and non-communicable diseases[32] while Bihar, Madhya Pradesh, and other backward states focused on building up their broken-down rural health system. However, during this period, two important ideas could not take root though the time was ripe: one, the integration of disease-control programmes that were being implemented as stand-alone vertical programmes into the NRHM framework; and two, the National Urban Health Mission (NUHM). Despite efforts to at least converge common components such as procurement, IEC, training, and so on, the integration of vertical programmes did not materialize due to the initial exclusion of concerned officials from the dialogue in the designing of the NRHM. Apprehensive of disruptions that might arise with the tinkering of well-established processes and national guidelines and alarmed at the eclectic manner of the functioning of the NRHM, the technical heads refused to part with what they felt was 'under control'. The urban health mission got held up due to bureaucratic indifference. Girish rued, '[T]he moment was gone and NUHM has been put on the back burner. It's important to seize the moments and opportunities when they come.' He was right as due to the shortage of funds for the NRHM initiatives the NUHM could find mention only in the Twelfth Plan. Conflicts over open-source technology could also not be resolved affecting the building of a solid information-and-monitoring system. Though the software was ready, its implementation was weak and, to this day, it continues to be one of the unfinished tasks.

National Health Systems Resource Centre (NHSRC)

Since the ministry had limited technical expertise to help design, formulate, and implement the various initiatives, a proposal was mooted to establish the NHSRC to help provide technical backup. Jalaja Sinha, as the MD of the NRHM, wanted to recruit an IAS officer in order to ensure better coordination with the ministry. Fearing the emergence of another power centre, the ministry appointed Dr Sundararaman, a medical doctor-cum-activist from the JSA, as the director of the NHSRC. A professor of medicine from JIPMER, Sundar, as the director of the State Health Systems Resource Centre (SHSRC) in Chhattisgarh, had been associated with the implementation of the Mitanin programme. This association had enabled him to gain experience of working with bureaucracies—both technical and administrative. That experience stood him in good stead in navigating the corridors of Nirman Bhawan and building up the NHSRC as the technical arm of the NRHM.

Registered as a society on 8 December 2006, the NHSRC was located within the premises of the National Institute of Health and Family Welfare (NIHFW). Unlike the SHSRC[33] in Chhattisgarh that focused exclusively on building the CHW programme in the first five years, the NHSRC was provided a wider mandate. It was handling all aspects of policy formulation and programme implementation, ranging from issues related to the NABH and ISO certification of district hospitals, recruiting and training health personnel, to developing guidelines and monitoring the implementation of the ASHA programme. It developed its own monitoring and data management systems through Common Review missions (CRMs), field visits, and operational research. All states were also urged to establish SHSRCs for which a seed funding of Rs 10 million was allocated. This was, however, not followed up and so, by the end of 2012, only a few states had SHSRCs.

The decrease in the number of public health specialists in the ministry at the national level and in state governments on account of attrition, non-recruitment, and disbanding of public health cadres adversely affected the availability of technical expertise within the ministry and at the implementation levels. Poor funding of public health institutions like the NIHFW at the national level and SIHFWs at the state level also consequently led to their decline. The new institutional mechanisms like the NHSRC and the SHSRC dealt a further blow to the already weak and struggling NIHFW/SIHFWs. The fact that these new institutions were evolving as parallel bodies impeded the growth of public sector capacity but that was not seen as a contradiction. To be fair, civil society did raise concerns. Thelma Narayan commented that 'the concept of creating SHSRCs was questioned as it would have been more prudent to strengthen the SIHFWs and the Departments of Health'.[34] The proposed SHSRCs were to be like the TSUs established by NACO to lend support to SACS in the implementation of the TI strategy. But the difference was that NACO had also alongside strengthened the SACS with manpower. But in the case of the NRHM, strengthening of the directorates was ignored and instead the SHSRCs were established to 'implement' the mission's activities.

As in other cases, the government and the NHSRC brushed these concerns aside and went ahead to promote these autonomous bodies. It is unclear why civil society made only a token objection to the creation of these autonomous bodies as it seemed to be an admission of the impossibility of reforming the public sector. Or was it that civil society considered itself to be the rightful representative of the people, treating the public sector and the people's sector as synonymous? Or was the objection muted only because the NHSRC, for example, was headed by one of its own? In other words, how would they have reacted if the government had appointed a private-sector IIM management executive instead or an ex-McKinsey executive as the head of NHSRC?

Establishing the NHSRC was an innovative idea, filling a long-felt need for an administrative mechanism to induct expertise to cope with the emerging challenges. Flexibility and autonomy enabled the NHSRC to appoint highly qualified and competent people to provide the NRHM with the required technical support. Operational autonomy allowed it to do some commendable work through data analysis and planning, lending clarity to the programme and helping to push the states to design their programmes and implement them. But over the years, while the dependence on the NHSRC grew, the thinking within the ministry began to wane. This was not a good development.

Policymaking requires policymakers to have their feet and ears to the ground with the capacity to absorb and internalize the various sources of information independently. In other words, to pass an examination, it does not help if the neighbour's son studies hard.[35] One way of overcoming this problem could have been establishing a division within the ministry for communitization or reform of primary care and have the NHSRC experts work directly in the ministry. This would have helped develop institutional capacity and memory, ownership and legitimacy, while the NHSRC could have continued to work on training, data monitoring and analysis, operational research, and innovation.

Some also contend that a greater impact might have been achieved if the NHSRC had been more focused on certain specific issues related to the revamping of the architectural design of the delivery system rather than on the broad mandate it was given.

The delivery systems were in a chaotic state and had no standardization. Each state needed to be stimulated to think of its delivery system based on its data and socio-economic context. Revamping it meant collection of data, analysis, and long-drawn negotiations that ministries at the state levels and in the central government typically never had the time to do. Such revamping would also have required community consultations and embedding the system within the community. Communitization and oversight of facilities by civil society as well as social auditing for enhancing accountability were areas most likely to be sabotaged by the system and were also those that required an enormous amount of financial and human resources to build capacity. Instead, the NHSRC developed a life of its own, handling an amazing array of subjects and blurred lines of accountability: communitization, technology assessment, recruiting and training personnel, development of standard guidelines and treatment protocols, quality assurance, infrastructure development, health financing, monitoring—each a complex and highly problematic area. It ended up weakening both the NIHFW as well as the ministry's policymaking ability. In fact, what happened was exactly what was feared in the context of an IAS officer heading the NHSRC. It became a parallel body 'influencing' the strategy. Tarun Seem strongly felt that by 'shifting the centre of technical expertise in program implementation, monitoring/evaluation matters out of the ministry to a self-empowered entity that recruited young consultants to do what the ministry should have learnt to do' not only did the quality and sustainability of the programme get hampered but the NHSRC as a concept also suffered.'[36]

Ambiguity still dogs the NHSRC with questions about its role and accountability. Is it a government think tank? A TSU to scale up implementation of specific priority areas of government policy through mentoring and close supervision to provide the critical feedback loops to the government? Or a handyman?[37] The SHSRC's position is equally confusing.

At the state level, the institutional design of the NRHM also created confusion. Imposing a mission director for the NRHM supported by an SHSRC, on the existing directorates of health and family welfare, generated interpersonal tensions that got resolved in some states but not in others, depending on the administrative leadership. In Tamil Nadu, the model worked well due to the seniority of the MD of the NRHM, who was also the former health secretary. So though the design consisted of the MD having control of the money and the director of health services governing the organization, Tamil Nadu reconciled the situation on the platform of shared responsibility. In Andhra Pradesh, however, there was a constant tussle between the MD and the commissioner of health and family welfare over the directorate of health, resulting in it being made accountable to the MD as well as the commissioner. In fact, such parallel structures all along the line down to the community level made the very goals of horizontal integration of vertically driven programmes deeply problematic.

Principles of the NRHM

The edifice of the NRHM was constructed on some basic principles. These principles unfolded into various programmes and instruments of action that highlighted the serious flaws plaguing the public health system. These gaps in the system such as excessive centralization of funding and policy formulation, the near absence of stakeholder involvement, weak management, dysfunctional institutional structures, infrastructure gaps, and poor monitoring had to be addressed urgently.

The following five principles defined the main architectural features of the NRHM that covered both the supply and demand side as discussed further.

Supply Side

Flexible Financing

Though healthcare service delivery is a state responsibility, yet due to serious fiscal problems, states depended upon central assistance that provided grants in cash and kind in the form of drugs, supplies, and equipment. This dependence gave the authority to the centre to fix targets, guidelines, and treatment protocols. Such top-driven and prescriptive systems left little room for the states to plan in accordance with their priorities or local conditions and cultural contexts.

Under the NRHM, the top-down model was to be reversed by providing flexibility to the states to plan in accordance with their needs. Implicit in this was the concept of decentralization that meant undertaking an elaborate process of planning upwards from the household/village level to block, district, and state level. To address the local needs arising from this new bottom-up plan, the NRHM budgets were unbundled into four pools: the RCH flexi pool, the NRHM flexi pool, polio pulse immunization, and disease-control programmes. Under each flexi pool, the ministry listed the components that were eligible for central assistance. For example, under the NRHM flexi pool, the states could utilize up to 33 per cent of the pool amount (25 per cent in non-high-focus states) to repair, refurbish, or construct health facilities, while the remaining amount could be utilized for providing incentives to the community workers, contracting human resources, engaging emergency transportation, and so on. Under the RCH pool, states were to ensure institutional deliveries, universal immunization, adolescent health, and cash incentives for institutional deliveries along with other smaller programmes like school health. The 18 high-focus states were eligible to receive 1.3 times more funding than the non-high-focus ones.

A systemic and landmark correction introduced in the NRHM was routing central assistance to states not through the states' finance departments but through a registered society established at the state and district levels. The concept of state and district societies was first piloted in the early 1990s under the Danish International Development Agency (DANIDA)-assisted project in Karnataka for the blindness control programme. The quicker absorption of funds and a higher level of performance led to its adoption on a national level under the World Bank-assisted National Programme for Control of Blindness (NPCB) launched in 1995. The 'society route', as it was referred to, soon became a standard norm for the World Bank-assisted projects, be it for strengthening the health system, control of malaria, or TB or HIV/AIDS programmes. Disease-specific societies with similar memberships and chaired by district collectors at the district level were constituted, leading to avoidable duplication and creating an anomalous position. Consequently in 2000, an attempt was made to rectify the situation by integrating them all into one health society but with no success. It was only under the NRHM that all these societies were brought under the ambit of the state and district health societies.

Implementation of primary healthcare under different disease-control programmes had resulted not only in fragmenting service delivery but also in substantial duplication of personnel and equipment, besides impairing integrated thinking and holistic care. For example, the ANM, while attending to a pregnant woman, also examines her for HIV or malaria. The vehicle to bring in an integrated approach was the State Health Society. This, then, was the rationale for the unbundling of funding and the provisioning of flexibility for states to plan in accordance with their disease and epidemiological profile.

True to intent, the states were asked to prepare their own plans. No targets or outcomes were strictly indicated. Nor any guidelines. In 2005, the states were provided funds for three to four selected activities, namely ASHA, CHC upgradation, and district planning. Consultants were sent to the states to help them prepare the plans.

The concept of PIP emerged in 2006. It was to be a five-year plan—a collation of district health action plans. This was to be prepared by compiling Panchayati-level plans that consisted of village-level plans based on household surveys. This idea was critiqued by civil society but a small experiment of participatory appraisal report (PAR) tried out in 'Karnataka and Rajasthan working with the poorest communities became the prototype. There was no ability or will to scale up such a process either.'[38] The idea of a long-term, household-based PIP was, however, to enable drawing up a list of interventions required, out of which some would be selected on the basis of priority and availability of funds.

The approach of the assessment of a household's needs as the basis for future planning was pure imagination. Planning depends on the availability of epidemiological information, longitudinal data, and trained people with the ability to triangulate information sourced from multiple data sets so as to strategize the interventions. For example, while information can be obtained about the number of children who need to be immunized—a data that is readily available—a one-time household survey cannot predict the number of children who may suffer from diarrhoea. But data on the quality of water being consumed and past data on the occurrence of diarrhoea could help model probabilities. Household-survey approaches work in sectors like education or water supply as the population to be served and the intervention to be made are stable and measurable. Basically, scaling this up would require substantial resources, human and financial, besides time for the process.

PIPs became wish-lists and only '3 percent of the PIP was approved since that was all that could be afforded out of the envelope available'.[39] As the idea slackened, consultants were once again sent off to the states to prepare annual plans. By 2009, the plans began morphing into 300-page documents. The two crucial months of December and January were taken up to prepare the annual plans for the next year's allocation of funds. These were also the months that form the peak period for implementing and grounding the activities approved in the current plan.

By 2009–10, the procedure for approval of state plans for release of funds evolved into a two-step process. The first step was the submission of the annual PIP by the state to the National Programme Coordination Committee (NPCC). The concerned divisions would then vet the relevant chapters and after incorporating their comments, the final plan would be submitted. The second step led to a meeting in Delhi followed by processing the agreed plan for approval and the issuance of the record of proceedings (RoP) based on which funds would be released. During the first two years, the secretary chaired the final discussions but since 2007, the mission director has chaired the meetings. The gradual disassociation of the secretary with the NRHM planning process inhibited the NRHM from getting out of the squared frame of the 'RCH agenda' into the health system paradigm it was meant to be. The states lost out on the guidance and broader perspective on issues related to human resources or drugs that were vital for the success of the NRHM but did not fall under the purview of its MD.

Up until 2010, the process adopted for the release of grants to states had three problems:

a. The RoP was not a monitorable instrument. It was neither possible to establish the linkage between the financial sanctions and actual achievements nor to detect deviations, if any. It was felt that providing an expected output for a given allocation was an infringement on the state's authority to determine its own goals and targets. However, in the absence of indicating outputs, it was impossible to get a sense of what was being achieved with the expenditures being incurred.

b. The planning process was centralized with consultants preparing the state plans, while the district officials were practically unaware of the plans and what was expected of them. Even today, say in Andhra Pradesh, district plans are a mechanistic and centralized exercise. A CMO says, 'We only fill up the prescribed columns with our data and send.'[40] This resonated Ashtekar's view that 'the district health plans were often a fill in the blanks for the local officer or a consultant. There was and is no scope to innovate local resource use or lateral thinking.'[41] Essentially, asking for district plans in the absence of any district-level data and training the district-level teams on data analysis was the equivalent of putting the cart before the horse.

c. The principle of flexibility was notional. The programme's divisions were bound by national targets already approved by the Planning Commission. For example, if a malaria-ridden state like Odisha desired to scale up focus towards reducing mortality and morbidity due to malaria and invest on procuring long-lasting impregnated bed nets by shifting allocations from other schemes—for example, the JSY, the school health programme, or the adolescent programme—it could not do so as the malaria budgets would have already been fixed and the state-wise allocation of bed nets would have been pre-decided for procurement by the central government.[42] Over time, the NRHM flexi pool developed rigidities. Most of its funds were committed to infrastructure-building, untied funds at various levels, annual maintenance grants, and ASHA remuneration, taking a vertical devolution shape.

Monitoring Progress against Standards

Monitoring consisted of two components—setting standards, known as Indian Public Health Standards (IPHS) and undertaking district-level facility surveys at periodic intervals carried out by the IIPS, a Mumbai-based institute of the central government. Facility standards laid down the area of the physical facilities, equipments, drugs, and human resources that are to be made available. To provide for emergency care round the clock, PHCs were to be made operational 24×7. Setting such standards enabled monitoring the deployment of personnel and other inputs, facilitating need-based budgets, and monitoring outcomes.

The location of health facilities and deployment of manpower in them were based on the expert committees constituted for the purpose. Norms were, however, applicable only for the primary health facilities—the sub-centres, PHCs, and CHCs. Since the central government funded only the salaries of the ANMs and some positions such as that of laboratory technicians, it was left to the states to follow the norms. Consequently, there was no uniformity—neither in location nor in nomenclature. In some states the 30-bed facilities were called block PHCs, while in others they were called CHCs. Some states like Karnataka had a PHC for a population of 16,000 against the norm of 30,000. There were no guidelines for district hospitals on either the services that should be provided or the manpower that should be appointed. The situation was made worse with almost all states except Tamil Nadu dissolving public cadres which adversely impacted the delivery of services. Thus, for example, a state like Andhra Pradesh had, till recently, posts by grade of appointment rather than by specialty for posting doctors in district hospitals. The result was that a district hospital could technically have three gynaecologists and no anaesthetist or surgeon and yet fill in all the civil assistant posts sanctioned to it. Likewise, a PHC that requires an MBBS doctor might have a specialist appointed even though the district hospitals might have a dire need for one.

Reducing such confusion and standardizing the delivery system was a need. Accordingly, the central government came up with the IPHS. But the standards set were unrealistic and aspirational. They were not linked with the capacity of medical colleges or the market to produce the required manpower and skills. It was therefore not surprising that by the end of seven years of implementation, there were still more than 75 per cent vacancies of specialists in the CHCs and of over 30 per cent doctors in PHCs.

Similarly, the linkage between the demand being generated under the JSY in which cash incentives were provided to pregnant women delivering in public facilities and the public sector capacity to meet the consequential demand was uneven. So even as the JSY was vigorously promoted, there was no strategy to link investments to facilities that would have to take on the burden of the increased load. In leaving the states to make choices, the optimality of the investment was not assured. For example, Uttar Pradesh's inability to scale up institutional deliveries is on account of low-bed capacity in government hospitals. The central government also did not particularly encourage contracting and co-option of private sector entities due to lack of confidence in the capacity of the state to do so in a fair and transparent manner.[43]

A calculation of the financial implications of implementing the IPHS, based on the costing data of the DGHS, showed a requirement of over Rs 1 trillion—70 per cent of it in the high-focus states. Against that, during the seven-year period from 2005–12, a sum of Rs 62.24 billion was spent on refurbishment and construction of facilities. Had a process of quantifying the financial needs for fulfilling the IPHS standards been carried out, it would have become evident that the current architecture was expensive and unaffordable to build up within one or even two plan periods. Not unsurprisingly, data showed that at the end of 2011, only about 742 CHCs, 3,633 PHCs and 23,940 sub-centres respectively conformed to the IPHS.[44]

Given the restricted resources, prioritization of investments would have been one option and the other would have been to give states the autonomy to innovate on the architecture most suitable for them. After all, an explosion of technology and an improved network of roads and communication had led to shortening distances. The old four-tier structure was neither necessary nor optimal any more. But in the absence of any such discussion, states had an ad hoc approach to the refurbishing, repairing, or construction of facilities.

For ensuring outcomes, the supply of all inputs—building facility, skilled personnel, equipments, and drugs—had to be synchronized. Inadequate capital investment and the reluctance of many states to lay down rational HR policies meant that there was little coordination. In other words, in the absence of guidelines to ensure a balanced mix of inputs under different heads—refurbishment of the building, contracting and training of staff, supply of drugs, and release of budgets—the outputs were suboptimal. Some health facilities got overcrowded with pregnant women due to the non-availability of beds. Besides, in several facilities, deliveries were conducted not by doctors, even if present, but by nurses or untrained ANMs, often adversely affecting the quality of outcomes.

Subsequently, in 2010, guidelines under the RCH programme were developed by the NHSRC, linking infrastructure with outcomes. As per these guidelines, facilities that conducted deliveries were identified, enabling higher allocations and closer monitoring. Such an analysis reduced the number of facilities to be monitored for institutional deliveries to about 18,000 out of over 0.15 million facilities. Such data analysis provided immense potential to rework the functions and outcomes of different facilities, a task that needs to be undertaken without delay.

Improved Management through Building Capacity

The NRHM fulfilled a long-pending need for management staff in health facilities and district health offices. This was a positive development as up until then, facilities consisted of technical staff and the ubiquitous clerical staff that played havoc most of the time quoting rules and procedures that medical doctors had little knowledge of. All blocks and districts were provided with additional assistance of a qualified management graduate and a chartered accountant. MBAs were recruited as district programme officers (DPOs) and block programme officers (BPOs). They were responsible for coordinating and monitoring the timely provisioning of all the various inputs required. This measure undoubtedly strengthened the CMOs. However, in places where the CMO was 'too incompetent or uninterested, the DPO filled in the space and acquired power. And often corrupt too.'[45]

Though the intervention was systemic, its full potential could not be realized for want of clarity on their roles and responsibilities and because they were not integrated and institutionalized into the formal structure. Success, therefore, depended on each individual's personality and their ability to get along with the CMO and their staff.

Monitoring the implementation of the PIP technical support at the national and state levels was to be undertaken by the NHSRC/SHSRCs. For monitoring the ASHA programme, a facilitator at the rate of one for every 20 ASHAs was to be provided for at the block level and by the ASHA Monitoring Committee, consisting largely of NGOs at the national level.

Innovation in Human Resource Management

Recognizing the importance of human resources for achieving health goals, the NRHM introduced a set of initiatives. The existing vacancies against sanctioned posts were permitted to be filled up with contractual appointees to be paid for under the NRHM. At that time, this did seem to be an innovative government measure. Prior to the NRHM, there were neither resources available nor any policy permitting permanent posts to be filled with contractuals, a relaxation that came with the Sixth Pay Commission allowing contractual appointments to be made at market rates.

While contractual appointees helped achieve short-term objectives, it also disincentivized states from creating new posts and filling up existing vacancies as it suited the finance departments to keep a control on non-plan expenditures. Being contractual, attrition was high and little investment was made to train them either. Some states were also hesitant to appoint people on contracts, since past experience had shown that contractuals nearly always succeeded in getting favourable orders from the courts to make them permanent.

A major disincentive was the uncertainty of central funding even after the plan period. With no exercise undertaken to assess the financial implications on the state budget if all the contractual appointees were to be made permanent, the states were reluctant to fill up posts as required under the IPHS. Yet this policy of contractual appointments did serve well as within five years, the NRHM was able to recruit over 1.40 lakh personnel—a task that would have been impossible if the regular recruitment rules and procedures had been followed. But then every state today is facing huge HR problems requiring priority attention.

To address the shortage in the availability of critical skills, an innovative approach was to scale up the multi-skilling of doctors in scarce specialties, such as anaesthesia or neonatal resuscitation techniques. But this was a short-term solution. What was required was launching systemic reforms towards the paramedicalization of primary care that implied a series of policy initiatives such as creating posts and a cadre of nurse practitioners to reduce maternal mortality. Scandinavian countries and Turkey had clearly demonstrated the value of strengthening the nursing profession by delegating drug-prescription powers to nurses or allowing them to take up complex procedures independently. Both reduced maternal mortality and improved women's health. Or, utilizing the huge army of doctors trained in the Indian systems of medicine by providing them training in public health and posting them in peripheral institutions. Or to implement the task force's recommendation of formulating policy to eliminate or contain the RMPs that, de facto, continue to be the first point of contact in the villages. Yet these architectural corrections could not make a headway and continue to be left unaddressed despite the availability of substantial evidence of primary-level care being provided by a network of informal providers and chemists (mostly unqualified) supplying over-the-counter dispensation of medicines.

The NRHM did not also leverage its persuasive power with states to restore the public health discipline by pushing them to take the hard decisions of earmarking certain posts only for those with public-health training. In the absence of such prerequisites, deployment of doctors in most states continues to be arbitrary and unrelated to the skills required for the functions to be discharged, largely because of political considerations. An anaesthetist posted in a PHC with no operation theatre enables him to attend to private practice, even while those having all the facilities would be lying unused for want of personnel. Thus, despite expending huge resources, the absence of an HR policy spelling out recruitment, deployment, training, incentives for motivation, and, most importantly, a policy on the issue of dual practice (doing private practice while drawing full salary and emoluments as a government employee) became a huge obstacle in the realization of several goals.

Notwithstanding the above, the NRHM lost its main mission of revitalizing primary healthcare and bringing in architectural reforms in the delivery of services in rural areas midway. Instead it got overwhelmed with the single-minded focus on pushing institutional delivery to reduce maternal and infant mortality. These were no doubt critical goals that had to be achieved. But such preoccupation with just one set of interventions did affect the larger agenda of providing need-based healthcare to all citizens—an issue elaborated in Chapter 6.

Priority Focus on Reproductive and Child Health

In theory, the aim of the NRHM was to provide comprehensive primary care as per need and in an integrated manner. In practice, however, it could not shed its family-welfare orientation and for all practical purposes, it got preoccupied with achieving the RCH goals of MMR and IMR.[46] Two interventions—ASHA and JSY—dominated all sense of achievement.

Impact of the JSY on Institutional Deliveries

The JSY was essentially a continuation of the Maternity Benefit Scheme sanctioned in the mid-1980s under which every pregnant woman was entitled to receive Rs 500. It has been reformulated into an impressive cash-transfer scheme under which, in the focus states, pregnant women are paid Rs 1,400 upon delivering in a public facility and an additional Rs 600 for defraying transport costs. Its aim was to reduce financial barriers to accessing hospital care and also incentivize behaviour change towards institutional deliveries that was positioned as the main strategic intervention for reducing MMR.

While the concept at the macro level was sound, the problems emerged at the micro level, particularly in the implementation details. Universalizing the push for institutional deliveries and giving up the approach of identifying high-risk pregnancies with differential incentives for those with a higher vulnerability to death was a serious omission. For example, a review of the number of C-sections conducted in district hospitals of Uttar Pradesh showed that less than 1 per cent of the deliveries were C-section though the norm was that 15 per cent of all deliveries required caesarean operations.[47] There was little idea of what happened to the remaining 14 per cent.

Similar distortions emerged with the transport subsidy of Rs 600 for coming to the hospital. Again in Uttar Pradesh, perverse behaviour was observed with reports of pregnant women in labour being transported in tractors, induced to deliver and taken back, all on the same day so as to avoid incurring additional transport expenditures. Since it was a one-time subsidy, expenditures incurred in going to a hospital in the event of false labour pains had to be incurred by households, deterring them to do so again. Such practical problems led to increasing the demand for inducing labour pains to hasten deliveries. Reports of increased mortality due to postpartum haemorrhage also emerged.

With the focus on promoting institutional deliveries, home deliveries were missed out from the policy radar and MIS formats as did the implementation of the Supreme Court order to pay Rs 500 to pregnant women irrespective of the place of delivery. The implication was serious. Women who delivered at home were perhaps the poorest and were probably from the deprived sections of society, requiring priority attention. Part of this oversight could have been addressed by differentiating incentives for the first-timers or based on residence that would have also enabled assessing the net incrementality in terms of behaviour change. The introduction of the electronic Mother and Child Tracking System in 2010—perfected over the years—has been able to partly address this issue.

Notwithstanding the above, the JSY did bring in an impressive behaviour change both among the women who came in droves to government hospitals and also among the care providers who came under pressure to improve quality. But in states that had serious supply-side issues, institutional deliveries had a weak impact on MMR that stagnated after a slight upward swing. In many hospitals, poor standards were observed with pregnant women being confined two to a bed or accommodated on the floor. Anecdotal evidence also indicated substantial scope for fudging and leakage.

Nevertheless, the JSSK policy of providing free care to all those delivering in government hospitals was clearly working. A recent study conducted by PGI, Chandigarh, in Haryana showed that the coverage of institutional delivery was 82 per cent, of which 65 per cent took place in public sector facilities. Approximately

63 per cent of the women reported no expenditure on delivery in the public sector. While this is encouraging, what is even more is that the mean out-of-pocket expenditures for delivery in the public and private sectors in Haryana were Rs 771 (USD 14.2) and Rs 12,479 (USD 229) respectively, which were catastrophic for 1.6 per cent and 22 per cent of households respectively.[48]

In 2010, three issues having clear programmatic implications emerged:[49] a) an absence of linkage between performance and financing, b) the absence of linkage between the training of skilled birth attendants (SBAs) and conducting deliveries, and c) the absence of linkage between facility upgradation and need. And most importantly, it confirmed the data available in the NHSRC facility reports that clearly showed that no more than 15 per cent of the facilities conducted deliveries.

Based on lengthy consultations, field visits, and data analysis, the NHSRC formulated the operational guidelines on RCH in October 2010. Facilities were graded in accordance with the expected package of services that would be made available there—a package that consisted of a list of entitlements such as tests, drugs, transport, and the rest that were to be made available and provided free of cost. States were encouraged to identify the 'delivery points', brand them as RCH centres, and provide financing and human personnel differentially and in accordance with the content of the package. This was later firmed up in 2011 as the JSSK.

Impact of Institutional Deliveries on MMR

Globally, during the period from 1990–2013, there was an impressive 45 per cent decline in MMR though the MDG target for the period from 1990–2015 was 75. The highest fall was registered in the South Asia region with 4.4 per cent compared to 2.6 per cent for the world. The average rate of decline of MMR in India during the period was 4.5 per cent and accounted for 17 per cent of the global number or 50,000 of the 289,000 maternal deaths.

India's period of high achievement was post-NRHM—2005–13—when the rate of decline of MMR averaged 5.7 per cent compared to 3 per cent during the period from 1990–2005. Impressive, yet lower than Bangladesh, Ethiopia, or Cambodia.

Because maternal mortality is a rare event, a very large denominator is required to assess its rate that is calculated for every 100,000 live births. To address this methodological problem, the data for three years is clubbed together to arrive at the MMR. A comparative analysis of the rates of decline taking the three-year averages of the years 2001–3, 2004–6, 2007–9, and 2010–12 provides a good idea on the real impact of the NRHM interventions:

TABLE 5.1 Maternal Mortality Ratio per 100,000 Live Births, 2001–12

Region	2001–3	2004–6	2007–9	2010–12
High-focus states	438	375	308	257
South	173	149	127	105
Others	199	174	149	127
India	301	254	212	178

Source: GOI, 2013.

As can be seen from Table 5.1, prior to 2006 (pre-NRHM) and in 2009 (post-NRHM three-year average of 2007–9) achievements have been modest—nearly constant at 24 and 22 for the southern states, 63 and 67 for the northern states, and 25 and 26 for other states. The maximum reduction of points has been in Assam that fell from a pre-NRHM rate of 10 to that of 90 post-NRHM. A worrying factor, however, is that during the three-year average for 2009–12, there has been a marginal reduction in the annual declines of maternal mortality in almost all the high-focus states of Assam, Madhya Pradesh, Odisha, and Bihar, though as a whole India crossed the 200 mark and came down to 178 per 100,000 live births. Such marginal to near-stagnant declines sharply brought out the limitations of the unidimensional strategy of promoting institutional deliveries for reducing MMR.

A cross-country study of 181 countries showed that maternal reduction is driven by four factors: fall in the total fertility rate, increases in per capita incomes, educational attainments, and proportion of women having skilled birth attendants.[50] It is therefore not surprising that the goal of less than 100 maternal deaths per 100,000 live births has been achieved only in Kerala, Maharashtra, and Tamil Nadu at 66, 87, and 90 respectively.[51] Table 5.2 shows a comparison of two southern and two northern states.

TABLE 5.2 Comparative Table of Indicators Impacting Maternal Mortality: Some States

State	Total Fertility Rate, 2011	Per Capita Income in Rs, 2011–12	Deliveries by SBA %, 2012	Female Literacy %, 2011 census	MMR 2011	MMR 2001
Tamil Nadu	1.7	84,058	92.4	73.86	90	134
Kerala	1.8	83,725	99.7	91.98	66	110
Uttar Pradesh	3.4	29,417	48.4	59.2	292	517
Assam	3	33,633	61.8	67.2	328	490
India	2.4	60,972	66.6	65.4	178	301

Source: MOHFW, GOI.

Such data shows the limitations of the one-dimensional focus on institutional deliveries (like sterilization in family planning) and the need for a multifactorial approach to maternal health by linking the health component with the programmes for female literacy, SHG under rural development, and programmes for women and child development.

In the last few years, the RCH programme has become sharper. To start with, mapping of delivery points has enabled focusing on those facilities that have a higher case load as has the policy intention of making every delivery totally free in government facilities. Though quality has improved and ASHAs have been useful in making a difference in several states such as Bihar, further acceleration in MMR reduction will require a more focused targeting of the low-performing districts. So instead of high-focus states, the NRHM needs to change to high-focus districts. After all, over two-thirds of infant and maternal mortality is concentrated in about 170 districts, while 222 districts account for three-quarters of child mortality. With district estimates now available under the AHS,[52] innovative and focused interventions in these districts could have amazing outcomes for reducing these burdens. The point to rue is that all this was known.[53] If only the NRHM had based its strategies on evidence and involved institutions like the IIPS in the designing of interventions.

In the absence of clearly costed operational guidelines for every intervention and due to the failure to link investments to outcomes, poor supervision, and weak coordination for channelizing and pooling resources, the ministry gradually lost control of the process resulting in sharp variances in state performances with some backward states continuing to fall further behind.

Demand Side

Communitization

Introduction: the Rationale

Communitization was the real landmark innovation of the NRHM. It was also the most critical. It had the potential to usher in profound changes in the architecture of governance in the health sector. Embedded in it was the principle of decentralization—understood to imply the transfer of funds, functions, and functionaries for health actions to local-level institutions in accordance with the constitutional mandate. PRI bodies and community organizations were to be the anchor on which such decentralized approaches to planning, implementing, and monitoring health interventions were to be constructed.

It was not just the downsizing of state instruments. Communitization also implied the principles of participatory decision-making through the active involvement of key stakeholders—taking responsibility for decisions made and monitoring outcomes, ensuring sustainability and accountability. Communitization underscored the belief that people are at the centre not the state. Such people-centred approaches facilitate problem identification, provisioning of solutions, priority-setting, financial allocations, and modes of implementation, thus ensuring that the health system becomes accountable to them. This was radical stuff.

Although communitization was on the civil-society agenda for a long time and got a strong mention in the NHP I of 1984, it was a neglected area. The health system had been guided by political choice, technical considerations, and administrative oversight with the state deciding what is good for the people.

The public health system soon went out of sync because there was no forum available for people's voices. For decades after

Independence, the only one-point agenda was family planning operations, and to be counted in a public health facility, a person had to suffer from one or the other notified disease, not body aches, fevers, snake bites, injuries, diarrhoea, or asthma. The hiatus between the availability and accessibility of public services was high, as in most states coverage under even routine services such as immunization or antenatal check-ups was low. The poor and marginalized often experienced denial of access to services because of several structural, geographical, and programmatic barriers as well as other unsaid barriers of discriminatory, corrupt, unempathetic, and often rude behaviour of the staff working in the public facilities. Because of these factors, most tended to self-treat unless the illness was serious. While some ignored or delayed availing of treatment, others, being wary of the treatment itself, resorted to the locally available and time-tested vaid or any quack. By 2004, footfalls to public facilities fell below 20 per cent. There was a clear gap between state action and people's needs and perceptions that required bridging.

Such conditions compelled civil society to fight vociferously for the incorporation of communitization into the NRHM design. Behind the simple-sounding phrase of placing people's health in people's hands was the aspiration for a socialized medicine to counter the emergence of the Western, technology-driven corporatization of healthcare, where treatment was seen as a technological fix. Viewing disease or ill health as the outcome of social conditions, values, and cultural practices called for an understanding of the societal dynamics at play, especially the social and caste connotations of power, for the positioning of health services. The ingrained social barriers to health cannot be addressed by merely positioning doctors or refurbishing facilities. NGOs demanded that communitization be the core of the NRHM so as to bring about the architectural correction of the health system from below rather than from above as has been the practice all these years.

Communitization was to be realized through a strategy consisting of four components: a) provisioning of an ASHA—a CHW—for every 1,000 population; b) establishing people's committees at the village level called Village Health and Sanitation

Committees (VHSCs); c) establishing patient welfare committees, called Rogi Kalyan Samitis (RKS), in all facilities; and d) community monitoring and social audit as a tool to make the public health system accountable.

CHW: the Historical Context

The health sector has had a tentative and halting experience with community-centred interventions. The pioneers in this field were the Aroles who believed that infant mortality was largely due to chronic starvation, contaminated water and poor sanitation causing diarrhoea, and respiratory infections. 'For all three, doctors are unnecessary' as such diseases were contextualized within the 'the traditions, the taboos, and the social injustices that are meted out to certain weaker sections of our society' with strong links between healthcare and poverty and access to basic goods such as water, nutrition, and sanitation.[54] Living on the same amount of money that an average family earned in that drought-stricken, impoverished taluk of Jhamked in Ahmednagar district of Maharashtra, they founded the Comprehensive Rural Health Project (CRPH), starting with eight villages and 10,000 people. The project now covers over a population of 0.5 million in 300 villages. The trained CHWs—married women from the Dalit communities—handle 80 per cent of the village's health problems.[55]

There were several such community-based initiatives[56] that, though small in scale, had one common thread running through them—a passionate belief in the demystification of medical treatment and active engagement of the community in healthcare through the medium of health workers.

The government was not unaware of these developments. In fact, in 1939, Subhas Chandra Bose constituted the Sokhey Committee that recommended a village volunteer service, followed by the Bhore Committee Report (1946) that suggested the formation of village health committees and trained voluntary health workers. Much later in 1975, the Shrivastava Report stated:

> What we need ... is the creation of large bands of part-time semi-professional workers from among the community itself who would be close to the people, live with them, and in addition to promotive and preventive health services including those related to

family planning, will also provide basic medical services needed in day-to-day common illnesses which account for about eighty per cent of all illnesses.[57]

The well-known ICSSR/ICMR Health for All report of 1981 and the NHP I of 1982 reiterated the need for community-based workers. The introduction of the Village Health Guide in 1977 by the Janata government has to be understood in this context alongside the fact that it was also to allay people's anger against the health staff for forcible sterilization.[58]

ASHA: the Design

The inspiration for the CHW on a scaled-up mode under the NRHM was due to the civil society advocacy led by Dr Antia, the support from the NAC that endorsed the million CHWs proposal of Jayaprakash Narayan, and the push from Gopalakrishnan in the PMO. The 2005 report of the NCMH had also endorsed the need for a CHW patterned on the Gadchiroli experiment. It was a low-hanging fruit waiting to be plucked.

ASHA emerged as an important intervention and rapidly became the symbol of the centre's intention to provide healthcare to the people at its doorstep. There was enthusiastic support from all quarters and substantial political attention as ASHAs gave visibility and with it political dividends.

Initially, ASHA was not intended to be a nationwide programme but rather a replication of the Mitanin experience in similar settings. But with time, the ASHA initiative caught the imagination of the policymakers and rapidly expanded in three phases: first in the high-focus states, then to the tribal areas of the non-high-focus states, and in its third phase, in the whole country, including Kerala but excluding Tamil Nadu that did not feel the need for ASHA as it had a good primary health system except in its tribal areas.

The eligibility criteria for ASHA included women of the village (married, divorced, and widowed) in the 18–35 age group with a minimum educational qualification of eighth standard to be selected by, and accountable to, the community and the panchayat. An ASHA was to be provided a medicine kit for attending to minor ailments. Subsequently, the criterion for educational qualifications that created problems in the most needy and backward areas where female literacy was low forced a retraction.

Though the ASHA was envisioned to be selected by, and accountable to, the community, the pressure to 'show results' led to the dilution of the community-based selection processes as was followed in the Mitanin programme of Chhattisgarh where selection was preceded by *jatras*[59] and campaigns to educate people on the importance of the CHW. Processes required trained facilitators. Since this was time-consuming, a majority of state governments left the selection to the district collectors: in reality, nomination by the ANM, the sarpanch, or anganwadi workers (AWWs).

Due to a lack of clarity or uniformity on what defined an ASHA, the type of training and mentoring to be provided was compromised with. As a consequence of the pressure to produce results, training at periodic intervals with focus on the job skills was substituted by a cascade-type training for three weeks by district- and block-level teams consisting of doctors and nurses working at the PHCs. Due to the non-availability of accommodation, training was mostly non-residential, impacting quality. Due to the patchy implementation of the supervisory and mentoring system, there was no on-site training of ASHAs either. Yet over the seven-year NRHM period, it was commendable that of the 848,940 ASHAs appointed, and a majority were trained for at least the first round of 23 days.

Right from its inception there were differences of opinion regarding whether the ASHA was a transformative agent making the health system accountable to the people, or a health worker treating minor ailments, ensuring early referral and counselling for behaviour changes while also encouraging community participation in decision-making. The government's perception was essentially focused on making her the delivery point for achieving programme targets and distribution of social goods, be it condoms, or mobilization of pregnant women for institutional deliveries and children for immunization, or distributing chloroquine tablets, or selling goods like sanitary pads.

Similarly, issues related to the payment systems for ASHAs invited heated discussions and a diversity of opinions that ranged from volunteerism and social solidarity, to payment of salary on par with the AWW, to a token remuneration in recognition of the value of time spent, to the concept of blended payments—a base-level remuneration topped with additional amounts based on performance. Abhay Bang, a health activist based in Gadchiroli of Maharashtra, 'stressed the need for increasing of benefits in incentive payment, with some payment from families/beneficiaries to bring in accountability and ownership of community'.[60] All had some merit but obviously trade-offs too.

Harmonizing these various viewpoints put the government in a dilemma. Not paying never works in a nationwide scaled-up model as sustaining motivation is hard and experience showed that programmes having no budget allocations nearly always fell off the shelf. But paying an honorarium was fraught with risks as the beneficiaries over time could seek permanent jobs, adding to the non-plan woes of the already fragile budgets. The concept of performance-based payments was thus considered a good solution to the problem.

Performance-based payments or P4P is an emerging market concept used for incentivizing higher productivity. Behaviour responses are awarded with cash by monetizing the functions performed. With monetary values accorded arbitrarily, they are often neither a measure of the cost to the government for generating that activity nor reflect the market value. Rather, the remuneration scales clearly reflected the government's priority, and so it paid Rs 200 for escorting a pregnant woman to the facility for delivery in non-high-focus states but Rs 600 for the same activity in the high-focus states, or Rs 50 for completing TB treatment but Rs 250 for completing the immunization schedule, and so on. Justified as a means 'to compensate for her time', every service provided or function performed was to be financially remunerated without reference to the outcome or quality or standard.

ASHAs' earnings were linked to caseloads. So to make the 'package' more attractive and worthwhile for sustaining interest and retention, more services were added with every passing day. In 2010, Rajasthan took a decision to provide a floor amount of Rs 500 per month as a state initiative. Quoting this, at the MSG meeting in 2010, Raghuvansh Yadav, the Panchayati Raj minister, asked for ASHAs to be paid a fixed monthly salary on the lines of the AWW. This suggestion was roundly rejected for fear that the ASHA may become yet another 'government servant'. Parties like the CPM would often raise the issue of giving fixed wages to the 'overworked' ASHA, though departmental reviews indicated a maximum workload of about four hours per day.[61] Undoubtedly, most ASHAs worked with the expectation and hope of becoming government employees.

ASHA Mentoring Group (AMG)

Concerns at the delinking of the ASHA from the community, the increasing grip of bureaucratic control over her, and the tendency to ignore tasks that had a lower remuneration were raised at almost every meeting of the AMG that was constituted in December 2005. The AMG consisting of 21 leading NGOs to provide technical support to this high-priority intervention met 10 times during the period from 2005–12. The NHSRC was nominated as the secretariat for the AMG.

A perusal of the minutes clearly reflects the growing frustration of civil society. At almost every meeting the members raised their apprehensions about the ASHA being reduced to a link worker where she has come to be 'defined by the targets of health department rather than based on community needs'.[62] The group called for policy clarity on her role to reiterate her primary responsibility as a mobilizer and an activist who is sensitive to the concerns of the community, development of measurable indicators to monitor outcomes, and the need to establish institutionalized supervisory structures. In fact, Abhay Bang suggested having a stand-alone state action plan for the ASHA—containing a long-term vision; role clarity; institutionalized training, retraining, and accreditation/certification processes; and an ASHA resource centre to look into all aspects of selection, skill development, training, supervision, monitoring, quality assurance, networking, resource mobilization, career progression, and budget. There was also concern that the euphoria and romanticization of the ASHA was resulting in the near-neglect of the ANM. Over time, some members became restive and gradually distanced themselves, while the 'critics' got sidelined and later removed. This was partly because the NHSRC felt that the members of the AMG gave no time to building the programme and met only when a meeting was called. Whatever be the reason, the environment deteriorated even as the guidelines issued on the role and functions of the ASHA in 2013 had no consensus, nor was any attempt made to build one.

ASHA in Operation

By 2010, ASHA had graduated to becoming the most visible 'achievement' of the government in every public document or speech made by the health minister. Every review of the NRHM started with, and was dominated by, ASHA-related issues. Yet clarity on what an ASHA is continued to be elusive. An assessment of the ASHA carried out by the NIHFW and an evaluation by the NHSRC in 2011 providing options for interpretation—as a facilitator, a service provider, or an activist. The fact that each role entailed a set of activities and each approach a different costing stream was not appreciated, such as the content, the pedagogy, and the type of trainers and skill sets required. Also, the supervisory, referral, and monitoring systems to be put in place would differ based on the functions ASHAs are expected to perform and the outcomes to be delivered.

For a government struggling to get its MMR and IMR down, debates of whether the ASHA should be an activist, or a service provider, or a mobilizer, or a catalyst were of secondary concern. What was needed was action on the ground since babies were dying unnecessarily for want of timely medical attention. Two-thirds of infants die within the first week of their birth and ASHAs could certainly have been an invaluable service to address this problem. To explain this, a small digression is necessary to discuss the issue of public policy for neonatal care.

With the disproportionately high focus on immunization, particularly on polio eradication, child health had been neglected since the late 1980s. While 40 per cent mortality of children under five was due to ARIs and diarrhoea, yet it took the ministry six years to clear the ARI strategy that was formulated in 1991, while little attention was paid to tackling diarrhoea till as late as 1993.

Likewise, even in 1990, neonatal mortality was considered a non-issue though it was responsible for more than two-thirds of the infant deaths. 'Newborn is never a public health issue. They are just a normal subset of young population' claimed the then assistant commissioner of the MOHFW. The Indian Academy of Pediatrics (IAP) itself had failed to produce public health evidence of the substantial contribution of neonatal mortality to infant mortality. Subsequently, with the launch of the Child Survival and Safe Motherhood Programme in mid-1990s, the AWW was asked to make household visits to the mother–baby pair three times within the first fortnight of birth.

In 2003, UNICEF developed the Integrated Management of Neonatal and Childhood Illness (IMNCI) protocol and undertook substantial training of the AWW since she was the only village-based 'health' worker. The IMNCI was seen as a technically sound, protocol-based strategy which ensured that errors in the early recognition of signs and symptoms are not missed out and immediate referrals of the newborns to a facility was complied with. Its implementation was, however, dependent on the availability of good roads and transport networks and a responsive, functioning health system, as evidence showed that babies died due to the delay in accessing appropriate treatments and most often, the facility itself would be found shut with no one to attend to them. Or, death would be caused for want of money to rush the child to a private facility or a higher-level hospital.

Between monitoring of nutrition, weighing of children, institutional deliveries, and immunization targets, particularly polio campaigns, neonatal care and the IMNCI were low on the scale of priorities. ASHA provided an opportunity to address this dire need of home visits to the mother–baby pair immediately after delivery—an opportunity acknowledged in 2010 inspired by the successful implementation of the 'Gadchiroli' home-based neonatal care (HBNC) model among the Mitanins of Chhattisgarh in 2009. Accordingly, attention turned to the idea of making the ASHA take up house visits of the recently delivered mothers and infants as a natural extension of the work she was doing. The NHSRC was directed to develop guidelines and draw up plans for the systematic training of ASHAs on HBNC.

Implementation of the aforementioned decision, however, was not easy. There was resistance from the concerned technical division of the ministry against allowing ASHA to be trained in what they felt were 'technical skills' considering she was 'just a housewife'. UNICEF was unhappy and it was rumoured that some of its officials exhorted state officers not to comply with the guidelines, inviting resistance from the states as well.

Meetings with state health secretaries and deputing their teams to Gadchiroli brought in acceptability for the HBNC strategy. UNICEF, too, gave up its misgivings and the technical objection within the ministry confined itself to making a justifiable demand to delete the provision authorizing ASHAs to dispense antibiotics.[63] Notwithstanding this, making the ASHA responsible for visiting the mother–baby pair for first-aid and early referral is, in the prevailing circumstances, the best option. As health systems develop and strengthen, the HBNC strategy can be replaced. In 2013, the latest guidelines have formalized the ASHA to undertake house visits as a part of her work description.

ASHA has been an important policy intervention in taking the system closer to the community. Programmatically, it has been a great success. The improvement of health facilities in terms of personnel, drugs, and general cleanliness has been accompanied by increase in the footfalls of pregnant women reporting for delivery escorted by the ASHA and the number of fully immunized children, timely dispersal of anti-malarial drugs, and reduced deaths.

The ASHA was the creation of civil society. Several civil society members felt let down as they envisioned the ASHA as an element of the 'rights-based approach' to make the system more accountable to the people and respond to the needs of the community, thereby helping it address the problems of poverty, hunger, and social exclusion. Instead the focus seemed on making her a contract agent working for a remuneration for the services rendered. Experts like Banerji felt that the approach adopted by the government was ahistorical making the ASHA yet another supply-side functionary rather than a demand-side protagonist.

A few key issues clearly emerged in implementing the ASHA programme: the compromising of processes that are a prerequisite for effective community participation as an instrument of change; the inattention to supportive supervision and institutionalized mentoring,[64] barring in one or two states; the overwhelming focus on the payment aspect that seemed to make monetary gain rather than social solidarity the motivating factor; the failure to engage civil society partners and NGOs to help implement this intervention and opting instead to do so through its own already overburdened and poorly trained staff; and so on. In fact, NGOs were also wary of working with the government, so much so that not more than three responded to the invitation to train ASHAs on the HBNC module that was launched in 2010.

Every year, the ASHA is being assigned more tasks. Clearly, the trend seems to be towards making her a multipurpose village health worker with a breathtaking span of functions and responsibilities. Time has come for the health system to recognize her as a field worker, remunerate her accordingly, and allow her to function as a departmental functionary as in Ethiopia (see Box 5.1).

Box 5.1   Health Workers in Ethiopia

In Ethiopia, the CHW (called the health extension worker [HEW]) is a 12th grader, who is provided a one-year training, is salaried, and—though selected (a mandatory requirement) by the community—is a government functionary, tasked to educate the families under her charge. The family in turn is also made to assume more responsibility by identifying one member who disseminates the messages to other family members, ensures full immunization, family planning services, and other benefits. At the primary health centres, one full-time supervisor is appointed with the single responsibility of supervising the HEWs. Its impact on reducing child mortality and other indicators has been substantial. What is also interesting is that donors in both India and Ethiopia objected to this community-based intervention.

Source: Author.

The one clear takeaway from the ASHA programme is that people desire and respond to village/community/close-to-household type of interventions for delivery of services. Time has, therefore, also come to focus on building a team of well-trained and qualified paramedics to provide primary care at the community level, which has been elaborated in Chapter 6. This would enable the paramedic to forge links with the community and be responsible for them through the trained, salaried, and accredited[65] ASHA worker provided with clear responsibilities, outputs, and accountability.

Institutionalizing People's Participation

A positive development in recent times is the emergence of what is referred to as the 'people's sector'. It is argued that the issue is not about the public or the private sector but the people whose opinions must matter and need to be central to all decision-making. The legitimacy of the people's sector rests on their satisfaction in being central to patient care. Be it the right to be informed or obtaining prior consent for undertaking invasive procedures, people's participation and patient rights are now not only a legal requirement but have increasingly emerged as a valued characteristic of modern medicine. In fact, in the UK, even in regulatory bodies like the British Medical Council lay people are inducted as board members.

In India, policymaking and priority-setting regarding financial, administrative, or technical matters related to health are centralized and operate in a closed-door system with limitations on entry. Institutional mechanisms are so layered that by the time people's voices reach the decision-makers, they get muffled or lost in the din.

Centralization often compromises the functioning of facilities. A health facility makes hundreds of decisions on any given day. In the absence of financial or administrative autonomy, the smooth functioning of a facility gets severely interrupted affecting patient care. How can the facility function when repairing an X-ray machine can take up to six months or fixing an electric plug needs to await permission from the district headquarters which can take over a month? Doctors in charge are blamed for lacking managerial capacity and subjected to innumerable trainings in management while the solution lies in laying down clear responsibilities and autonomy for decision-making and delegation of powers for financial decision-making. Besides, reporting systems need to focus on ensuring accountability to the patients in the first instance.

Such a situation was the backdrop against which the NRHM had to incorporate elements of decentralization and people's participation in planning and implementation processes at the village and facility levels through the Village Health Sanitation and Nutrition Committee (VHSNC) and the RKS.

Village Health Sanitation and Nutrition Committee

The VHSNCs were to largely comprise women chosen from various castes of the community and elected members of the panchayats. Their task was to undertake household surveys to help the ASHA prepare the village health plans (the bottom-up approach) and assist in, and monitor its, implementation. To facilitate taking up local action, Rs 10,000 was also placed at the disposal of the gram panchayat and the ANM.

From the guidelines, it was clear that the VHSNC was an advisory body without any powers of effective oversight over ASHAs who were selected by and paid for by the ANM. It also did not have access to financial resources to take up works it considered priority as the money was allotted to the panchayat to be spent by the sarpanch/panchayat secretary and the ANM, without any obligation to refer to or seek advice from the VHSNC. More importantly, VHSNCs were also not given any training for the functions they were expected to discharge or to have their capacities built.

The utility of VHSNCs varied in accordance with the importance and understanding it received from the respective states. In some states VHNSCs did receive a positive response and were used effectively to further the agenda of immunization and antenatal care. In Andhra Pradesh, a limited experiment was carried out for using the village councils of the SHGs for converging programmes that impacted the well-being of women and their children—health, education, nutrition, security, water supply, and so on—by bringing coordination among all the related departments at that level. It was greatly successful but later sabotaged as it meant greater accountability that was resented. In other states like Tamil Nadu or Karnataka, NGOs were able to get an effective response from the community through VHSNCs. Thus the VHSNC, as an idea, had great value. Its sustainability and true value as a people's institution was stymied due to an inadequate design and ambiguity on the various inter-institutional relationships at the community level.

The system issues that arose while rolling out and monitoring VHSNCs was whether it was a parallel body to the panchayat that had its own subcommittee for health and its relationship with the panchayat itself—one a constitutional body and the other constituted by a government fiat? And was constituting a VHSNC a tacit admission of a lack of trust in the panchayat's capacity to deliver the NRHM agenda? On what basis was this body authorized to prepare a plan—that, too, an inter-sectoral one—much less monitor its enforcement? What is its power over the ASHA? If recommendatory, what is its scope and what are the resources at its disposal for local action?

Rogi Kalyan Samiti (RKS)

The first patient welfare committee was constituted in Indore, Madhya Pradesh, during the plague scare that hit India in 1995 to secure people's cooperation to shut down the general hospital for a few days to clean up the thousands of rats roaming freely there. Earlier in the late 1980s, Andhra Pradesh constituted an autonomous organization for managing secondary-level hospitals and later hospitals were also encouraged to have their own development committees. The idea of such committees was twofold: a) to mobilize resources to bridge the fiscal deficit that nearly always plagued all hospitals, and b) to take appropriate action for providing essential services or amenities for the welfare of patients. So the hospitals were by law authorized to rent out or sell their properties; levy user fees; and mobilize donations in cash or kind towards diet for patients, building a ward, contributing equipment, constructing toilets, and the rest.

According to the guidelines, the RKS was to recruit members representing all sections of society. They were provided with untied grants of Rs 0.1 million in PHCs and Rs 0.5 million in district hospitals. The RKS was to meet once a quarter to plan and monitor the functioning of the hospital for patient welfare. But the policy to not levy user fees and a restricted scope to mobilize resources pushed the facilities to function on shoestring budgets.

In the literature on hospital management, two issues are often discussed: a) to establish systems of oversight by the users and patients to ensure that the facilities implement official policies and guidelines, and b) to develop appropriate rules and systems of governance to make it patient-friendly. Such supervision is considered essential as information asymmetry has the potential to abuse and exploit the patients' vulnerability. But for an RKS to play such an oversight role, the first prerequisite is to have the members trained and made competent for the roles they are expected to play. Understanding medical needs, priorities, budget statements, audit reports, government guidelines, and policy documents are all important skills and as essential as participation in meetings, reading of minutes, raising questions, and so on, probably more so since the subject is complex and the doctor's position and technical expertise can more often than not overawe the lay members. As none of these institutional systems are in place, the RKS exists only on paper in some places, is relatively redundant in some, but extremely innovative and vibrant in states like Kerala that combined the other finances available under the RSBY to improve their hospitals.

Community Participation and Monitoring

The fourth element of communitization in the NRHM programme implementation was community participation. The NRHM also had a cabinet approval to expend 5 per cent of its budget for civil society initiatives. Therefore, to implement this policy, in 2006 the NRHM established, the Advisory Group on Community Action (AGCA) with its secretariat in the Population Foundation of India (PFI), an NGO established by J.R.D. Tata for supporting the population stabilization programmes. This committee had 21 members—prominent civil society activists, many of whom were also members of other committees established under the NRHM. Its main function was to advise on developing community partnership and ownership for the mission, community monitoring, suggesting norms for funding schemes to be implemented by NGOs, and examining proposals received under the NRHM for community/NGO participation.

From its inception until 2015, the AGCA met 27 times. But right from the start, the AGCA adopted a wider vision of reforms that were not to be restricted to promoting the NGO sector. Discussions reflected in the minutes were rich in content in terms of the issues they brought to the table. Yet a perusal of these minutes reveals a certain tension that the AGCA faced all through due to a clash in perceptions regarding its purpose between the government and the civil society members. In the government's view, the AGCA was meant to further the communitization agenda, particularly relating to community monitoring and spending the NRHM budget (5 per cent) earmarked for NGOs. It wanted NGOs to 'play a participatory role, not only advisory'[66] and sustain the several policy initiatives the government had undertaken at the behest of civil society—the VHSNC, the RKS, and the ASHA.

The members of the AGCA had a different perception of their role: advise, develop models, and provide feedback. They saw themselves as a body meant to provide inputs related to health delivery that ranged from increasing access and utilization of quality health services by all, to the promotion of equity and social justice and inter-sectoral convergence. They wanted a resource centre to be established for community monitoring with a system of interface with the NHSRC, which was seen as an institution engaged with supply-side issues.

The tasks they had set for themselves were ambitious and far beyond their capacity. On the other hand, government policy-making and implementation were already being reviewed and relentlessly followed up by the NAC, the Planning Commission, the PMO, the PSC, and the media. They were not in the mood to wait for the wisdom of the AGCA or its feedback, which they felt was only focused on picking holes rather than helping to solve the problems by joining hands as partners.

And the government was justified in its wariness of the AGCA. What the government desperately needed was the building of social capital and scaling up of community-based initiatives acknowledged to be of critical value for the success of the NRHM. The initiatives were to be implemented by identifying suitable NGOs; building their capacity; drafting operational guidelines; training and building capacity at the state, district, and block levels; building supervisory capacity; and so on instead of just advising and finding fault. But despite a passage of five years, the AGCA was still trying to find its feet.

One important initiative that unfortunately did not get much traction was the concept of community monitoring and social audit. Of all initiatives, this was the most powerful means to enhance accountability and transparency in the implementation of public policy.

Community monitoring envisaged community oversight of the functioning of the health system. Its effectiveness depended on the delivery system being in place and the community having adequate resources of its own to opt for alternatives available in the event of an unresponsive public system, or to fill the gaps in cases of genuine systemic bottlenecks.

The idea of community monitoring and social audit never got traction with the NRHM that virtually signed it off by 2009, informing civil society to go to the states and market their concept to get included in the PIP. The NRHM's denial of direct funding resulted in this idea falling off the policy radar. The hesitation was because of the knowledge that public facilities were facing serious shortages and challenges and the NRHM feared the risk of this monitoring becoming a fault-finding mechanism further alienating the community and widening the chasm between them and the service providers, besides inviting resistance from the health authorities.

NGOs, however, continued to implement the concept independently. Implementation by the CEHAT in nearly 300 villages of Maharashtra and an equal number by PFI in Bihar has shown that while initially community interaction with the local authorities did raise arguments, it also helped find solutions. Overall, there is adequate evidence in the country to demonstrate that trusting and partnering with the community always helps in smoother implementation and promotes better outcomes. Such trust is what is valuable.

As the infrastructure falls into place and community awareness expands, it is a matter of time before community monitoring will come into being in the current format or some other form of grievance redressal. Hopefully, this is only a pause in the process of making the public systems accountable to the community and the people they are expected to serve.

The agenda of communitization was extremely important. However, the full realization of the interventions fell short on account of lack of clarity and overlooking the importance of training and capacity-building, nurturing and mentoring, and constant monitoring and supervision. In an institutional sense, there were three key areas where the NRHM fell short:

a) In having the technical committees—the AMG and the AGCA—more intensely involved in preparing guidelines, monitoring, and providing feedback, much like what the TRGs did in NACO. These committees should have been 'located' within the ministry so as to be linked to policy.

b) In not having established a division for communitization within the ministry with the mandate of having the four-pronged strategy implemented with the help of the NHSRC and other institutions and making it a part of the daily routine of the secretary or the minister, for whom it was enough that ASHAs had been appointed as per target. This would have helped keep the intangible issues within the policy radar and also enabled scaling up. The NGOs in dealing with the mid-level officials[67] missed an invaluable opportunity in the actual process of policy planning and formulation.

c) In not institutionalizing the process of communitization—the ASHAs, the working of the VHSNC, and community social audit— with the appropriate technical support staff. In all departments (education, nutrition, rural development, or NACO), such community-based interventions have been provided with an institutional structure. Thus, for example, the *saheli* of Mahila Samakhya, the village organizations of the SHGs, the anganwadi worker under the ICDS, or the TI programme under NACO had supervisory and mentoring structures. Under the TI programme of NACO, every ten TIs had a supervisor with a monthly remuneration of Rs 25,000 per month, while the sahelis had *sahayogin*s and the SHGs had community coordinators. In short, community empowerment and processes cannot be carried out in a void. This was a serious omission and continues to be so.

※

The shift from welfarism to liberalism sharpened disparities and inequalities but also enabled the emergence of NGOs and an articulate civil society demanding equality and social justice. The original concept of the ASHA and communitization was a means of empowering the most marginalized—not by handouts or targets to achieve but through intensely process-driven strategies that entailed a series of meetings and extensive dialogues during the initial stages. Such participation implied problem identification and solutions coming from within and owned by the community. Processing such a dialogue required communication skills, patience, and experience necessitating facilitators. For poor women hitherto tied to their gender roles of wives, mothers, sisters, or daughters, belonging to a group meant gaining an identity and a voice. And a voice emerging from the process is what led to empowerment.

The NRHM had all the articulation of empowerment and it provided for the VHNSC and the ASHA at the community level in good faith. But in reality, the institutional structures required to facilitate and nurture these ideas were never focused upon. ASHAs were initially mere instruments to get pregnant women to hospitals for delivery and over time their engagement got influenced by the money they could earn by rendering services for the department. The departments of health at the national or state levels did not understand the complexities of the process of communitization. The grand vision thus floundered for want of an understanding of the building blocks. It disregarded the process of learning from ground experience within and outside health and consequently paid the price of patterning the ASHA and community empowerment on the sole experience of the Mitanin as the perfect model, even as the Mitanin itself was getting 'undermined' with the change from volunteerism and solidarity to services against payments.

The design and processes applied to the communitization and the ASHA agenda would have been different had they been based on an understanding and a recognition of the existence of social constructs and barriers that inhibit women, especially from availing of health services for themselves and their children. If only prior to its launch, extensive consultations had been held to develop models to suit the diversity of this country's social landscape, pilot them, identify partners, and provide institutional structures before scaling up, the trajectory of the NRHM would have been different.

This was not done for two reasons. First, the community worker was a concession to the civil-society vision but in reality, she was a mechanism for delivering services to the community, which the system was unable to do with ANMs. The second was the sheer lack of imagination to balance processes essential for bringing in transformative change and the severe pressures to show results. These pressures and concerns bureaucratized the processes.

Run up to the Twelfth Five Year Plan

During the seven-year period from 2005–12, a total of Rs 714.7 billion was released by the central government to the states, while the actual expenditure was Rs 744.62 billion—a more than threefold increase from the earlier time periods. Of this, Rs 203.13 billion (27.8 per cent) was spent under the RCH pool, Rs 207.94 billion (28 per cent) under the NRHM pool, Rs 46.98 billion for polio (6.4 per cent), Rs 57.24 billion (7.7 per cent) for disease control, and Rs 229.31 billion (30.79 per cent) under the treasury route towards salaries of regular staff and miscellaneous details.[68]

Additional resources helped accelerate reductions in maternal and infant mortality rates (see Table 5.3); expand total immunization coverage; upgrade and improve the quality of infrastructure; assure an expanded availability of critical inputs such as manpower, equipments and drugs, emergency transport; and, most of all, stimulate and revive interest in primary care, providing an opportunity to state health departments to innovate and scale up. Above all, as Thelma Narayan, a health activist from Karnataka, notes, 'there has been a democratization of the health system during this period, even if it is cacophonic and speaking in different voices. Health is also now much higher on the public and political agenda as is evident in the political manifestos of all parties before the 2014 elections'.[69]

Over the years, many improvements set in. Some learnings of the NACO experience also got co-opted into the NRHM—more use of data and more focus and issuance of operational guidelines spelling out the vision, mission, objectives, and so on. The RCH

TABLE 5.3 Rates of Decline among Key Indicators Pre- and Post-NRHM (%)

Indicator	IMR	NNMR	U5MR (2008/2012)	MMR
Pre-NRHM: rural (2000–5)	74 (−2.9)	49 (−3.5)	76 (−6.6)	NA
Post-NRHM: rural (2005–12)	46 (−4.6)	33 (−3.1)	58 (−4.9)	NA
Pre-NRHM: urban (2000–5)	44 (−1.9)	27 (−3.2)	43 (4.7)	NA
Post-NRHM: urban (2005–12)	28 (−5.0)	16 (−5.1)	32 (−7.3)	NA
Pre-NRHM: all India (2000–5)	68 (−3.1)	44 (−3.4)	69 (−7.2)	301 (−4.1)★
Post-NRHM: all India (2005–12)	42 (−4.5)	29 (−3.4)	52 (−5.5)	178 (−5.7)†
Highest acceleration during the years 2000–12	−8.8 (2010)	−10.5 (2011)	−7.8 (2010)	Reduction from 79,000 to 47,000 deaths per year.

Source: Review of Selected Demographic Indicators—Levels and Trends, January 2014, MOHFW, GOI.
Notes: ★ 2001–3.
† 2010–12.

programme got out of its narrow shell of institutional deliveries to a more comprehensive reproductive healthcare to be provided free of charge in all government facilities, even as the agenda expanded to address problems of disability among children and concerns of adolescents. Expenditure management processes that were poorly handled at the start of the programme in 2007 substantially improved with better oversight and closer monitoring, vastly contributing to better utilization at the state levels. Likewise, the statistical wing that had earlier been kept out of the NRHM came to the centre stage with a far better HMIS in place and data sets to enable focused planning.

With the help of the NHSRC and a laborious interactive process, the ministry undertook the task of identifying lagging districts and the current status of infrastructure. This enabled differential planning among and within the districts and also helped carve out areas requiring special attention—financial, human, and material resources on differential norms. Besides, reviews were also more systematized and monitoring was intensified with the development of electronic tracking of maternal and child health indicators. By 2012, there was a greater streamlining and a measure of confidence and momentum at the national and state levels to achieve the broad goals of the NRHM. The midterm review of the Planning Commission and the working group reports prepared by the ministry for the Twelfth Plan clearly laid down the challenges and tasks to be addressed. On 15 August 2011, the prime minister had also announced from the ramparts of the Red Fort that the Twelfth Five Year Plan would be a 'health plan'. A mood of optimism thus prevailed in the ministry before the unfolding of the Twelfth Plan period.

The Bolt from Above

The reality was, however, different. In 2009, when the UPA was back in power, the growth rate was a dizzying 9 per cent. It was believed that in addition to the farmers' loan waivers, other policies like the Rajiv Aarogyasri had somewhat helped the Congress win in Andhra Pradesh, as did the RSBY in some other states. Besides, the Left parties had also left the UPA. The NRHM and with it the concept of the state's dominant role in healthcare and public provisioning of health services slid in importance. Instead the Congress manifesto talked about expanding health insurance.

Thus, even though the midterm review of the Planning Commission called for the continuation of the UPA I policy, the spread and popularity of the RSBY and the Rajiv Aarogyasri and the rapid manner in which these programmes were able to co-opt the private sector for delivery of services was not lost on several important policymakers, particularly in the Planning Commission. The fact that UHC was essentially a political issue that could entail significant political dividends was also being recognized.

Soon after the release of the midterm appraisal, the Planning Commission, indicating its impatience at the performance of the NRHM, constituted, an HLEG in October 2010. The HLEG was to provide an architecture for UHC. In 2009, the Rockefeller

Foundation had flagged UHC as a global priority. UHC was the flavour of the season and the intention was to include it into the forthcoming Twelfth Five Year Plan.

The HLEG was chaired by Srinath Reddy, a cardiologist by training and the president of the PHFI in India. It consisted of 15 members, of whom barely six had any idea of the functioning of the health system either as practitioners or as long-standing researchers. The ministry got to know of the constitution of the HLEG only through the media.[70] Initially, the health ministry was kept out but subsequently the PD of the NRHM and Yogesh Jain of Jan Sahayog, an NGO from Chhattisgarh, got included due to the intervention of the PMO.

The HLEG got a substantial grant from the Rockefeller Foundation and was able to access several international consultants who helped in preparing the report. For validating its preliminary findings, the Planning Commission did not look at Indian academicians or people working in the Indian health system. Instead it sought the opinions of foreign academicians, representatives of the corporate sector (Naresh Trehan of Medanta, Kiran Mazumdar of Biocon, and Devi Shetty of Narayana Hrudayalaya), and donors, namely the World Bank that enthusiastically endorsed the HLEG.[71]

The report was to be submitted by November 2011 but was delayed. It was consequently not in the public domain and available for discussion in the working groups established by the health ministry or the Steering Committee established by the Planning Commission for preparing the Twelfth Five Year Plan vision. The report was therefore released as a parallel to the report of the steering committee and not so much as an input to it.

The Planning Commission incorporated much of the HLEG report into its Twelfth Five Year Plan chapter on health. According to the Planning Commission's officials, the chapter was sent to Srinath Reddy and Shiv Kumar[72] for their approval. The ministry was not taken into confidence and clearly, it did not seem to matter what the ministry officials thought as they were seen as people lacking vision or competence. The Twelfth Plan ignored the many findings and recommendations of the ministry made in the working group reports that could have meaningfully overcome the weaknesses of the NRHM in particular and public service delivery in general.

On 13 March 2012, the deputy chairman of the Planning Commission wrote to the health minister drawing his attention to two recommendations being proposed for promoting 'accountable care'. One was the recommendation of the HLEG to have governments purchase care from managed care organizations (providers) constituted as integrated networks as delivery nodes operating within a geographical area to provide a continuum of services—primary, secondary, and tertiary—to the registered populations. Payment to these networks was to be on a per capita basis. Closely drawing from the US model of managed care,[73] it was to be implemented over two-to-three plan periods.

The second recommendation was to release grants directly to the states, bypassing the central health ministry, under the Additional Central Assistance route (ACA) as is being done under the Rashtriya Krishi Vikas Yojana (RKVY). It was felt that this would incentivize the states to purchase these services and bring in the required reforms. The final draft of the Twelfth Plan document continued to include both the recommendations made in the initial draft despite the reservations expressed by the ministry.

The health chapter was sent to the ministry for the first time a few days before the meeting of the Full Planning Commission. It caused dismay. Senior officers of the ministry were clearly upset and questioned the very foundation of the recommendations that seemed to suggest a health-insurance model to provide services through the private sector while undermining the public sector. They questioned the basis for promoting health insurance when even a scheme like the RSBY, notwithstanding all its computerization, could not provide basic data such as district-wise information of surgeries conducted type-wise and the balance of money pending against each patient at the end of care. Not to mention that the RSBY had increased utilization but had no impact on reducing out-of-pocket or catastrophic expenditures. They were concerned that the chapter on health contained irrelevant examples of PPP rather than successful ones like the 108 under which data showed how a majority of the patients had chosen to go to government hospitals.

Many health activists who were members of the HLEG are reported to have stated that they felt let down as the recommendations were clearly aimed to 'destroy' the public sector that they were committed to.[74] Sundararaman who was very intensely involved in this whole process stated:

> Yes, the 12th plan proposal in its original form, (before it was modified by a strong intervention by the health minister Ghulam Nabi Azad), was all about outsourcing healthcare. Building only around para 3.1.10 of the HLEG report, the 12th Plan was proposing outsourcing block or district health systems as a singular package to corporate agencies. These agencies were to lead what was called an integrated network, but what in effect was placing public facilities under a different ownership, and shifting the government's role from a provider to a purchaser. There was no doubt a section of health leadership, at least Srinath and Nachiket Mor were driving this ... Some civil society activists on the HLEG like Yogesh Jain were unaware of the interpretation of this paragraph and quite aghast at the turn of events.

Those were strong assertions and clearly brought out a complete breakdown in the understanding of issues between the ministry, the Planning Commission, and the HLEG itself. The minister was briefed about the HLEG report that was the basis of the Planning Commission's largely unacceptable recommendations. Palpably livid, he is reported to have taken a very strong stand against the health chapter at the Planning Commission meeting and refused his endorsement. The prime minister requested the Planning Commission officials to meet with the minister and sort it out.

The meeting was held the next day. The deputy chairman of the Planning Commission, his senior officials, and the ministry officials met in the minister's chambers but the outcome was inconclusive. The minister felt it was premature to consider direct funding of block grants to the states as proposed. He also felt that managed care-type of models that implied releasing block grants to providers to supply services through a network of private providers/hospitals was flawed, if not outright premature at the current level of development of the health system. He is reported to have commented: 'We are just now beginning to learn and run the system; we are just learning to break in the horse and ride it and one year before [the] election, you want me to change the horse midway? How?' To be fair, Azad was generally sceptical of private sector engagement without appropriate safeguards being put in place in the first instance.

> I receive people who have been asked to pay Rs 1 million for a surgery—I refer them to AIIMS, and AIIMS tells me that there is no need for any surgery in the first instance.... We are not able to get data on OPD and IPD numbers from private medical colleges ... what is our capacity ... we are not even able to do basic primary care properly and here you want us to track every disease ... every encounter to be tracked?

While the Planning Commission wanted to engage the private sector, the minister wanted funding for public sector facilities on a per capita basis in order to strengthen them. Unable to arrive at a middle ground, the proposed chapter of the Planning Commission was dropped. There were clearly three concerns about the further expansion of the private sector: a) that the public health system must not be undermined and instead be made to play the key role, with private providers supplementing it on a PPP basis; b) the limitations of the private sector in delivering public goods and its negligible presence in the rural (hard-to-reach) areas need to be squarely acknowledged; and c) establish, in the first instance, a regulatory framework that would address issues related to excessive billing and complaints of malpractice. Clearly, there was an enormous amount of simplification and the implications of this strategy had not been thought through.

Having failed to get the global agenda of UHC approved by the ministry, the proponents of the HLEG report tried the NAC route. An endorsement from Sonia Gandhi would have been powerful enough to overrule the ministry. A presentation by Srinath Reddy was organized, but Sonia Gandhi and the NAC refused to endorse it without hearing the ministry's viewpoint. The ministry, too, gave a counter presentation making a strong case of how the NRHM was making a difference on the ground and how they needed some more time, money, and, above all, trust. They also pointed out how many essential services—be they drugs, basic diagnostics and treatment against all infectious diseases, family planning, or reproductive health services—were being universally provided free of cost. In some ways, UHC for primary care was already being realized in large swathes of the country and was comparable to other developing countries. Subsequently, the NAC came up with a health plan. Its plan was, unsurprisingly, almost the same as the HLEG report since two NAC members were also members of the HLEG.

Though the authors of the HLEG report blamed the health ministry for 'lack of enthusiasm' for UHC and for not having 'actively engaged'[75] the states on the report, the fact is that it is the authors who have to blame themselves. While writing a report and formulating recommendations, the ministries at the central and state levels—the natural recipients of the recommendations—ought to have been taken into confidence. In other words, had the HLEG consulted and worked with the ministry and perhaps been a bit humbler, it might have gained insights into the operational problems faced in the implementation of programmes and provided a road map and solutions regarding how to usher in the much-needed transformative change.

In addition to an already complicated situation was the miscommunication between the Planning Commission's officials and those of the ministry. Overall, the tragedy is that for the first time ever a prime minister had proactively agreed to raise the health budget to 2.5 per cent of the GDP. The Plan did provide it but due to confusion regarding the strategies and communication gaps, the impact got diluted. Piqued with the health ministry, the Planning Commission also failed to provide the required budgetary support in the first two years of the Plan, seriously denting the momentum in the implementation of the NRHM.

Thus, the HLEG report, quite unintendedly, undermined the NRHM that, given all the constraints and problems, had been so impressively rolled out in the states.[76] With no clarity on what the future must hold and the sequencing of the operationalization of the strategies proposed by the Planning Commission in the Twelfth Plan, the health ministry was left directionless, not knowing which way to proceed.

The HLEG report was a well-written document that brought to the fore many issues of importance. The concept of UHC was first articulated by Bhore in 1946, reiterated in the Shrivastava Committee Report in 1975, constantly promoted by civil society since the 1990s, elaborated in the NCMH Report of 2005 that called for universally available, free, comprehensive primary healthcare and subsidized secondary care targeting the poor. Yet official policies refused to recognize the principle of universalism and the obligatory role of the state to provide healthcare to all citizens. Drawing heavily from earlier reports and publications, the HLEG report strongly advocated equity and providing a continuum of services—from primary to tertiary—in a seamless manner as well as the dominance of the government's stewardship role as a regulator, financier, and guarantor. It argued against using commercial private insurance to purchase care or as a means of health financing. Instead it called for architectural corrections in the administration and management of the health system at the national, state, and district levels.

But the report was ahistorical. Though several of its recommendations were similar to those made in earlier reports like the NCMH's, and though India was struggling to revive for the past five years just one part of the health system under the NRHM, it did not analyse why some of the recommendations of the NCMH, which was after all co-chaired by the finance and health ministers (no report ever before had such a high-level chairpersonship), had not been implemented or why the NRHM was finding the implementation of assuring universal access to even essential goods so tough.[77] In rejecting the history and the context and in not addressing the question of *how, who, and at what cost*, the HLEG report seemed to be an aspirational document, divorced from the realities of the rough and tumble of realpolitik. Besides, UHC is all about financing. In advocating for it and demanding a public spending of 3 per cent of the GDP, no analysis of the macroeconomic environment was made to assess the feasibility of such an open-ended definition of UHC. For, after all, UHC was politics—deciding who is to get what care, from whom, and at what cost and that, too, within financial constraints. In ignoring the tension between the public and private sectors, the overwhelming capacity of the private sector to undermine the public sector that continued to be the refuge of the poor, and in seeking to brush away the contradictions by saying that private sector could be 'contracted-in', the HLEG was being simplistic.

Positioning the HLEG report just at the start of the Twelfth Five Year Plan period without examining the programmatic, legal, and operational issues involved and pitching it as an alternative to the ongoing NRHM did more harm than good. It was a tactical blunder. It lost its case as being a serious option to be considered.

To bolster its argument, the HLEG listed the best practices of 16 countries—Thailand, the UK, Turkey, Brazil, Mexico, and so on. But there was nowhere an honest examination or analysis of on what elements and within what time frames and under what fiscal circumstances did these countries build their health systems, making them capable enough of implementing the UHC policy. For example, Thailand's journey to UHC started 30 years ago, not in 2001. Turkey went through a decade of implementing radical reforms such as banning private practice by government doctors, to cite one example, that enabled the launch of UHC. Most importantly, all these countries had strong public health systems that, in terms of quality, were on a par with the private sector. Nor were the implications of the implementation in China (which came closest to India in terms of a 'messy health system') examined. Evidence showed that under UHC, China had over 95 per cent of its population covered but barely half the population had access to services resulting in no impact on catastrophic expenditures, clearly and loudly pointing to the fact that UHC will have no effect if the supply side is dysfunctional.

Such an examination would have enabled the report to sequence the reform process and provide a road map for implementing its strategy. In leaving out key issues like the benefit package unaddressed, it left the field open for various interpretations of what UHC could and must mean in the Indian context. Besides, the lack of clarity on this fundamental issue thrust the whole question of the fiscal implications of this policy initiative into a black box. Nor did the report take a stand on what precisely the government must do and not do while coordinating with the private sector. For example, it recommended that medical colleges should be linked to district hospitals that ought to become knowledge hubs, but did not specify whether these colleges would be private or government. This entailed its own implications as on the basis of this logic, the MCI has now permitted private promoters to establish medical colleges provided they have an MOU with the government leasing out 300-bed facilities for 33 years or on a 99-year lease. And read with the recommendation that primary care centres can be outsourced to private providers, it was unclear as to how the costs would be contained if virtually the whole supply chain was to be contracted out. In the UK, the GP is private but wholly 'owned' by the government. The government also owns nearly all the hospitals and all medical education is within the university structure. This has enabled it to keep control on costs and the quality of care.

For all these reasons, the HLEG report generated controversy like no other report had. The debates and arguments between the Planning Commission and the health ministry basically reflected two viewpoints that continue to persist even today. One viewpoint believes in investing and strengthening the public sector, using the private sector to supplement its efforts, and a health system built on the foundations of a strong primary care that would prevent disease, promote wellness, and treat sickness in its early stages.

The other viewpoint, advocated by the then Planning Commission and now NITI Aayog, is to privatize healthcare and sustain it through a web of financing mechanisms and subsidies. Already the private sector is the pampered child with extensive custom- and excise-duty exemptions, 30 per cent tax exemptions on private insurance premiums, and credit from financial institutions. There are no regulations on where, how, and in what way to practice. Also, there is now a ready market through government-sponsored insurance policies with weak redressal mechanisms, no accountability, no risk, besides being focused on the profit-making inpatient care (some only provide surgical treatment).

Between these two views, the HLEG ought to have found in the government its natural ally. Unfortunately, it seemed to be pitted against the latter, even as the ministry stood alarmed and concerned at the selective manner in which the Planning Commission took advantage of some of its recommendations to push its privatization agenda. This huge miscommunication cost the NRHM dearly.

The harsh truth is that India has huge supply constraints in terms of the availability of doctors, paramedics, other supporting infrastructure and resources, rules, laws, regulations, implementing agencies, and enforcement mechanisms. If in urban areas almost every street has a diagnostic centre and a provider with all kinds of competencies, almost in half the country (where the poorest live and where the disease burden, particularly infectious diseases and RCH, is also highest) there is neither a public nor a private sector capable of providing even a modest package of essential services cash-free and, more importantly, hassle free. Secondly, there is also no clarity as to where the money will come from and the fiscal implications for the government in the medium term. For, after all, there is adequate evidence available that when the financial barriers are removed, there is a sharp increase in utilization that again needs to be managed. Thirdly, the assumption that there is a huge surplus capacity and all that is needed is to stimulate demand is not borne out by any evidence. Yet it is this assumption that seems to drive the policy for UHC/NHA.

For implementing UHC, India needs to undertake deep reforms in its macroeconomics as well as the health sector that it has little stamina for as repeatedly demonstrated by the political system. As addressing the supply imbalances call for taking hard decisions and making substantial investments of nearly 1 trillion, it is repeatedly overlooked. Instead, since politics in India is all about perception, it is so much easier to allocate some funds for insurance or schemes and leave it on the people and the states to make sense of it.

It was in this backdrop of confusion and 'betrayal' that there was a change of government. As has been argued all through in this book, health policy is closely linked to the fortunes of political parties. The priorities, perceptions, ideologies, and compulsions of the political leaders in power matter deeply to which way the pendulum swings.

NDA, May 2014

The general elections of 2014 brought the BJP to power on its own strength to form the government. The NDA's manifesto laid out an ambitious vision for health. Appointing an experienced minister who was also a doctor as the cabinet minister augured well. The minister flagged critical issues facing the health sector for his priority attention: reform of medical education; eradication of kala-azar and controlling infectious diseases; launching a national health assurance scheme; launching aggressive campaigns to contain non-communicable diseases by starting with anti-tobacco; and integrating Indian systems of medicine, particularly yoga, for overall wellness. Even while he held discussions, set up expert committees, and toured villages, he was suddenly dropped within a few months, bringing to a halt many of the initiatives he had started. A new set of priorities emerged, namely expansion of immunization coverage and the list of vaccines to be administered.

The two years under the NDA witnessed some rapid changes. In August 2014, the prime minister announced the abolition of the Planning Commission that was replaced by a three-member NITI Aayog by a cabinet resolution dated 1 January 2015. In February 2015, the report of the Fourteenth Finance Commission was submitted that enhanced the share of untied resources to be transferred to the states, promptly followed by the slashing of all central budget allocations for programmes that directly impacted the lives of the poor—the SSA, the MGNREGS, and the ICDS. While health, for the third year in a row, saw no increase in budgets, allocations for HIV/AIDS that again affects the survival of many poor were slashed and in September 2015, the department wound up instead of being expanded into a department of public health, thereby fulfilling a long-standing demand. Around this time, the RSBY was shifted to the health ministry, without its budget but for good measure. Disassociated with the health ministry, the RSBY had undermined the efforts being made by the NRHM in strengthening the functioning and quality of care delivered in public hospitals. By accrediting all and sundry private hospitals with a disregard for the quality or standards, the impact was weakened in terms of reducing out-of-pocket expenditures.

Even as the report prepared by some of us at the request of the ministry for rolling out the NHA was shelved, a hurriedly prepared NHP was put on the website in January 2015. Reportedly,

5,000 comments have been received. In February 2016, the draft health policy was approved by the CCHFW, while in the budget the NHA was rolled out for the BPL families, enhancing the sum assured under the RSBY from Rs 30,000 to Rs 100,000. Guidelines to implement the NUHM and UHC in a few districts have also been 'issued'. Clearly, this is a case of several darts being flung into the air in all directions.

NRHM: Current Status

The Twelfth Plan brought in some important changes. The NRHM is now called the National Health Mission (NHM). The NHM consists of four components: the NRHM, the NUHM, disease-control programmes, and non-communicable diseases. Second, the funds are no longer to be released to the state and district health societies but routed through the state finance departments. As of now, under the NUHM some guidelines have been issued that essentially appear to suggest a model similar to what was implemented in the rural areas. It is not clear whether there is any attempt at sharpening the design features based on evidence related to the epidemiology, health needs of the urban poor, infrastructural gaps, options to utilize alternate providers, and building the appropriate institutional capacity to implement and forge partnerships with the urban local bodies, or civil society, or social enterprises.

While there is a deafening silence on undertaking any reforms, the 2016 budget announced some new initiatives with far-reaching implications. Besides the NHA for the poor mentioned above, a new scheme called the National Dialysis Programme (NDP) has been launched. Under this scheme, district hospitals will be provided funding support to supply these services in a PPP mode. To further this scheme, custom and excise duties have been waived to facilitate import of the required equipments, going contrary to the government's 'Make in India' policy. The expenses for the NDP are to be met out of the NHM budget, further straining the already underfinanced mission that has over the last five years received about half the amount allocated under the Twelfth Plan as shown in Table 5.4.

TABLE 5.4 Budget Allocations for NRHM: 2007 to 2016–17 (Rs Crores)

Year (Rs in crores)	BE: NHM+ Health	RE/AE: NHM+ Health	RE/AE for NHM: Only NHM	NRHM during Eleventh Plan Year	NRHM during Eleventh Plan AE
2012–13	27,127	20,908.18 (AE)	16,763 (AE)	2007–8	10,380.40
2013–14	29,165	22,476.66 (AE)	18,215.44 (Est)	2008–9	11,239.33
2014–15	30,645	23,684.66 (AE)	18,039.30	2009–10	13,305.76
2015–16	24,549	25,799 (RE)	18,295 (RE)	2010–11	14,696.42
2016–17	31,300	–	19,000	2011–12	16,509.36
Total for Twelfth Plan	142,786	92,868.50	90,312.74		66,131.27
Total plan allocated in the Plan document	268,551		193,405		90,554
Release to total Plan (%)	53.17		46.70		73.03

Source: MOHFW, GOI. Does not include NACO.

Note: 100 crores equal to 1 billion. AE: actual expenditure, BE: budget estimates, and RE: revised estimates.

This is an important time and continuity of leadership would have helped. Instead there is a change in leadership in the NHSRC, even as the NRHM has its fourth minister, eighth health secretary, and the fifth mission director.

❧

The NRHM had too many objectives and too much rhetoric. It lacked clarity as it sought to take on more issues than it was capable of handling. The NRHM mandate of bringing in 'architectural corrections' to the rural health system resulted in a whole set of disparate activities being taken up. In soft-pedalling contentious issues pertaining to human resources, corruption, and governance and the failure to engage with, and encourage, a large number of research institutions to undertake operational research for providing evidence to make policy choices, the NRHM made itself vulnerable. The closed-door approach and failure to institutionalize the processes was the undoing of the NRHM, putting it in danger of being wound up in the Twelfth Plan. A missed opportunity was its inability to forge sound inter-sectoral linkages and making it an area of foundational importance—as over 0.4 million children under five continue to die due to waterborne and sanitation-related diseases—or to envision in real terms the roles of the public and private sectors among the several models offered by the NCMH and other publications.

The NRHM was the government's first serious and long-overdue attempt to revamp the rural health system. It injected substantial funds of the magnitude never witnessed before. By all counts and given the circumstances of frequent changes in leadership,[78] it has done well and covered substantial ground. What was needed was that the Twelfth Plan should simply have continued it with greater resources and better clarity based on the rich experiences gained in the actual implementation of such an ambitious vision. No system in any country has been revamped within five years. Instead of consolidating the gains made in the strengthening of the delivery system and expanding the efforts further based on the lessons learnt, the debate got diverted by the UHC issues, leaving one to wonder whether this was deliberate or the result of a poor understanding of how health systems evolve.

A close and critical review of the NRHM could provide valuable lessons. The first is the need to pay attention to detailed micro-planning with the implications for finances and human resources clearly mapped out, and building in interventions to address them. Malaysia, for example, pays significant attention to this aspect, referring to the process as 'bringing down planning from 300 feet to 30 feet'. The second is to ensure clarity about what is to be achieved by whom and by when and have guidelines that would enable standardization of the quality of services while scaling up the interventions. The third is to acknowledge the past so as not to repeat mistakes, understand and listen to the present, and read the future. The fourth is to focus on data analysis, evidence, and monitoring and accept its foundational importance while designing policy. And finally, expand the dialogue and listen to the voices of the stakeholders and key population groups who will be most affected by what the government does or does not do.

A last word: whatever be its shortcomings, one needs to understand the NRHM within the context of the huge challenges it was asked to face. The NRHM was a great experiment implemented against huge odds with a lot of dedication by several individuals. It is for the new leadership to build upon it and take the programme of NHM further to achieve the vision laid down in 2004.

NACP III and NRHM: Any Lessons to be Learnt?

I was posted as secretary in the Department of Health in 2009. Learning from the rich experience of NACO, I found the design of the NRHM confusing—too many objectives and too much rhetoric. Contrary to my expectations, I neither found the urgency of a mission nor a clarity of purpose. After all, the NRHM was to bring in 'architectural corrections' to the health system. Instead I found a range of a disparate set of activities that were not necessarily coordinated. The HMIS was concentrated in the hands of one individual and divorced from the statistical monitoring cell of the department, while the finance division was under a director-level officer, functioning with a set of consultants who had little experience in public health financing or audit. Both reported to the joint secretary of the NRHM and not to the mission director. The RCH flexi funds were being used in the RCH division whose joint secretary was an officer with no field experience in health at the state level and had been promoted from the post of director only the year before. The mission director, who was also new to health, coordinated the project.

There were no institutionalized fora that brought the states, civil society, experts or academicians, and other stakeholders together, nor were there any operational guidelines at that time. The 'thinking' came from the NHSRC, which in turn possibly consulted others, organized the CRMs, and so on. It was an atmosphere very different to the hands-on approach of NACO. The mood was celebratory all the way and even a question was seen as being 'anti-NRHM'. The approach smacked of an inexplicable air of arrogant fundamentalism that was intimidating.

Since then, there have been improvements: more use of data; greater focus and clearer operational guidelines spelling out the vision, mission, objectives, and so on; and a flood of interventions. Focus districts indicating the current status of infrastructure have been identified, enabling differential planning among and within districts and carving out areas for special attention: financial, human, and material resources on differential norms, outcome-linked funding alongside systematic reviews, and intensive monitoring.

All this sounds familiar and looking back, I wonder if NACO did have some lessons for the NRHM. Globally, it is acknowledged that the physical and financial efforts to mobilize a response to fight HIV/AIDS had several lessons for the health sector as a whole. In India, however, any attempt to learn from the NACP III experience was limited to the understanding that HIV is but one infection. Besides, the scale and sweep of both the programmes being vastly different, it was argued that drawing any comparisons between the two programmes would not stand scrutiny. This section challenges this understanding.

Questions arise as the NRHM was a far more complex and multidimensional programme covering the wide span of rural healthcare, promoting the well-being of the population as a whole living in highly varied geographies and circumstances. Besides, this vision had to be implemented with the states that owned the staff and other variables. Every state had its own ideas and preferences. It was not a vertical programme to be implemented on priority and at the risk of overlooking patient needs.

While so, the HIV/AIDS control programme was a vertically funded programme where the expenditures incurred on staff and other incidentals were fully funded by NACO. There was also a uniform understanding and clarity on the objectives and strategy of the HIV/AIDS programme. Though focusing on one particular disease, it had varied aspects. However, the central theme and causal factors being the same, it enabled forging cross-linkages, standardization, and scaling up.

The point, however, is not in the content and bandwidth of the issues being addressed, but that both had their own dimension of complexities and were, in the ultimate sense, management challenges. In other words, the principles of management do not vary whether you are selling just Coke or, with it, the chips too. And management is as much about leadership as it is about the work culture, accountability frameworks, and monitoring the systems put in place. Besides, in actual reality, the NRHM was never a movement and due to the manner in which it panned out, it soon became yet another centrally sponsored project with defined budgets and terms of reference. From the start, it was focused on one single programme of promoting reproductive and child health, which became, inter alia, the proxy for the revival and functioning of the primary health system. This then narrows the incomparability factor between the NACP and the NRHM. And what makes such comparison interesting is that though both the NACP III and the NRHM were launched at the same time, within similar political contexts and constraints, they had two different outcomes—one a success and the second a work in progress. The question is why?

There are six broad reasons that could possibly help provide a productive hypothesis.

Use of Evidence

The NACP strategies were based on evidence originating from various and multiple sources that helped identify the target groups and the states and districts to concentrate upon. Nearly half-a-dozen institutions were engaged in this effort and NACO itself had over a dozen people monitoring data. The NRHM, too, had various sources of data and evidence but had no mechanisms to actively incorporate the IIPS and other institutional apparatus to analyse and interpret the data so as to identify districts and map the vulnerable population groups requiring focused attention. Based on a set of criteria, the states and districts could have been categorized and graded in order of criticality to arrive at the nature and quantum of resource support required for achieving the goals. Such categorizations were possible as data was available that showed that three-quarters of maternal and child mortality were concentrated in one-third of the districts just as malaria was predominantly prevalent in half-a-dozen states, while kala-azar was confined to a few blocks in two states and so on. Grading based on the capacity of the health system and epidemiology could have helped in differential planning for the purpose of allocating human and financial resources, besides providing special management structures to monitor closely. Funds would then have followed need than be frittered thinly all over and utilized by states having a higher ability to absorb and make use of. Such approaches of prioritization become vital when funds are limited, time is short, and disparities on certain key indicators are wide.

Related to the use of evidence is the value of mapping as a means of bringing about architectural correction—one of the primary goals of the NRHM. NACO used various strategies for mapping out key population groups and facilities and juxtaposing that data with the prevalence levels for guiding investment decisions. Mapping of all health facilities would have helped identify not only which services and capacities were available and where but, superimposed with epidemiological information, it would have also helped point out the gaps that need to be filled on priority. The linkage between programme needs and availability of funds for infrastructure under the NRHM flexi funds would have demonstrated the necessity of prioritizing investments. Mapping would have yielded information on the existing inefficiencies, gaps, the duplication within the system due to wrong siting of facilities, or the absence of the availability of even the bare minimum of inputs, making them non-functional. It would have given information on the spread of not-for-profit and missionary institutions to co-opt and widen the delivery base. The three-tier model of primary care had been structured over five decades ago. Much has changed with improved road connectivity and technology making many facilities redundant. In other words, mapping enables an evidence-based gap analysis for enabling greater efficiencies of resource-use and optimizing outcomes. But this was not done and absence of such vital data for planning and prioritizing is still not seen as a handicap.

Stakeholder Involvement

Given the global concern and the stigma attached to HIV/AIDS, the approach had to be inclusive with all stakeholders actively involved. The NACP was an open participatory effort. Such participation was institutionalized through the TRGs where the sex workers or people living with HIV/AIDS were involved, alongside donors, state governments, and civil society, in the finalization of the design of the interventions and also in all the implementational processes: data collection, ART centres, and the STD clinics. They advised, implemented and monitored, and shared responsibility, such as mopping up those lost to follow-up for treatment. If NACO had 18 TRGs with over 300 experts reflecting on programmatic issues, the NRHM also had several platforms—MSG, EC, AGCA, AMG, and so on—but had almost the same group of people rotate in them. Besides, the two fora for NGO engagement that were set up were relegated to two institutions outside the ministry, engaging with mid-level officials. There were no platforms for the chief policy and decision-maker to interact and understand the issues and constraints for bringing in the desired corrections. The design of such dialogue was faulty as the engagement with civil society was perfunctory. This was unfortunate as a reading of the minutes of the AMG and AGCA meetings show that several excellent suggestions had indeed been made but were never addressed. Over time, even this limited engagement petered out.

Technical Support

Communitization was a goal that was common to both the programmes. Yet while the NACP provided 25 per cent of its budget to NGOs and collectives, the NRHM spent none. Even the funds that were mandatorily released to village panchayats and hospital committees were inadequate and not followed up with reviews and guidance. In the NACP, community participation was structured and capacity-building of the recipients as well as implementers a key activity. For this, NACO innovated the establishment of TSUs to build such capacity. Under the NRHM, the SHRCs were expected to do the same and focus on the ASHA, just as the

Chhattisgarh SHSRC did on the Mitanin. But such was not the case and not every state had an SHSRC. Besides, while TSUs had a clear mandate and were monitored, SHSRCs did everything and were responsible for nothing. Most often they duplicated or supplemented the directorate. Few, however, brought greater competencies than were available with the directorates. The concept of TSUs as implemented by NACO was, however, adopted for the immunization programme under which the BMGF positioned some 40 to 50 people in the PHFI to work with the ministry on the various aspects of the roll-out and scaling up of immunization. This is in addition to the WHO-funded polio eradication group that is now engaged with routine immunization as well.

Communitization is a process and a resource-intensive activity that is heavily focused on training on a concurrent basis. In addition to the TSUs, NACO had a network of 11 institutions training the NGOs and community members and 45 schools of social work capacitated for training counsellors. Such systems were weak in the NRHM and with low priority for reviving the training institutions, it became impossible to train male workers for the sub-centres and a great challenge to train ASHAs for HBNC.

Standardization for Scaling Up

Simple and easy-to-read operational guidelines were the key to communicate the goals, objectives, and content of the interventions. NACO had over 40 such guidelines that the state and district teams were trained upon and were familiar with. The NRHM had no such guidelines, which resulted in every state and district functionary interpreting the mission in their own way. In 2010, this concept of operational guidelines was introduced into the NRHM programme and since then several guidelines have been issued. Barring a few, most are difficult to read and understand as they are complex with too many objectives and lack clarity. Besides, the NACO guidelines were used for budgeting resource allocations, since all activities were protocol-driven and costed. That was not the case with the NRHM guidelines, making it difficult to implement the many actions indicated therein.

Monitoring

The NACP was intensively monitored and such monitoring was also structured with a view to inculcate habits. For example, in fixing the weekly meeting, it got the division heads hold their own reviews two days before. Likewise, indepth tours on a monthly and quarterly basis were also routinized. Every review was minuted and action taken reviewed. Bimonthly meetings with the PD of SACS helped iron out pendencies and clarify operational issues. The NRHM had no such formalized systems of review and monitoring. Much of it was outsourced to the NHSRC that conducted a structured annual review of the NRHM implementation called the CRM. In the initial years, the NRHM also held several workshops, but largely for sharing ideas and experiences. It was only in 2010 that the practice of holding structured reviews with the state health secretaries on the implementation of the various programmes started. Such reviews also brought back attention to infectious diseases-control programmes that until then were operating outside of the NRHM though integrated on paper. Structured reviews have a different purpose than workshops for experience sharing. Reviews are the most important instrument to get feedback on how the programme is doing, on the understanding key functionaries at the implementation level have of the schemes, on the difficulties they experience with the central guidelines, and so on.

Organizational Structure

Structures reflect intent and priority. The management organization is the main instrument for implementing policy. Realizing the importance of this aspect, NACO provided an organogram consisting of nine divisions, each having a full-fledged team at NACO and in SACS. This helped in ensuring accountability. For one infection, NACO (of the ministry) had 150 people working alongside scores of others in donor organizations and institutions. The NRHM office in the ministry had one mission director assisted by two joint secretaries and two directors who in turn had a couple of doctors, consultants, and clerical staff. The organizational structures were not aligned with the responsibilities, accountabilities, and reporting systems. For example, infectious diseases were to be 'under the MD of the NRHM' but the programmes were being monitored by another joint secretary and the DGHS directly under the guidance of the secretary. Likewise, even while communitization was a core principle—the main feature of the architectural correction—it was outsourced to the NHSRC and the PFI with no team within the ministry dedicated to monitor and convert into policy the many actions required. Such dysfunctionalism was present in the states as well, as the NRHM sought to become a vertical but integrated programme where the MD of the NRHM had the money and the mandate but not the power over those implementing the programme activities.

Leadership

The culture built in the implementation of the NACP was very different to that prevailing in the NRHM. Not only were all stakeholders—key population groups, media, judiciary, civil society groups, sectoral departments, state governments, academic institutions, professional organizations, and so on—directly engaged but most were also active participants in policymaking and the implementation of the policies. The wide, open, and transparent culture enabled building in a host of leaders at all levels. In fact, the success of the HIV/AIDS battle was largely because of the consistent leadership provided to the cause by several dedicated leaders, who were committed and knew the history. This was not the case with the NRHM. Participation was restricted not only in terms of the people but was also confined to meetings. There was no consistent leadership committed to what the NRHM stood for and ensure that the political will stayed focused on the goals and promises. This was its biggest shortcoming and the reason for the fall in momentum and enthusiasm. For example, in the supplementary budget of 2015, HIV/AIDS was the only programme that had its budget restored, largely because of media editorials and the persistent efforts of PLHAs and civil society leaders. No such activism or pressure was seen when the budgets were being cut for the NRHM. That, then, is the difference. In other words, the

NRHM did not invest enough resources on building a constituency of stakeholders.

The aforementioned seven aspects of programme management highlight the need for the ministry in the centre and states to expand and open their systems to co-opt the talents and expertise outside the government, restructure their own organizations to meet the emerging challenges, and focus on laying down systems that provide stability and resilience to the organization. In the recent past, NACO has faced some challenges, yet because of the systems put in, there is a certain resilience that can make recovery under a good leader possible. That is not the case with the NRHM programme where in outsourcing data management and monitoring functions to the NHSRC, the ministry appears to have lost touch with reality giving the impression of being out of control.

Notwithstanding this, the implementation of both the programmes highlighted a common limiting factor. Neither a vertical nor a horizontal 'integrated' approach can scale up efficiently unless the underlying issues related to the health system are not resolved, such as private practice by government doctors, posting and transfer of human resources, the policy pertaining to the private sector, and so on. Clearly, while deep reforms in health financing and governance are urgently required for bringing about transformative changes in the health sector, the two studies of the NACP III and the NRHM implemented during the period from 2005–12 showed how much can be done even with an incremental increase in funds and political support. The outcomes relative to the size of the problem and constraints of history were impressive. Yet they were inadequate calling for a higher ambition.

For two decades India has been faced with an inability, bordering on paralysis, to take decisions and to provide a direction. The country's public policy is confused and lost in its own rhetoric. On the one hand, it persistently denies any attempt at 'privatization' of the health sector, while on the other its every policy helps in strengthening the private sector and weakening the public sector.

But this strategy of starving the public sector of resources and allowing it to be haemorrhaged is not sustainable. Similarly, the policy of refusing to regulate the sector is also going to be problematic due to the externalities, information asymmetry, missing markets, and other types of market failures that are inherent to the health sector. In no country has a pure private-sector model in healthcare worked and India simply cannot be naive enough to think it can be an exception to this rule. The continued neglect of, and the inability to address, serious challenges facing the health sector by successive governments seem to suggest that policymakers are either not realizing the gravity of the situation or perhaps have no will for the long haul of reform.

Notes and References

1. The Right to Education, the Right to Food, and banning of scavenging were products of the UPA II (2009–14).
2. The NAC had no real power but it had the prestige that proximity to Sonia Gandhi gave it. Following from that, it had access to all policies and authorities to lobby for people or ideas.
3. The wife of Montek Singh Ahluwalia who was the then deputy chairman of the Planning Commission. However, Isher Ahluwalia is an internationally well-known economist in her own right.
4. R.L. Misra, who was the health secretary in 1992, Rachel Chatterjee, and I co-authored this book. It was the first comprehensive diagnostic of India's health system.
5. NCMP, available at http://nceuis.nic.in/NCMP.htm (accessed on 31 August 2016).
6. Javed Chowdhry, the former secretary of health and family welfare, prepared an internal report for the ministry on why and how these three institutions were shut down. It was only under intense pressure of the PSC that they were revived and made functional.
7. The health minister's letter to the PM, dated 29 September 2004.
8. Letter of secretary, dated 25 October 2004.
9. The Rural Health Services (RHS) division was a very insignificant part of the ministry with barely a couple of people working in it.
10. Post 1995, the family planning programme had changed to Reproductive and Child Health (RCH) programme. It was an important programme headed by a joint secretary, while another joint secretary (Policy) looked after family planning.

11. Dr Antia was a well-known plastic surgeon-turned-health activist from Mumbai where he established the Foundation for Research in Community Health (FRCH); Dr Imrana was professor of Community Medicine in JNU; Abhay Shukla was a health activist from Maharashtra and was working with an NGO called the Centre for Enquiry into Health and Allied Themes (CEHAT), and Dr Mira Shiva was a Delhi-based health activist (discussion with Mira Shiva).
12. Around this time, there were several small experiments coming up for furthering community-based approaches. The chief minister convened a high-level meeting with some NGOs. I was also invited to one such meeting. Ravi Narayan of the Community Health Cell in Karnataka later evaluated the JSR that influenced the designing of the ASHA programme.
13. In an interview with Thelma Narayan (2014).
14. In an interview with Mira Shiva (2014).
15. In 2012, I met Gopal an hour before he left for Kerala. I asked him who had conceived the idea of the NRHM. Too physically weak to answer, he pointed his finger at himself. I bid him goodbye and promised to await my interview with him. I never knew that I would not see him again. A few days later he died of cancer.
16. The JSA was at the forefront of promoting community-based approaches to health. Their People's Health Charter of 2000 advocated a CHW for every village.
17. Minutes of the meeting (September 2005).
18. Minutes of the meeting (September 2005).
19. Minutes of the meeting (2006).
20. Sundararaman in an interview, Delhi (2013).
21. Personal interview with Sundararaman, New Delhi (2013).
22. Sundararaman in an interview (2013).
23. Abhay Shukla, 2005, 'NRHM: Hope or Disappointment', *Indian Journal of Public Health*, 49(3): 127–32; D. Banerji, 2005, 'Politics of Rural Health in India', *Indian Journal of Public Health*, 49(3): 113–22.
24. Quoted in the *Telegraph* on 8 February 2004. Romesh Thapar used this phrase to ridicule Rajiv Gandhi's government which, he alleged, was formed of Western-educated elites.
25. 'These issues were repeatedly discussed in the AGCA—often not minuted and also therefore not acted upon' (Thelma Narayan of CHC, Bangalore, in an interview in Bangalore [December 2014]).
26. Shukla's email dated 13 October 2005.
27. In fact, one of the task forces was specifically meant to oversee the role of the private sector and the recommendation was for strict

regulation. This, however, was not pursued as an equally critical part of the strategy to strengthen the public sector.

28. Admittedly, the public and private roles are linked to political economy and are discussed in the context of financing and provisioning of services in the three domains of primary, secondary (specialist), and tertiary (super specialist) care. The NCMH had sought to provide some demarcation—a dominant role of the public sector in primary care as both provider and financier, a mixed one in secondary care but funded dominantly by public revenues, and a tertiary sector dominated by private sector and social health insurance with public funding to protect people below the poverty line. These issues merited discussion and debate but were ignored as the views of civil society prevailed over the government that continued to be in denial of the private sector.
29. Tarun Seem, the former director the NRHM, in an interview (2014).
30. Ashtekar Shyam, 2008, 'The National Rural Health Mission: A Stocktaking', *Economic & Political Weekly*, 43(37): 23–26; Ravi Duggal, 2009, 'Sinking Flagships and Health Budgets in India', *Economic and Political Weekly,* 14(33): 14–17; Vikas Bajpai and Anoop Saraya, 2012, 'NRHM—the Panacea for Rural Health in India: A Critique', *Global Journal of Medicine and Public Health*, 1(3): 24–30; Ashish Bose, 2010, 'Whither NRHM', *Economic & Political Weekly*, 45(6).
31. Jalaja in an interview (2013). Such centralization was inevitable as in the early stages, there can be only one leader. Besides, Hota was involved with the NRHM since the first day of its inception.
32. Kerala, for example, trained ASHAs right from the start in counselling and actively engaged them in the District Mental Health Programme (DMHP).
33. The SHSRC in Chhattisgarh was constituted by Alok Sinha, the health secretary of the new government of Chhattisgarh, and facilitated in 2002 under the EU-assisted Strategic Implementation Plan (SIP) that roped in Action Aid, a well-known international NGO, to help set it up. It made sense as Chhattisgarh, being a new state, had no SIHFW of its own.
34. Thelma Narayan of CHC, Bangalore, in an interview (2014).
35. In fact as a secretary, I tended to look more towards the NHSRC to operationalize some of my thoughts and ideas than to my joint secretary since the former was quick on the uptake and agile. The quality of examination of issues that was done by the director and the joint secretary-level officials in the late 1990s has reduced, partly

due to an overload of work and partly because of the availability of the lazy options of having the NHSRC do the analysis work—an option we did not have in the past when we had to do all analysis by ourselves.

36. Tarun Seem in an interview (2014).
37. Seeing this anachronism, at one time, I did think about keeping the identity of the NHSRC intact but merging it into the NIHFW and SHSRCs with the SIHFWs. That might have resulted in institutionalizing the work and impacted government thinking and work culture over time. This was much needed as both the NIHFW and SIHFWs continue to be 'associated' with family planning and training in the old style. The chairman of the board of the NIHFW is the minister of health. In terms of attention or resources, it is of least importance, reflecting in some way the priority we accord to institution-building and fostering knowledge.
38. Discussion with Tarun Seem. This idea and rhetoric of health plans based on household surveys was borrowed from the Sarva Shiksha Abhiyan. But the differences in the two sectors were not taken into account.
39. Tarun Seem, the former director of the NRHM, in an interview (2014).
40. CMO, East Godavari District, Andhra Pradesh, 2014.
41. Shyam, 'The National Rural Health Mission'.
42. This, I believe, is an important issue. Odisha, for example, has a substantial number of malaria cases, which is also the reason for high levels of child and maternal mortality. Preventing malaria by investing in long-lasting impregnated bed nets may have been better value for money and would have achieved better outcomes as was witnessed in Ethiopia.
43. The then health secretary would keep requesting for permission to co-opt the missionary hospitals and other nursing homes for Rs 3,000 per delivery. My site visits showed that the charges for a normal delivery were Rs 600. In hindsight, our hesitation was providential as with time massive corruption unfolded in Uttar Pradesh.
44. Rural Health Statistics, 2012, Statistics Division, MOHFW, GOI.
45. Tarun Seem in an interview (2014).
46. Undoubtedly, disease-control programmes got a stepmotherly treatment. Among those suffering from malaria were young illiterate males in rural areas who spent over Rs 213 per episode getting treatment if they survived since 80 per cent of all malaria was the deadly P. falciparum. Yet surveillance was weak and budget expenditure reduced

between 2005 and 2009. See Indrani Gupta and Shamik Chowdhury, 2014, 'Burden of Malaria in India: The Need for Effective Spending', *Journal of Public Health*, 3(January–March): 95–102.

47. A study conducted by Tej Ram in 2013 showed that in Madhya Pradesh—a high-focus state—while no data was available for 20 per cent of the district hospitals, 56 per cent of them were found to be functioning suboptimally. Tej Ram Jat and Miguel San Sebastian, 2013, 'Technical Efficiency of Public District Hospitals in Madhya Pradesh, India: A Data Envelopment Analysis', *Global Health Action*, available at http://www.globalhealthaction.net/index.php/gha/article/view/21742 (accessed on 15 September 2016).

48. S. Prinja, P. Bahuguna, R. Gupta, A. Sharma, S.K. Rana, and R. Kumar, 2015, 'Coverage and Financial Risk Protection for Institutional Delivery: How Universal Is Provision of Maternal Health Care in India?', *PLoS ONE*, 10(9): 1–15.

49. Provocation from a visit to a sub-centre in Madhya Pradesh that had a labour room, a ward, three staff, a telephone, and a full-time van to rush a case to the district hospital and was conducting 70 deliveries a month. Due to the rush of cases, the staff was not deputed for SBA training. The PHC located in the interior with no case load had highly trained staff and a higher budget.

50. Margaret C. Hogan, Kyle J. Foreman, Mohsen Naghavi, Stephanie Y. Ahn, et al., 2010. 'Maternal Mortality for 181 Countries, 1980–2008: A Systematic Analysis of Progress towards Millennium Development Goal 5', *The Lancet*, 375(9726): 1609–23.

51. Sample Registration System Bulletin (2012).

52. As per a decision of the prime minister's task force in 2007, 18 million households have been surveyed by the RGI on an annual basis since 2010–11.

53. The NCMH Report of 2005, for example, had clearly brought out evidence for a district-based differential approach.

54. CRHP website (accessed in 2014).

55. According to a 2008 evaluation, childhood mortality showed a 30 per cent reduction in risk, infant mortality fell from over 200 to 20 per 1,000 live births, malnutrition dropped to less than 15 per cent, and immunization rates were 99 per cent for measles, DPT, and OPV.

56. The Coordinating Agency for Health Planning (CAHP), the VHAI, the MFC, and so on.

57. Shrivastava Committee Report, 1975. This recommendation later led to the appointment of the Village Health Guide Scheme in 1977.

58. This was followed by several attempts by different states: the CHW in the tribal areas of Andhra Pradesh; the Jan Swasthya Rakshak (JSR) in Madhya Pradesh, Mitanin in Chhattisgarh, Saathi in Rajasthan, Saheli in Jharkhand, and so on.
59. A jatra literally means a journey. It signifies dramatic campaigns involving songs, street theatre, and the like.
60. At the ASHA Mentoring Group meeting (4 August 2009).
61. NHSRC, 2011, 'ASHA: Which Way Forward? Evaluation of ASHA Programme', available at http://nhsrcindia.org/download.php?downloadname=pdf_files/resources_thematic/Community_Participation/NHSRC_Contribution/ASHA_Which_way_forward_-Evalaution_of_ASHA_Programme_Report_NHSRC_417.pdf (accessed on 31 August 2016).
62. Abhay Bang, a doctor from Gadchiroli, Maharashtra, stated this at the fifth meeting held on 4 August 2009.
63. Recently, the government has permitted ANMs to administer injectable gentamicin. This is a positive step as weak transportation and non-availability of authorized personnel to provide antibiotics continue to be one of the major reasons for the large numbers of neonates dying of respiratory failure.
64. In NACO, for every 10 TIs, a supervisor paid Rs 25,000 per month was appointed and monitored. Under the NRHM, I do not recall having ever reviewed the implementation of this aspect of the programme.
65. The NHSRC is in the process of designing a course for ASHAs and have them accredited by the National Institute of Open Schooling. This will help weed out those who have no aptitude and also ensure standards.
66. S. Jalaja, the mission director at the inaugural meeting of the AGCA in October 2006.
67. 'The AGCA was negotiating with me and through me in these matters.... If only the AGCA had negotiated with the JS directly, perhaps the gains of the pilot phase could have been preserved and scaled up' (personal communication with Tarun Seem [2014]).
68. These are actual expenditures incurred and include expenditure against the state share, so there is a discrepancy between the figures of expenditure and those relating to 'releases' by the GOI.
69. Thelma Narayan in an interview in Bangalore (2014).
70. At that time, I was the secretary of the ministry. Normally, when governments constitute committees, the procedure is that the concerned department be consulted, informed, and perhaps even

included, so that there is a greater chance of 'ownership' at the time of implementation of recommendations. This process was not followed. Besides, the departmental representative to such committees is also normally appointed by the department after seeking orders of the minister or secretary depending on the level and importance of the committee.

71. Many of them, however, related to me that they had no time to read the report and they supported it only because it called for a greater commitment of government resources to health.

72. A member of the HLEG and also of the MSG, the PHFI, the NAC, and so on.

73. [A] managed care organization is responsible for managing the care of a population through a health care system that: monitors and coordinates care through the entire range of services (primary care through tertiary services); emphasizes prevention and health education; encourages the provision of care in the most appropriate setting and by the most appropriate provider (e.g. outpatient clinics versus hospitals, primary care physicians versus specialists); promotes the cost-effective use of services through aligning incentives (e.g. by capitation of providers, cost-sharing by consumers).

See Neelam K. Sekhri, 2000, 'Managed Care: the US Experience', *Bulletin of the World Health Organization*, 78(6): 830–44.

74. Sundararaman in an interview, New Delhi (2014). This was also confirmed to me by some of the members like Yogesh Jain and others.

75. Srinath Reddy and Mathur Mani Raj, 2015, 'Universal Health Coverage: Question of Workability in India', Public Health Foundation of India, unpublished.

76. This was sadly ironic as many of the vocal members of the HLEG were also members of almost every committee set up under the NRHM and had, in a way, 'fathered it' all along.

77. The complete blank on the NRHM was surprising considering that the HLEG had several members who were in all the committees of the NRHM and were, or at least should have been, aware of the problems of the implementing policy.

78. During the period from 2005–12, there were two health ministers, five health secretaries, and four MDs of the NRHM.

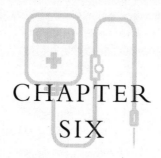

CHAPTER SIX

Making Our Future

*I*n the first part of the book, three arguments were offered to explain the current crisis in India's health sector: low funding priority for health in the development agenda, weak governance, and an indifferent leadership. The two narratives in Part II of the book added one more to the aforementioned list: the lack of stability in policy that seems to be in constant motion only to stay in the same place. It has been the case of taking two steps forward and one step back, adding new schemes, and shifting goalposts year after year. Yet, notwithstanding the continued weak political support and knee-jerk, patchy responses to the crisis, the future does hold potential, which *if* taken advantage of, can be beneficial, but *if not*, can cause more human suffering, widen disparities, and hurt the economy in the long run.[1] In matters of health, the price of neglect can have long-term consequences that can be quite devastating.

From the point of view of public policy, there is an urgent need to move away from incrementalism and acknowledge the complexity of rebuilding the existing inefficient health system. The policies and strategies should be evidence-based, embedded within the socio-economic context of the country, and devised on the basis of a close study of the past failures and an uncompromising commitment to equity and fairness.

All through the text, and particularly at the end of the chapters on finance and governance, suggestions on what needs to be done have been made. Arising from those set of issues, I list out five areas that, I think, India needs to attend to comprehensively: a) strengthening the process of decentralization and cooperative federalism, b) revamping the delivery system—both public and private—for achieving the objective of Health for All, c) strengthening the people's sector, d) expanding the use of technology, and e) acknowledging the value of evidence and knowledge. Building a consensus around these issues can be tedious but is vital. But then, shaping the future has never been easy.

Strengthening Decentralization and Cooperative Federalism

The impact of excessive centralization in distorting priorities, particularly in terms of resource utilization and better quality of implementation, is widely recognized by most scholars. It is for this reason that the recent policy focus on strengthening of the notion of cooperative federalism is seen as a step in the right direction, setting a wrong right. The actualization of this notion implies shifting the arena for planning, designing, and implementation to the states. The challenge lies in managing the transition of the power of decision-making to states while ensuring at the same time that all states stay faithful to the script of achieving the laid out national goals.

But such decentralization is easier said than done. Despite the commitment to strengthen cooperative federalism (an argument used to justify the slashing of central grants in the 2015 budget on subjects that fall in the states' domain), in the 2016 budget, the central government unilaterally announced two national schemes: the National Dialysis Services Programme, that is to be implemented in district hospitals in a PPP mode (accompanied by custom-duty waivers for importing the required equipment and consumables), and a threefold increase in the sum assured for hospital treatment from Rs 30,000 to Rs 100,000 under the RSBY. Neither of the two initiatives addresses the core issues plaguing the health sector. Instead, the announcements do curtail the states' autonomy to decide what is best for their people. For, what does a dialysis unit or a health voucher worth Rs 100,000 mean to the people of, say, Shravasti (the most backward district of Uttar Pradesh) that has a building which is an apology for a district hospital, or Vaishali in Bihar with a district hospital that has eight beds? Likewise, where is the evidence to show that the RSBY has been useful in terms of reducing out-of-pocket expenditures? Giving up the power of patronage is not easy, particularly when such policies benefit powerful constituencies such as the for-profit private sector, which in the current environment of lax regulations and weak competition from the public sector stand to benefit the most.

On the other hand, the states have the historical legacy of neglecting and according low priority to health, causing understandable anxiety and some apprehension. Health per se does not get votes, building a world-class capital and flyovers do. And within the health sector, the hiatus between what needs to be done and what yields political dividends is an even more serious problem. An expensive cochlear transplant provided free-of-cost to the child of an agricultural labourer in a corporate hospital grabs media headlines, not the fact that millions of children are today safe from a lifelong disability like polio or premature death due to measles. The same optics focus on earmarking seats in a private school for the poor instead of demanding that government schools be substantially improved and brought on par with the private ones.

Limited resources force looking at issues in binary terms: public or private, prevention or medical treatment, tertiary care or primary care, and so on. Choices are made in accordance with political expediency. In such a scenario and in the absence of well-defined national goals based on norms and principles, the apprehensions about whether the mere availability of additional funds will indeed stimulate states to redraw their priorities seem real.

Addressing these apprehensions will then require paying attention to two important aspects: a) providing a national vision with goals guiding what needs to be achieved by when, and b) building data and information to guide such goal-setting and policy directions.

National Vision and Goal-setting

Both the central and state governments then stand challenged. To realize the benefits of cooperative federalism, states need to be committed to a set of national goals. These goals cannot be only in terms of aggregate targets, such as reducing maternal mortality to less than 100 per 100,000 live births or infant mortality to below 30 per 1,000 live births by 2010.[2] Such targets mean little as the disparities between Kerala and Bihar or Uttar Pradesh are very wide since these states have different socio-economic contexts and capacities to deliver. Aspirational goals set within unrealistic time frames and poor resources are not taken seriously.

Given the substantial inter- and intra-district differentials, both in terms of implementational capacity and epidemiology, goals and targets should be based on an assessment of state and district data. Besides, qualitative targets need to also reflect a national vision based on values, such as assuring equal treatment to all citizens or ensuring non-denial of care in an achievable, understandable, and measurable manner. Such differential planning will enable ranking under key indicators—both quantitative and qualitative.

Such meaningful goal-setting requires reliable data; expertise in epidemiology, biostatistics, health economics; an understanding of the resource capacity to implement interventions aimed at achieving the laid-down goals at the state and district levels; and state- and district-wise assessment of fiscal capacity. Costing of interventions will enable estimating the fiscal implications. Modelling of options that may include the impact of procrastination on the economy and social stability will help understand the trade-offs.

Equalization of Funds

Goal-setting along the aforementioned lines defines and drives the agency role of the central and state governments. And when costed, goals not only help measure the relative distance from the national mean—a distance that the fiscally weaker states and districts will need to traverse—but also help determine the additional resources that will need to be mobilized for bridging the gap.

The principle of differential treatment by the central government was indeed acknowledged while designing the NRHM by prioritizing 18 states requiring additional assistance from the centre. Accordingly, these high-focus states were eligible for 0.3 per cent more funds than the rest. But in the absence of any idea about the resource gap, this policy was ineffective in making the desired impact.

In other words, in the face of the wide interstate differentials in resource needs and endowments and given that the health sector has significant interstate externalities and a strong redistributive element in terms of enhancing equity, ensuring a certain essential standard of services for all citizens irrespective of their place of birth needs to be the basis for the discourse on cooperative federalism and decentralization. This, then, takes the dialogue and the complexity of policy to a much higher plane than the simplistic approach of the NRHM. Adopting such a policy will, however, not be easy and would require a consensus. This would be required in view of the fact that the low-performing districts account for three-quarters of the country's disease burden and have weak delivery systems.[3]

Political expediency influences resource allocations more than is often acknowledged. In low-resource environments and with competing demands, the politics of prioritization get even more accentuated and take on a much more intensive political character, particularly if there are elections around the corner. The process of negotiation in plural political systems is tough. Transferring huge amounts to states where the ruling party is not aligned or denying funds to a potential ally can be problematic for the political party in power at the centre. But this is precisely where the national vision and evidence-based goal-setting can help the centre rise above partisanship in order to alleviate the welfare and well-being of the weakest sections of society. Besides, forging consensus towards promoting values of sharing and concerns for equity is what leadership is all about.

Canada, for example, earmarks financial transfers to states for health and education.[4] Such transfers are conditional to states achieving certain normative benchmarks aimed at universal access and uniform quality of health services. The fact that the 14th Finance Commission erred in not earmarking a certain proportion of the enhanced devolution for health and education is indicative of the absence of such values determining our national discourse. The commission was technically right that it is the elected state governments that have to make choices and lay down priorities. But it is equally right that in unequal societies, the voices of the poor are barely heard and thus there has to be a national vision that defines development and binds all states as equal partners to be held accountable. Or else, what explains the woeful neglect of providing tap water or toilets or clean air to all citizens? Aren't these the most basic needs that elected governments should have felt obliged to provide on priority?

Revamping the Delivery System

One of the core principles of the NRHM was making architectural corrections to the delivery system, which it did but only partially—institutionalization of some sort of community engagement, providing for people's oversight in the functioning of facilities, bringing in some management changes, and so on. It was tinkering—merely strengthening the existing government delivery system in the primary care space and that, too, in an ad hoc, patchy fashion. The revamping of the delivery system within the context of achieving access to affordable healthcare should have been the driving factor.

Revamping the delivery system, then, must consist of three distinct components on which the government needs to construct a comprehensive vision: a) to universalize access to comprehensive primary care and public goods free-of-cost; b) in view of the resource constraints, to ensure fully subsidized treatment in secondary and tertiary hospitals and institute some amount of co-sharing of expenditures by those who have the capacity to pay; and c) to enforce a rule of law to check the current laissez-faire environment and ensure that the provider practice is ethical and rational.

Primary Care and Public Goods

The WHO has defined primary care as the first level of contact for individuals, the family, and the community with the national health system, bringing healthcare as close as possible to where people live and work; primary care also constitutes the first element of a continuing healthcare process.[5] Drawing from this, scholars have made a distinction between primary care and primary healthcare. While primary care implies family physicians providing individual care on a long-term basis, primary healthcare consists of individual care alongside population health and includes concepts of equity and universality. Such a definition is further broken down to define primary care to consist of person-focused health services that are accessible when first needed and are comprehensive, integrated, and coordinated with the other components of the health system.[6]

On the face of it, this definition sounds simple, logical, and reasonable. But in terms of implementation, it is far more challenging and complex than running a nursing home. Primary care deals with a large amount of uncertainty and a wide range of variables and possibilities that may range from genetic, behavioural, and environmental to cultural, calling for alertness and timely referrals. This is why primary care is neither low-cost nor is it something that paramedics can provide all by themselves without the support of the medically qualified. In programmatic terms, such care implies access to a qualified provider in times of need—someone who has the capacity and authority to refer to higher levels of care as and when required. Such a definition, then, has to be, ideally, the basis for designing the health system architecture.

In the absence of such thinking, capacities, and ambition, and with the NRHM having a tenuous linkage with social determinants and an obsessive concern about institutional deliveries and RCH, the services being provided in the primary-care settings in India are few and fragmented. Consequentially, there is little evidence to empirically demonstrate the effectiveness of primary care and that it is deserving of resources and policy attention. For example, US data shows that over a decade of focusing on primary care, there was a 36 per cent reduction in hospital days, 42 per cent reduction in emergency, and a 25 per cent increase in childhood immunizations, besides substantial improvements in the process of care measures, and so on.[7] Similarly, in a study of Brazil, it was seen that after taking into account improvements in literacy, sanitation, urbanization, and so on, there was a drastic improvement in the health of Brazilians during the period between 2000 and 2009 due to the effective implementation of primary care. Data showed that for every 100,000 population in the age group of 24–74 years, there was a reduction in the number of cases of cardiovascular diseases from 40 to 27 and heart diseases went down from 23.3 to 12.4. Also, the family health programme coverage increased from 21 per cent to 68.6 per cent and there was a reduction in hospitalization from 3.32 per cent to 2.83 per cent.[8] Likewise, studies in Denmark and the UK have also shown that mortality on account of cerebrovascular and other heart diseases fell from 42 per cent to 37 per cent during the period from 2000–9 due to primary care. Since high costs are making hospital care unsustainable, comprehensive primary care to prevent, avert, and manage disease at the early stages is once again emerging as a global priority.

The importance of primary care also emerged within the context of calling upon countries to ensure UHC. Country-wise analysis showed that barring about 40 countries, most are unable to provide universal access to all medical care and healthcare. And even in these 40 countries, there are exclusions, gaps, and limits to what the state can afford to provide. It is for this reason that the Sustainable Development Goal (SDG) also calls for UHC of essential services and not all care as was defined by the HLEG.

Secondly, no country has ever provided high-cost hospital care without first providing a full and liberal access to primary care. This is for two reasons: a) cost, and b) the concept of public goods. The vision of Alma Ata was for a broad-based primary care that included medical treatment as well as access to social determinants. These public goods then fall within the remit of the state to provide. Investing in them alongside information campaigns on changing behaviours and lifestyles, and promoting hygiene to prevent sickness is cheaper in the long run, both in terms of saving investments for hospital infrastructure and providing costly in-patient treatment. Besides, almost 80–90 per cent of all illnesses can be treated in primary-care settings. Therefore, good economics makes a strong case for investing in comprehensive primary care as the first charge on public finances.

India has seriously reneged on that. Right from the start, it has spread its scarce resources over a range of activities. Due to inadequate funding, primary care continues to be fragmented and focused on a few national health programmes implemented vertically. Treatment for routine ailments like fevers and body pains are provided by the peripatetic quack, poorly qualified solo practitioners, or costly hospitals in urban environments. Out of a list of about 30 activities that constitute primary care, hardly a dozen are being provided fully or partially (See Box 6.1).

Box 6.1 Current Status of Primary Healthcare in India

Provision of services: fully/partially

a) Identification of pregnant women for ANC
b) Promoting institutional deliveries
c) Preparing birth plans and escorting to higher facility
d) Nutrition counselling and listing of children with medium and severe malnutrition.
e) Listing of eligible couples: contraception/birth spacing, different methods, vector control measures
f) STI Treatment
g) HIV and TB Control programmes
h) Identification of leprosy
i) Immunization of children
j) Surveillance programmes
f) Provision of curative care

Provision of services: negligible or requiring substantial strengthening

a) Identification of high-risk pregnancies
b) Natal services
c) Early identification of post-natal complications and escorted referral and follow-up
d) Health Education on menstrual hygiene and RTI
e) Identification of adolescents and counselling on personal hygiene/health promotion
f) Promoting use of safe water and toilets
g) School health programme
h) Advocacy against tobacco, alcohol, and substance abuse
i) Active surveillance, early detection, referral of NCDs: heart, cancers, diabetes, hypertension
j) IEC for education relating to rabies and snake bites
k) Surveillance and early detection of blindness and refractory errors
l) Surveillance and early detection of congenital deafness
m) Oral hygiene education
n) Identification of elderly and escorting for treatment
o) Mental health
p) Promoting wellness and counselling

Source: Report of the expert committee for National Health Assurance, MOHFW, GOI, 2014.

Given below is an illustrative list of primary healthcare activities and the current status of their implementation in the country.

This needs to be reversed. Alongside reorienting the training of medical students and reworking payment systems to incentivize personnel to work in the primary care space, the government needs to invest 1 per cent or so of the GDP on strengthening the required infrastructure and another 2 per cent or so on the social determinants. These investments need to go in tandem and on priority in order to lay the foundation for an equitable health system.

Box 6.2 Reorganization of the Primary Healthcare System

Reform and Suggested Restructuring: A Vital Prerequisite for National Health Assurance

- Village Health Unit: The village with a 1,000 population to be the lowest health unit with a team made up of an ASHA, an anganwadi worker, a traditional dai (if available), and a less-than-qualified practitioner (if available). This team would be remunerated based on performance and achievement of the package of tasks and services to be performed.
- Above the Village Health Unit would be the FHC[9] located at a population level of 5,000. The FHC should have a team of a junior health assistant (F), a junior health assistant (M), a counsellor, a pharmacist, and a laboratory technician—all working under a doctor with a diploma in family health (an AYUSH doctor trained for a year on public health can be a good alternative as well) or a nurse practitioner.
- The third rung is the CHC located at a population level of 100,000. This will provide curative services, screen for NCDs, and stabilize and refer serious cases. It will also act as a gatekeeper. All public and private hospitals will be required to treat patients only on referral from the CHC for availing subsidized or cashless treatment.
- In urban areas, the government needs to directly provide or arrange to provide primary care services to the entire population: the affluent, middle classes, and the poor.

Source: NHA report of the expert committee, MOHFW, GOI, 2014.

Reorganizing the Public Delivery Structure: Need for Diversity

The existing three-tier primary-care delivery structure is old, costly, and, in many instances, redundant. Reorganizing the delivery system on the principle of decentralization implies taking healthcare closer to the people. Since primary care is provided on the principle of universalism, the government will need to be the dominant if not the sole provider. The sub-centres in rural and urban areas must have the capacity to provide emergency care, treat minor ailments, and offer a comprehensive package of preventive services. To signal the centrality of, and focus on, family health, they should be renamed as Family Health Centres (See Box 6.2). And in hard-to-reach areas that entail huge distances and where populations are fragmented into unviable units, the institutional design of primary care will need to factor the availability of village health units for providing first aid and maintaining disease surveillance and information. Rather than population as the only norm, facilities should be sited in accordance with the functions to be performed, based on population needs, geographies, and epidemiology.

Remodelling the delivery structure is long overdue and there is no scope for lazy options or the luxury of continuing to strengthen the existing structures that are not functioning despite the provisioning of all inputs. Such 'health movements' took place in other countries in the initial stages of building their health systems. In the early decades of its independence from colonial rule, China established the barefoot doctors who lived in the midst of the community and also launched several public health campaigns such as promoting the drinking of boiled water. Brazil focused on primary care through family health teams, and Thailand invested nearly wholly on building a strong community-based public health infrastructure alongside accompanying policies, such as making it mandatory for every doctor to work in a provincial 30-bed hospital during the first three years upon recruitment into government service, and so on.

The first set of steps for stimulating such a transformative process of change will require mapping of facilities, involving the community in planning the optimal utilization of available resources in a consultative and transparent manner, and establishing supervisory–mentoring structures. Such re-engineering in the siting of primary healthcare facilities—public or private non-profit—would require immense energy and mobilization of human resources with almost 150–200 people working at the state levels and no less than 50 people at the district level for offering technical support to the field workers and other stake holders such as the communities, local bodies, and related sector personnel. As of today, the availability of this scale of human resources, expertise, and effort is absent at the state and district levels.

Given the complexity and size of the task, the governance of primary care needs to be organized by an appropriately instituted department of public health.[10] For handling the substantial resource gap[11] and building infrastructure and maintaining standards, appropriate institutional mechanisms need to be put in place as these functions are far beyond the ability of a chief medical officer with meagre competencies and his staff.

The question is: can India also launch such a movement? Whether it has the imagination and the will is in doubt.

Secondary and Tertiary Care: Public Sector

As indicated in the previous paragraphs, primary care is the first point of contact with the focus on preventive care and handling nearly 80 per cent to 90 per cent of patient needs by a network of family physicians. Scholars have made a further distinction by adding two more tiers. One is secondary care that consists of short-term hospitalizations, routine surgeries, specialist consultations, and rehabilitation addressing about 10 per cent to 12 per cent referrals. The other tier is tertiary care. It is 'institution-based, highly specialized, and technology-driven…. In some instances, tertiary treatment may be extended, and the tertiary care physician may assume long-term responsibility for the bulk of the patient's care.'[12] It is largely provided by teaching hospitals and includes services of super specialists. At any given time, not more than 5 per cent to 10 per cent of patients will need such care. Tertiary care guzzles money. In the US, about 60 per cent of the total health spending is incurred on 1 per cent of the sick in tertiary hospitals.

Due to the varied cost streams, it needs to be kept in mind that the hierarchy of service-delivery units is in tandem with the hierarchy of health needs. A simple appendicitis performed in a secondary hospital will cost two to three times more in a tertiary-hospital setting and four times more in a corporate hospital. Such are the cost structures. It is for this reason that cost-effectiveness analysis should be the basis for planning the architecture of the delivery system, more so when money is not fungible. The idea of converting district hospitals into medical colleges, which is rapidly gaining ground, needs to be evaluated in this context. For, if all district hospitals become tertiary care centres, then which level will provide secondary care and what is the investment needed for that?

As in the case of primary care, hospitals, too, are in urgent need of capital infusion. Most hospitals and the older-generation medical colleges are treating two-to-three times the patient load as against the capacity they are designed for. A majority of hospitals require relaying of sewerage and waste-disposal systems, electrical systems, and full-fledged systems for routine maintenance of costly equipment, infrastructure, and laboratories. In fact, many district hospitals are old and impossible to maintain. A majority of them do not even have the staff to maintain basic sanitation.[13] The availability of such a workforce at the facility level is non-existent in most cases. While the timely supply of drugs and consumables has vastly improved in several states in the recent past, the issue continues to be problematic, as seen in the media reports on the non-availability of diagnostic kits or life-saving drugs for HIV patients.

Revamping secondary and tertiary care should start with freeing them from political control and interference of the ministry and departmental heads. Constant interference in postings and human resource management have sapped the hospitals and also, to a large extent, politicized the doctors themselves who have created a vested interest in letting the status quo continue. Besides, a surgeon may be competent in the area of his training but he need not necessarily be a good hospital manager.

This needs to change. Management should be professionalized. This is yet again a recommendation that has been made often but not acted upon. Running hospitals is like fighting a war. Autonomy and operational space need to be given alongside adequate resources and the management be held accountable for health outcomes[14] measured in terms of quality parameters. Currently, we have no such benchmarks to evaluate ourselves by.

Hospitals also need not be solely dependent on government budgets. Instead they should be given the flexibility to raise a proportion of the resources from community donations, or even user fees or other demand-side instruments from those who can afford to pay, particularly for non-essential services or expensive diagnostics and so on. The proportion of budgetary support and the hospital's own fund mobilization should, however, be capped so as to ensure that fundraising does not dominate the agenda. Governments should also shift to need-based financing. In other words, protocol-driven accountability frameworks; adequate and timely resource flows; and operational flexibilities alongside close, outcome-based monitoring are the only ways hospitals can be turned around to fulfil the expected functions.

Currently, as per the latest NSSO data,[15] public hospitals provide 40 per cent of all treatment. This is an average, as in tertiary care, provisioning of treatment by public hospitals may not be more than 10 per cent. Can the government aspire to provide 50 per cent of the total treatment in the secondary- and tertiary-care markets, say, within the next 10 to 20 years so as to contain costs and lay down the benchmarks for rational-quality care?[16] Investments to strengthen district hospitals and super-specialty hospitals and establishing AIIMS-like institutions need to be understood in this background.

Private Sector

As already noted in the introductory chapter of this book, India always had a private sector. It was ubiquitous and though based on fee-for-service, financial considerations were not the dominant factor in taking clinical decisions. That has changed. India's health sector is privatized and highly commercialized. Though not a homogenous entity, the private sector consists of a large component of unqualified quacks, solo practitioners, nursing homes, small hospitals, and a highly visible corporate sector.[17]

While there are no reliable estimates or data available on the extent, spread, or nature of private-sector service deliveries, some scholars have made some projections. Hooda estimates that the share of private hospitals in health delivery is '54.3 per cent of the medical institutions, 75 per cent of the hospitals, 51 per cent of the hospital beds, 75 per cent of the dispensaries and 80 per cent of all qualified doctors'.[18] Two to three per cent of hospitals are reported to have more than 200 beds while an estimated 6 per cent have a bed range between 100 and 200. The rest are all small hospitals.

The 71st round of the NSSO survey estimates that the private sector provides about 58 per cent of care in rural and 68 per cent in urban areas and is growing at 15 per cent per year. The corporate sector is reported to constitute about 2 per cent of the private sector but provides three-quarters or more of tertiary care in urban areas and accounts for a sizeable amount of the money spent on healthcare. It is trying to expand with mergers and acquisitions, though not always successfully. Over the past two decades there has been a change in ownership patterns from owning hospitals to corporate entities to now becoming part of multinational chains. The main modes of finance are also changing from private funds to institutional borrowings to private equity and venture-capital-type investments to foreign direct investments. And all this in an unregulated environment with the government oblivious of the enormous impact such shifts towards high-end and more sophisticated care will have on its fiscal and human resources, even as it rushes in to partner with them for providing services to the poor.

It is important to rein in the private sector to achieve the goal of improved health and reduced impoverishment. A regulatory architecture to ensure transparency and accountability on the lines recommended in the NCMH and HLEG reports needs to be put in place. It is often argued that the creation of new institutions is a drain on the economy. It is not realized that ineffective monitoring, poor coordination, and weak oversight are costing the government much more. This narrow thinking needs to give way to recognizing the fact that health is a complex sector that requires a network of management bodies. Just adding consultants in the ministries of health is not the solution.

Universal Health Coverage[19]

Conceptually, UHC is embedded in the concept of fairness and equity, where health is a human right. Due to the overpowering presence of the private sector and the woeful, resource-starved condition of public hospitals, the need to co-opt the private sector entered the policy dialogue and became the default position for expanding access to services.

Public–Private Partnerships

In India, the term 'PPP' is loosely used to cover all forms of outsourcing—be they laundry, sanitation, transportation, or laboratory services. The largest examples of PPP are those that were entered into under the various government-sponsored insurance programmes, starting from the CGHS to Yeshasvini to the RSBY.

PPP is defined as sharing risks and responsibilities.[20] Against that in India, evidence shows that PPPs have been more loaded in favour of the private sector with the government bearing a disproportionately higher risk.

Mention has been made of PPPs in Chapter 2 under which instances have been cited of district hospitals being handed over to corporate entities without proper and clearly specified contractual obligations, patient-redressal systems, systems to enforce penalties for reneging on contractual obligations, and so on. Therefore, PPP arrangements must consist of clearly worded contracts that are professionally negotiated and enforced stringently in order to avoid unnecessary and expensive litigation where only the private sector benefits. The private sector has an edge with its strong lobbying power. Some examples are the World Bank, the IFC, the CII, FICCI, insurance companies, and so on that are able to offer convincing data and have ready access to the political leadership.

Key information regarding the kind of services, their quality, prices, and providers is a big black box. Some mapping studies taken up on a sporadic basis are all that the government has.

Without such data, formulating policies for forging partnerships is impossible, if not fraught with serious consequences. For example, mapping of facilities in Malappuram, the most backward district in Kerala having a population of four million, showed that there were 113 hospitals in the private sector compared to 10 in the government, while all dental (150) and ophthalmic care (11) was available only in the private sector. Private sector also accounted for three times the number of beds (6,937 against 2,514 in the government) and laboratories (244 against 61 in the government). More serious is the unregulated proliferation of X-ray units (250)[21] and medicine shops (2,028) and, in general, their uneven spread.[22] Similar data has emerged in other mapping exercises as well. With such data, how can the private sector 'complement' government provisioning or 'contract-in' arrangements as suggested in the HLEG report? More importantly, how does one choose which private provider is to supply what services when price is also influenced by volume? In such environments, how does one foster competition and ensure that there is no cartelization?[23]

In most countries, there are laws for establishing hospitals or diagnostic centres. India has no such requirement, which has led to an unabashed proliferation of hospitals, nursing homes, and diagnostic facilities wherever convenient to the promoter. This has resulted in the haphazard spread of services. Clearly, what is required is to have all states mandate compulsory registration of private providers and undertake the mapping of all facilities. Such data will help the government bring in some order and rationalize the supply side, besides enabling the government to decide where to enter into a partnership and where to invest in building its own facilities, what to close down and what to support on a long-term basis, and so on. For instance, as in the US, laws to mandate 'certificates of need' for locating facilities and services are sorely required.

Government Role

The key objective of UHC is to reduce impoverishment of individuals and families on account of medical bills. It has been argued[24] that in the Indian context, efforts made so far to realize UHC have only strengthened the private corporate sector and the insurance industry. There is some truth in this assertion. In the absence of a reform agenda and a strategy for achieving UHC, the manner in which state governments have enthusiastically sponsored health insurance as central to public policy in the name of pursuing the goal of UHC has given rise to such misgivings. Such enthusiasm for the private sector is also, in no small measure, due to the inability or unwillingness to pay the political price that may follow in disciplining public sector doctors to become more accountable and banning private practice. I know of political leaders who feel that that they can sidestep and substitute governance of public systems by bringing in the private sector to provide the services. This is shortsighted as, in reality, managing the private sector is more difficult and complex.

The problem is centred around the dichotomy between reason and politics. Reason states that for containing costs and given the level of incomes as well as social, economic, and epidemiological disparities, investing in ensuring universal access to comprehensive primary care will in itself reduce over half the disease burden and out-of-pocket expenditure among the poorest quintiles. But the Planning Commission's definition of UHC aiming to cover all the population with all services—primary, secondary, and tertiary—in a 'seamless manner' through managed care networks is a different concept altogether. To justify such an approach, examples of the UK, Turkey, Thailand, and so on are often cited.

But the comparisons are erroneous and misleading. The UK introduced such a vision of universalism when the middle classes were impoverished as a result of the World War II. Besides, universalism was defined as a minimum:

> Individuals should recognize the duty to be well and restoration of a sick person to health is a duty of the state and the sick person. And so universal coverage as a minimum—a solid and level floor, no interior walls and a roof that need not be level but whose height is determined only by people's own wishes and means.[25]

Germany, on the other hand, introduced social health insurance in 1860 to counter the rise of communism and assuage the trade-union movements. So both the UK and Germany founded their health systems on the principle of social solidarity that continues to be a very priced value and the bedrock of health policies in all European countries.

Thailand, Sri Lanka, Turkey, Brazil, on the other hand, have invested in establishing not only a strong primary health care system but also public hospitals that provide three-quarters of hospital services, making it easy to contract private sector to fill gaps and address specific needs. Besides, these countries have had a strong and consistent public policy committed to promoting health and well-being, so much so that when Turkey launched the health transition reform programme in 2003, its first policy was banning private practice by government doctors.

In India, the situation is materially different. The aspirational middle classes that include the elite political class and trade unions have already created their own corporate hospitals and private public schools that fulfil their aspirations of quality. They will not now want to pay taxes in order to create a general system of healthcare on grounds of promoting equity. Nowhere have middle classes been known to give up their privileges for others.[26] Instead, the support for UHC from among these classes is more in the nature of extracting additional subsidies and benefits from the state. For example, anecdotal and survey data show how the RAS has really benefited the middle classes disproportionately more than the poor. Social solidarity does not seem to carry any traction in India.

Politics is all about perceptions. It is also about electoral votes. As the cabinet resolution establishing the NITI Aayog shows, middle classes and NRIs are a very important constituency for the current government. It follows from this that the current government may give a higher priority to National Health Assurance (NHA). Under the NHA, cashless treatment through subsidized insurance will be provided in all public and private hospitals, albeit for the poor that in most states are liberally defined.

While the policy to provide health assurance to all is laudable, there is an apprehension that in the absence of the required investments to set right the supply-side distortions in the public health delivery system, coverage may get limited to only those with access to hospitals whose availability is higher in developed states and the urban areas of the poor states. Due to the anxiety to cover large swathes of rural populations, standards and eligibility criteria for providers may also be compromised with as we have seen in the RSBY. Given the stagnant budgets and a continued reluctance to build the primary health care system, the NHA will further widen disparities, particularly in terms of quality and access to essential care, without having any impact on catastrophic expenditures.

So given these objective conditions, what options does India have for UHC and how can policies be so designed that the poor can also be benefited? The expert group constituted by the current government in July 2014 suggested universal primary healthcare for all people and that 60 per cent of the poor and not-so-poor population be covered for secondary and four select tertiary care services (heart ailments, cancers, pediatric surgeries, and emergency care) with no financial cap for cancers that will follow a treatment plan as approved by an expert board to be constituted for the purpose. It also recommended investment in public health infrastructure, particularly in the space of primary and secondary care. Furthermore, services were to be procured from public and private sector providers through a government trust as is the current practice in most states.

It is incorrect to assume that constituting a government trust to procure services from the private sector is an adequate response to privatization. Price inflation and out-pricing will continue so long as the providers' treatment practices are not regulated stringently and payments are based on fee-for-service, even if lumped as package rates and topped with insurance caps of eligible limits. Such cocktails are easily gamed by the players who are smarter than the government. Instead the government needs to think strategically, keeping control on those areas that are susceptible to profiteering, having tight regulations, and the machinery to enforce them.

A serious handicap in assessing the implications of the aforementioned recommendation was the absence of vital data on quality and costs, particularly if outpatient care and all secondary care are to be included. A recent study conducted by Prinja Shankar for PGI, Chandigarh, that reviewed all the literature on government-sponsored insurance showed three findings: a) the overall utilization has gone up, b) out-of-pocket or catastrophic expenditures have not come down at all under the RSBY, and

c) there is evidence of some marginal impact on out-of-pocket expenditures under the state-sponsored schemes.

Any financing model for UHC/NHA will therefore need to be comprehensive as well as distribute risk among all stakeholders—the government, providers, and consumers, making them accountable for responsible utilization and non-collusive behaviour. Protocol development, standard formulation, costing and pricing of services, accounting, and so on are all technical functions that ought to be undertaken by a full-fledged body. An autonomous authority established at the national, state, and district levels along with strong but uncomplicated systems of grievance redressal with powers to penalize fraud or mistreatment within strict time periods could be one option.

Achieving the two goals of improved health outcomes and reducing impoverishment due to medical costs is a substantial challenge as in dual systems of delivery and finance containing cost is difficult, if not impossible. There are enough studies to show that health insurance—private or government-sponsored—has had an inflationary impact. Yet every government is keen to fund such insurance programmes that make one wonder whether the motivation is people's welfare or promoting the commercial insurance and private hospital industry.

In light of the above, it has become even more imperative that strong primary healthcare systems are established for containing costs and disincentives to hospitalizations without referral enforced. Managed care as a model proposed by the HLEG under which private networks will provide a single-window facility for primary, secondary, and tertiary care services may be problematic as they are known to avoid taking on the very sick and high-risk patients to keep their costs low. The fact that costs have not been contained in the US that has managed care is conclusive evidence regarding the limitations of this model. Applying it in India would require deeper study.

Before the narrow bandwidth available closes irretrievably, the government needs to decisively assert itself as the market leader and lay down benchmarks for rational quality care. It needs to build institutional capacities to compete with the private sector on quality and price and safeguard its interests and those of the patients. This is not easy. Retrieving the public sector needs an extraordinary political will, good governance, and a well-trained technical manpower.

The alternative narrative to the organized private sector is muted. Civil society; patients groups (like those witnessed briefly for HIV/AIDS); and proponents of prevention, ethical practice, and rational treatment are unequal in their media reach and ability to influence political leaders.[27] The countervailing impact, then, can only be through good data 'exposing the commercial interests, the malpractices and exploitative conduct of the commercial private sector'. The government, for this reason, should invest on research—a need that continues to be least appreciated. Even today most research is donor-funded and conducted by private foundations.

The government's ability to build knowledge capital among academic institutions and research organizations will determine the effectiveness of its control over what is clearly a runaway situation. Since such capacities do not exist in most states and given the general perception of health being synonymous with hospital care (that too, corporate) and health insurance, the centre has a great responsibility to build data systems and analytical capabilities in all states for helping evidence-based policymaking.

Notwithstanding the need to build competencies for constructing a health system on the principle of universalism, the task is much harder and more complex than what has been detailed previously. Constructing a single health market with a single payer is difficult, if not impossible. India has, in reality, missed the bus, so to speak. For over 60 to 70 per cent of the people, 'markets' and 'choice' are fuzzy concepts. They are more worried about getting their next meal and their everyday needs of schooling, health, and housing that have to be paid for from their meagre incomes. More than choice, it is affordability and convenience. So the poor have made their arrangements for going to the local quack or practitioners who often provide them relief on credit, sending their children to a private school that claims to be teaching English, and eating what they can afford to buy. India needs to step up on its social welfare functions and build appropriate social security nets in order to achieve UHC.

UHC costs money. Unless the current spending patterns and macroeconomic fundamentals do not undergo changes, money for health will continue to be scarce. In other words, policies that support doling out subsidies benefiting the middle classes, not taking action to arrest non-performing assets of banks, foregoing tax revenues to 'incentivize industry' that amounts to almost 6 per cent of the GDP, 'incentivizing' corruption with low rates of conviction, and non-investment in supervision and institutional oversight need to be reversed. Spending also needs to be more efficient. The WHO estimates that in low- and middle-income countries, almost 40 per cent of the total health spending by the government is wasted or siphoned off. Improving tax systems for increasing the tax-to-GDP ratio beyond the current 17 per cent, arresting leakages and evasion of taxes through illicit financial flows to tax havens that is estimated to be about 4 per cent of the GDP, adopting innovative forms of taxation, and widening the tax base by increasing and diversifying jobs are measures to mobilize additional resources. Viewed against this backdrop, there is scope for India to provide the required resources for health and social determinants. It is always the will that is needed.

It is estimated that for providing universal access to essential services as laid down in the Sustainable Development Goals (SDG), countries would need to spend USD 85 per capita or 5 per cent of the GDP. Against that, India is currently spending about USD 18 per capita or a little over 1 per cent of the GDP for all health. It is for this reason that I do not subscribe to demands for spending of 2 or 3 per cent of the GDP. Instead the health discourse should move away from such demands and hold the government accountable to the implementation of the stated policies, no matter what that takes—1, 3, or 8 per cent of the GDP.

Institutional Reform and Enforcing the Rule of Law

Strengthening Technical Capacity

New diseases have emerged and crowded the landscape. Non-communicable diseases (NCDs) are a burden that the system needs to build the capacity to cope with. The NCD initiative launched in 2010 has barely taken off and many states have no capacity to handle chronic conditions or even common ailments like hypertension, diabetes, and asthma on a long-term basis. While the problem is complex, the institutional architecture is the same—it only has additional hands, that, too, taken on an ad hoc, temporary basis. There is an urgent need to build the technical capacity of the ministries at the centre, state, and district levels and fresh recruitment of technical specialists should be taken up. The language that is spoken in Delhi and international seminars is incomprehensible to the officials working at the floor level and being held accountable for outcomes. This hiatus needs to be bridged by simplifying words and concepts.

The argument that there is no value addition in establishing more bodies and assuming that the thinking can be outsourced to agencies or committees or yet another joint secretary in the ministry is a misconception and the result of an enormous amount of simplification of difficult processes. As suggested in several reports, new institutions need to be established to address the multifarious requirements and emerging challenges of the sector: an independent food and drugs authority, utilization of IITs and other research bodies to regulate medical devices, an independent authority to procure essential commodities, a health promotion and data repository agency for promoting positive lifestyles and public information, a health infrastructure corporation to mobilize resources for constructing facilities and maintaining them as per standards, and a national authority to coordinate insurance programmes and harmonize the different government-sponsored insurance schemes, to name just a few.

Strengthening Regulatory Capacity

The logic of markets and privatization drive the need for regulators and regulatory systems. Enough has been written on the urgency of strengthening and professionalizing the regulatory bodies—the Food Safety and Standards Authority of India (FSSAI), the Drug Control Authority, and the MCI. All of them lack enforcement capacity and muscle.[28]

Take the example of the MCI that has been in the news of late. Parliamentary committees and the Supreme Court have adversely commented on its poor functioning as the regulator charged with the responsibility of ensuring standards in medical education and physician practice. Over the years, the MCI has failed to establish transparent processes of granting recognition to medical colleges, update curricula, curb high capitation fees, or ensure quality and credibility of the products emerging out of the institutions. Such failures have adversely affected our national reputation and the quality of patient care. This aspect is not captured as there are no quality standards to measure outcomes.[29]

Much of the problem is rooted in the Act that provides for an elected body to govern the MCI, giving rise to sharp conflicts of interest and vast room for corrupt practices. It is for this reason that there have been consistent demands to revamp the MCI. With this in view, in 2010 a draft bill was readied providing for the National Commission for Human Resources for Health that was finally tabled in Parliament only in December 2011. When the 60th PSC returned the bill to the ministry on 23 November 2012, no action was taken to address its concerns.[30]

In 2015, the PSC took suo moto cognizance of the Ranjit Roy Chaudhury Committee report (February 2015) and submitted a scathing report on the non-functioning of the MCI, calling for a radical architectural correction. The 92nd Report of the PSC was tabled in Parliament on 8 March 2016. Instead of taking advantage of this second opportunity to set aside the current MCI by establishing a transition team and forging a transformative process, the government constituted a three-member committee under the chairmanship of the deputy chairman of the NITI Aayog.

The committee has since placed its report along with a draft bill in the public domain proposing the disbandment of the MCI and replacing it with an architecture as proposed by the Ranjit Roy Committee and endorsed by the PSC. Accordingly, the report has recommended establishing a national medical commission (NMC) to devise policy and plan human resources based on geographical and epidemiological needs and instituting four divisions to deal with curriculum development, teacher training, and standard-setting for undergraduate and postgraduate education. The other recommendations include instituting accreditation and assessment processes of colleges and courses for ensuring uniformity in standards, registration of doctors, licensing, and adherence to ethics. The NMC is to be assisted by a medical advisory council (MAC) consisting of state representatives.

The draft bill is likely to invite much comment. Removing the process of elections and replacing it with nominations without adequate checks and balances against the arbitrariness of executive action has raised apprehensions that the cure may be worse than the disease. Nominations to the MCI by the UPA II and to the National Board of Examination by the current government of persons having no teaching credentials, deep conflicts of interest, or questionable integrity, and in a non-transparent manner, have given rise to legitimate fears that the nomination process may politicize the MCI even more. With the draft bill providing extensive powers to the ministry to issue directions to the MCI, there is a concern that the council's autonomy may be compromised. Besides, with the dilution of penal provisions, allowing private medical colleges freedom to levy fees as they deem fit, and permitting the for-profit private sector to establish medical colleges, there is a worry that the current trend of commercialization may only deepen further. There have also been concerns that such policy shifts that entail profound implications for the health sector are being made with minimal consultations. If these widespread misgivings are not taken into consideration, yet another review by the PSC will become inevitable, taking the reform to 2018 or beyond. Such events only go on to demonstrate how deep the rot is and how difficult it is to address the crying need for a strong regulatory body consisting of people having a high moral standing in the profession and selected in a transparent and open manner. Until the prevailing crass commercialization of the profession and corruption are not weeded out, there is little one can expect in achieving health goals.

Reforming the MCI is only part of the story. States must be sensitized and incentivized to formulate HR policies and they should institute transparent systems for recruitment, appointment, deployment, promotion, and professional enhancement. Payment systems need to be worked out keeping in view the circumstances.

Alongside the MCI, there is an equal urgency to make the FSSAI and drug regulation more effective as detailed in Chapter 3. There is a general reluctance to enact laws and enforce them. Andhra

Pradesh enacted a hospital regulation Act in 2000, rules were framed in 2005, and it is still in cold storage. The same is the fate of other states that have similar laws. Regulations are seen as bringing back the 'Licence Raj' and the tyranny of the inspectors. Partly true, but still a facetious justification for inaction. The truth is otherwise.

It is also time for the government to seriously deliberate two issues: one is to bring in a constitutional amendment revisiting Schedule VII that provides for the functions and responsibilities between states and the centre. Part of the reason for the chaotic environment of poor-quality education and increasing drug resistance is the dual responsibility of the centre and states over these matters, nullifying any attempts of the central government to introduce radical and transformative reforms.

The second is enacting a comprehensive public health law made applicable to all states and its implementation made conditional for central resources. Such a public health law needs to cast certain obligations on the states, all caregivers, and hospital entities to adhere to protocols and standards. Also, there should be public display of prices being charged for the various procedures, details of the personnel employed, and the rights of the patients. It should be made mandatory for facilities to furnish returns to the government on laid down indices and outcomes achieved, computerization of records, and grievances settled. Such a law should be binding on public as well as private hospitals with patient safety being its primary purpose.

A close reading of this section will make it clear how 'unready' we are for introducing UHC or any of its variants. No doubt the special interest lobbies will hustle the governments in this direction. But for ensuring we do not end up with a fragmented and iniquitous health system entailing heavy costs[31]—both human and financial—like the US's, it is prudent to adopt a systematic and deliberate approach, while, at all times, focusing on the goal of UHC and the Right to Health as the ultimate destination.

Strengthening the People's Sector

The people's sector consists of three components: the elected local bodies in rural and urban areas, the communities and patient groups, and civil society organizations that work for and on behalf of them. It is a sector well recognized under the NRHM, but whose potential was not fully exploited.

Local Bodies

In India, unlike in Brazil, locally elected bodies are not accountable for, or involved in, providing universal access to basic goods, a responsibility they can discharge as they have taxation powers. Local bodies can do little if they are going to be grant-dependent bodies. They need to raise their own resources that they are empowered to do, at least to some extent. To fully utilize their potential, reforms should be undertaken, making health functionaries accountable to them, stipulating what they need to achieve, and releasing grants based on performance. Accordingly, decentralization of functions to the level of local bodies will imply provisioning of budgets for the functions they are expected to perform—such as the incentive money to ASHAs, grants for mobilizing children for immunization, and so on—and that they will be held accountable for outcomes. In other words, in addition to releasing grants, decentralization and involvement of urban bodies and panchayats imply a shift in financing and governance structures with investment in capacity development through intensive institutionalized training and supportive supervision on the lines of Kerala.

In this context, it is argued that the NUHM must have full and active participation of the departments of urban development and the urban bodies. I strongly believe in involving other sectoral ministries as equal partners. With this in mind, when I was the central health secretary I had two or three rounds of meetings with the Department of Urban Development that were attended by state representatives too. The idea was to have them build capacity and utilize the existing infrastructure to deliver primary health care services in lieu of resources to be made available to them under the NRHM. This would have been a win-win situation since the Jawaharlal Nehru National Urban Renewal Mission (JNNURM) had created infrastructure conveniently located in the midst of slum populations that could have been appropriately utilized for establishing the primary health centres.[32] This is only one example—the scope for synergies is substantial as I had learnt during my stint as the special officer and commissioner of the Municipal Corporation of Hyderabad.[33] Unfortunately, the matter was not pursued after I left. The whole issue is about sharing power and having control over resources. As a rule, the health ministries at the national and state levels have not demonstrated (except somewhat under the HIV/AIDS control programme) a work ethic of sharing resources or working with other sectoral ministries—an attitude that is a major inhibitor in achieving health goals.

Notwithstanding the above, in the Indian context, community-based approaches have brought to the fore conflicts at two levels that need to be managed and resolved as a first step. Empowerment of the poor demands a shift in the power structures, conflicting with the constitutionally mandated PRIs that are party-based and often reinforce the existing inequities and status quo within the village community. The second arena of conflict pertains to the NGOs, which, on the one hand, may be challenged by the PRI bodies while advocating community problems and, on the other hand, be in confrontation with the communities themselves as they tend to keep control on those they have empowered. Since empowerment itself can be a disruptive process entailing political ramifications, community engagement and participation needs to have the full backing of the government until such time that the community is not strong enough to provide the leadership.

Importance of Social Audit

We saw the value of engaging with communities and civil society organizations in the two case studies of the NACP and the NRHM. As the primary stakeholders, communities need to be made active participants in policy formulation and implementation at all levels. They need to be trained on how to discharge their functions, what questions to ask, and how to keep vigil to ensure there is no siphoning off of the benefits meant for them. Social audit was one such means of holding governments accountable and was successfully implemented under the MNREGS in Andhra Pradesh. In a similar fashion, some NGOs have conducted social auditing for health in Maharashtra, Bihar, and Chhattisgarh, among others, and demonstrated its value in resolving community needs. This, then, has to be the foundation of the health system. The implications of the extensive use and nurturing of civil society organizations that have a commitment towards enhancing ideals of equity and fairness were amply demonstrated in the HIV/AIDS programme and under the NRHM in several parts of the country. The democratization of health policy formulation and its implementation are vital for the alternative narrative to be heard, besides being consistent with our democratic credentials. Thailand, for example, organizes national and provincial assemblies on an annual basis where the ministers and officials talk with citizens and civil society groups. Can we expect that without the discourse becoming partisan and acrimonious?

The Use of Technology

The immense importance of technology in ensuring a better quality of life and furthering equity in access cannot be overemphasized. In the health sector, technological improvements are a paradox. On the one hand, technological advances have saved lives but also increased costs, while on the other hand, they have shrunk borders and distances, improved efficiencies, and reduced operational costs. In this dynamic situation, for poorly resourced countries, technology can be, and is, a boon. With telemedicine, mobile connectivity, and easy electronic transmission of medical records, there is really no need to have to physically locate a specialist in a rural centre to provide access to those populations. Likewise, many diagnostics can be self-administered or conducted by lay health workers without requiring expenditures on laboratories or highly trained laboratory technicians to be located in every small facility. As seen in the MCTC programme, computerization has made vast quantities of information easily available, making monitoring easier and more purposeful. Portability of patient records is a reality and a great help for ensuring the continuum of treatment for mobile patients. Medical colleges can now access self-learning modules for updating their technical knowledge in addition to being taught by the best teachers. These are all profoundly valuable and in many states, there has been a beginning. The only danger is that technology does give the impression that it can be a substitute for human interaction. One needs to guard oneself against that and recognize that technology is but a tool, not the mind itself.

But more than the uses of technology in improving physician competencies and practices, the phenomenal growth of social media can be a game changer and can help in bringing in a transformative change in our policies. What people, particularly the poor and the underprivileged, lack is knowledge and access to information. Social media can provide that to build the pressure on governments to bend policies towards promoting equity. Accompanied by policies like the Right to Information, accountability of governments and health providers can be ensured.

Role of Evidence and Knowledge

Contrary to common perception, health is a knowledge-intensive sector. It is for this reason that countries with advanced health systems invest in research and evidence. India has a poor record in this aspect. Chronically strapped for funds, governments have always depended on donors for providing the research and evidence for policy formulation or policy correction. The implications of this are realized when we also understand that evidence need not be value-free. Lack of capacity has hindered us from analysing even the substantial amount of data and information available. Non-use of data and evidence is the reason for the poor quality of the policy. And more worrying is the gradual decline in undertaking evaluations to study the impact of policy in order to bring in the necessary corrections. Neither at the central nor the state levels is any budget earmarked for this purpose or monitored for its utilization either. This is one reason why India has few institutions with the capacity for operational research in health.

In Mexico, it is a legal requirement for all new schemes/ideas to go through a pilot phase based on a baseline. The further expansion or continuance of new schemes is subject to the outcome of a rigorous evaluation. Besides, the concept of research and evaluation is fully embedded in the ministry that has a full-fledged department under it dedicated for this purpose.

India has no such institutional mechanisms or legal requirements. Often, policies[34] are introduced, continued, or scaled up in accordance with prevailing perceptions, hunches, or political expediency. For example, there is no explanation as to how policies like the RAS or the RSBY or those to promote PPP are being continued with and scaled up without adequate analysis of benefits, costs, fiscal implications, long-term impacts, and so on. Such ad hocism needs to stop.

The issue staring India is how to provide equitable and universal healthcare with inadequate funds. With the multitude of problems India faces, there is a need to keep focus and base policy on evidence. But being rational and evidence-based also implies taking decisions that may be inconvenient, which is why Keynes said, 'There is nothing a government hates more than to be well-informed; for it makes the process of arriving at decisions much more complicated and difficult.'[35]

༄

Societies that have transited from welfarism to neo-liberalism have shifted from welfare, patronage, and dependency to empowerment, entitlements, and rights.[36] But unlike them, India seems to be 'caught between welfarism and neo-liberalism—large doses of populism mixed with blatant privatization'. Despite the rhetoric of socialism and constitutional pronouncements, India's development story continues to be based on a model of privilege and inequality of opportunity, safeguarded by an array of institutional arrangements and value systems. Though a democracy, people are uninformed and not trusted to be active partners in development. This is much more so in the health sector.

This needs to change as the democratization of health is vital for health security. In the past decade, infectious diseases like SARS, H1N1, Ebola, and so on that rapidly raced through village and country boundaries finally got contained only by community action, not by the billions that petrified countries poured in as aid to the affected countries. Besides, people's participation is vital for ensuring that policy is aligned with what they really need. Achieving this vision would require leadership that is committed to the values of human equality and a belief that health has an intrinsic value and is worthy of being pursued for its own sake.

But if India does not want to be known as the 'sick country' of the world, then it has to take tough decisions and get started on the long road of reform. And reform does not mean tinkering around the existing system with new ideas and schemes.

Reforms are painful processes—they hurt some, benefit others. But they need to be undertaken—revamping regulatory authorities, rebuilding anew the broken health system, and fixing it in a manner that makes all stakeholders accountable to serving the last person standing in the line. This calls for thinking. For careful assessment of options. For a decisive leadership. Other countries have done this and achieved better outcomes. India has not been able to do so as yet, but it most certainly can as it is a country with huge potential.

I have spent over two decades of my life in this sector. Sometimes when one reads of people and even children dying due to diarrhoea or measles or TB or malaria, I cannot but feel that time has stood still in India. There is so much to be done and so much that can be done, but only if our governments care and rise above partisanship and political squabbling!

We, as a people and a nation, need to look ahead. The past is over. Today we have the future in our hands to mould and shape. We must not let this opportunity slip by. We owe that to the future generations.

Notes and References

1. Weak health systems with poor community-based primary care systems were the ones most affected by Ebola, leading to substantial economic losses. Even China suffered a 0.5 per cent loss in its GDP due to SARS and India lost an estimated Rs 5 billion of exports during the 1995 plague.
2. These were goals indicated in the NHP (2002) and were to be achieved by 2010.
3. A study showed that 247 out of an estimated 650 districts in the country accounted for three-quarters of maternal, infant, and under-five child mortalities alongside communicable diseases. Also, three-quarters of the estimated infrastructure gaps in terms of facili-

ties, beds, and personnel were in these districts—47,166 facilities out of 62,876; 33,384 beds out of the total requirement of 42,344; and 28,000 personnel. See NHSRC, 2010, 'Accelerating Maternal and Child Survival: The High Focus Districts Approach', MOHFW, GOI..
4. C. Rangarajan and D.K. Srivastava, 2004, 'Fiscal Transfers in Canada: Drawing Comparisons and Lessons', *Economic & Political Weekly*, 39(19): 1897–909.
5. *Primary Health Care* (Geneva: WHO, 1978).
6. Leiyu Shi, 2012, 'The Impact of Primary Care: A Focused Review', *Scientifica*, available at http://dx.doi.org/10.6064/2012/432892 (accessed on 31 August 2016).
7. From a presentation by Jonathan R. Sugarman on primary care presented at the Global Partners Forum in Seattle, USA. See also Katherine Gottlieb, 'The Nuka System of Care: Improving Health through Ownership and Relationships', *International Journal of Circumpolar Health*, available at _ http://www.circumpolarhealthjournal.net/index.php/ijch/article/view/21118 (accessed on 31 August 2016).
8. Davide Rasella, Michael O. Harhay, Marina L. Pamponet, Rosana Aquino, and Mauricio L. Barreto, 2014, 'Impact of Primary Health Care on Mortality from Heart and Cerebrovascular Diseases in Brazil: A Nationwide Analysis of Longitudinal Data, *BMJ*: 348, doi: 10.1136/bmj.g4014.
9. Based on the NHA Report where the FHU was recommended, the central government changed the name to call them wellness units. The two have different meanings and a different association of services and functions. What is needed is family health, not individual wellness.
10. Primary care requires expertise in disease surveillance and family health, linkages with social determinants, communication with communities and the marginalized sections of society, home nursing, and so on. This needs laboratories and a range of skills—epidemiology, nurses, counsellors, physiotherapists, laboratory technicians, entomologists, opticians' community, social psychology, and so on.
11. Estimated to be Rs 1.4 trillion as per GOI consisting of the IPHS standards provided for the three tiers of primary care. District hospitals and medical colleges will need to be added.
12. Shi, 'The Impact of Primary Care'.
13. In 2009 or so, the Andhra Pradesh government contracted out the sanitation of all its 23 district hospitals to a Mumbai-based

contractor. Weak and poor enforcement had left many hospitals with accumulated filth.

14. In the UK, an element of internal competition was introduced by having GPs buy care from competing hospital units. This needs to be studied to see if such incentives can be applied in India.
15. NSSO, 71st Round, Key Indicators of Social Consumption in India (2014), GOI.
16. I have no doubt that the existence of AIIMS acts as a great price holder and has also forced an amount of rational care.
17. Besides hospitals, private sector in health-related areas is substantial—pharmaceuticals, medical devices/equipment, diagnostics, telemedicine, health insurance, and so on.
18. Shailender Kumar Hooda, 2015, 'Foreign Investment in Hospital Sector in India: Trends, Patterns, and Issues', Working Paper 181, available at http://isid.org.in/pdf/WP181.pdf (accessed on 31 August 2016).
19. Though some scholars do use the words 'coverage' and 'care' interchangeably, the implication is different. Thus, China may have achieved 98 per cent of coverage but not care that implies services. Likewise, under the RAS Andhra Pradesh may have covered 85 per cent of its population but access is low for want of facilities. Here it implies financial coverage and physical access.
20. A. Venkat Raman and James Warner Bjorkman, *Public–Private Partnerships in Health Care in India: Lessons for Developing Countries*, Routledge Studies in Development Economics (Oxford: Routledge, 2009).
21. This gives a ratio of one X-ray machine per 16,000 people. Overexposure to X-rays can cause cancers. Likewise, medicine shops should be run by qualified people. So many medicine shops in such a backward district are suggestive of an indiscriminate sale of drugs that can cause drug resistance.
22. Sunil Nandraj, 2015, 'Private Healthcare Providers in India are above the Law, Leaving Patients without Protection', *BMJ*, 350.
23. I am reminded of an instance in Kolkata. A group of well-meaning doctors took a bank loan and established a CT scan diagnostic centre charging prices that covered actual costs. A liquor baron opened a similar centre across the road, charging nominal rates and thus drawing away the client load, resulting in the doctors defaulting on their loan and forcing closure. The liquor baron then hiked prices.
24. Anil Gupta et al., 2011, 'Universal Access to Health Care: Threats and Opportunities', *Economic & Political Weekly*, 46(26 and 27): 27–30.

25. Beveridge, *Social Insurance and Allied Services*.
26. As a sequence to the recommendation of the NCMH report of 2005 that suggested the creation of a social health insurance corporation by merging all government-sponsored insurance programmes, namely the ESIS and the CGHS, to create the required velocity for an insurance pool to launch a UHC, the non-gazetted employees who constitute the major chunk of the CGHS membership refused to do so. So did the ESIS.
27. As I write, it is learnt that the state plan for health is being written by a committee headed by Dr Devi Shetty, who is a known protagonist of the corporate private sector and specialist care and is believed to be not supportive of redressal systems like the ombudsman. The alternative voice is not available despite the presence of a large number of public health activists who were responsible for preparing an exhaustive plan of action over a decade ago that is yet to be implemented. In Andhra Pradesh, too, rumours have it that it was the corporate sector that fixed rates and designed much of the RAS in the initial years.
28. I recall an incident of a drug inspector who was sent to the 'Agra Market' for checking the manufacture of spurious drugs. When he went there, the owner sat down to discuss the matter, placing a gun on the table. The inspector exchanged pleasantries and returned. States have barely half-a-dozen such inspectors. How are they expected to handle mafias?
29. Dr G.N. Rao of LV Prasad Institute, Hyderabad, observed that even the gold medalists they recruit need training. This was a telling statement on our educational system.
30. The Supreme Court adversely commented on this lapse in its judgement (Civil Appeal No. 4060 of 2009) stating: 'In its 60th Report, the Committee had recommended to the Ministry of Health and Family Welfare to re-examine the concerns expressed by it and bring forward a fresh Bill. Rather than seizing the opportunity to come up with a better Bill, the Ministry remained apathetic to the state of affairs and did not respond with vigorous corrective measures.'
31. The US currently spends 18.5 per cent of its GDP on health. It is reported that a state like California spends 30 per cent of its government budget on health at the cost of education. Health spending is creating several distortions in the US that India can ill afford.
32. Land/space in urban areas accounts for 30 per cent of the unit cost of services. Providing this in itself can be leveraged to offer services at reduced costs as compared to the private sector.

33. As the special officer (there was no mayor) and commissioner of Hyderabad, I was able to sort out and implement the World Bank-funded India Population Project within a year which was hanging for over two years for want of attention from the municipality.
34. Donor-funded projects are an exception as they have exhaustive evaluation processes as a mandatory requirement for continuing financial support.
35. John Maynard Keynes, *The Collected Writings of John Maynard Keynes: World Crisis and Policies in Britain and America*, vol. 21 (London: Macmillan, 1982), p. 409.
36. Aradhana Sharma, *Paradoxes of Empowerment in Neoliberal India* (New Delhi: Zubaan, 2010).

Select Bibliography

Ainsworth, M., Chris Beyrer, and Agnes Soucat. 2003. 'AIDS and Public Policy: The Lessons and Challenges of "Success" in Thailand', *Health Policy*, 64(1): 13–37.
Andrew MacAskill, Steve Stecklow, and Sanjeev Miglani. 2015. 'Rampant Fraud at Medical Schools Leaves Indian Healthcare in Crisis', available at http://www.reuters.com/investigates/special-report/india-medicine-education/ (accessed on 27 September 2016).
Appleby, Paul H. 1953. *Public Administration in India: Report of a Survey*. New Delhi: Manager of Publications.
Arora, P., N.J.D. Nagelkerke, R. Moineddin, M. Bhattacharya, and P. Jha. 2013. 'Female Sex Work Interventions and Changes in HIV and Syphilis Infection Risks from 2003 to 2008 in India: A Repeated Cross-sectional Study', *BMJ*, 3(6), DOI:10.1136/bmjopen-2013-002724.
Ayyar, R.V. Vaidyanatha. 2009. *Public Policymaking in India*. Delhi: Pearson Education.
Balarajan, Y., S. Selvaraj, and S.V. Subramanyam. 2011. 'India: Towards Universal Health Coverage', *The Lancet*, 377: 668–79, available at http://www.thelancet.com/series/india-towards-universal-health-coverage (accessed on 27 July 2016).
Baru, Rama V. 2012. 'A Limiting Perspective on Universal Coverage', *Economic & Political Weekly*, 47(8).
Basu, I., S. Jana, M.J. Rotheram-Borus et al. 2004. 'HIV Prevention among Sex Workers in India', *Journal of Acquired Immune Deficiency Syndromes*, 36(3): 845–52.
Bennett S., S. Singh, D. Rodriguez, S. Ozawa, K. Singh, V. Chhabra, and N. Dhingra. 2015. 'Transitioning a Large Scale HIV/AIDS Prevention Program to Local Stakeholders: Findings from the Avahan Transition Evaluation', *PLoS ONE* 10(9), DOI: e0136177. doi:10.1371/journal. pone.0136177.
Bergkvist, Sofi, Adam Wagstaff, Anuradha Katyal, Prabal V. Singh, Amit Samarth, and Mala Rao. 2014. 'What a Difference a State Makes:

Health Reform in Andhra Pradesh', Policy Research Working Papers, Washington, D.C., World Bank.

Bernal, Victoria and Inderpal Grewal (eds). 2014. *Theorizing NGOs: States, Feminisms, and Neoliberalism*. Durham, NC: Duke University Press.

Beveridge, William. 2000. 'Social Insurance and Allied Services', *Indian Joural of Public Health*, 78(6): 847–55.

Bhat, Ramesh and Nishant Jain. 2006. 'Analysis of Public and Private Healthcare Expenditures', *Economic & Political Weekly*, 41(1).

Brown, Garrett W., Gavin Yamey, and Sarah Wamala. 2014. *The Handbook of Global Health Policy*. Oxford: Wiley-Blackwell.

Choudhury, Mita, H.K. Amar Nath, and Bharatee Bhusana Dash. 2012. *Distribution of Public Spending Across Health Facilities: A Study of Karnataka, Rajasthan, Madhya Pradesh and Assam*. New Delhi: NIPFP.

Choudhury, Mita. 2012. 'Health Care Financing Reforms in India', Working Paper No. 100, NIPFP, New Delhi.

Commission on AIDS in Asia. 2008. *Redefining AIDS in Asia: Crafting an Effective Response*. New Delhi: Oxford University Press.

Dandekar, Vikas. 2015. 'Capping Cardiac Stents Gets NHSRC Backing', *The Economic Times*, available at http://economictimes.indiatimes.com/industry/healthcare/biotech/healthcare/capping-cardiac-stent-prices-gets-nhsrc-backing/articleshow/48446217.cms (accessed on 26 September 2016).

David, Peters H., A. Yazbeck, R. Sharma, G. Ramana, L. Pritchett, and A. Wagstaff. 2002. *Better Systems for India's Poor*, Human Development Network. Washington, D.C.: World Bank.

'Demand for Grants', 19 major states, 2007–8 and 2011–12, Ministry of Finance, GOI.

Duggal Ravi. 2001. 'Evolution of Health Policy in India', CEHAT (unpublished).

'Evaluation of the Janani Suraksha Yojana: Recommendations', National Health Systems Resource Centre, MOHFW, GOI, available at http://nhsrcindia.org/pdf_files/resources_thematic/Public_Health_Planning/NHSRC_Contribution/Programme_Evaluation_of_Janani_Suraksha_Yojana_-Sep2011.pdf (accessed on 27 September 2016).

ESCAP. 2005. 'Minding their Business: Women Sex Workers' Actions to Prevent HIV/AIDS', Part II, in Community-level Good Practices in HIV Prevention, Care and Support for Policy Consideration: Two Case Studies, United Nations.

Finance Commission Reports, 6th–13th.

Forgia, Gerard La and Somil Nagpal. 2012. 'Government Sponsored Health Insurance in India: Are You Covered?', Directions in Development, World Bank, Washington, D.C..

Forgia, Gerard La, Shomikho Raha, Shabbeer Shaik, Sunil Kumar Maheshwari, and Rabia Ali. 2014. 'Parallel Systems and Human

Resource Management in India's Public Health Services: A View from the Front Lines', Policy Research Working Paper 6953, Health, Nutrition and Population Unit, World Bank, South Asia Region.

'Framework for Implementation'. 2013. National Urban Health Mission, MOHFW, GOI.

Framework for Implementation, 2005–12, National Rural Health Mission, MOHFW, GOI.

Garg, Suneela and Anita Nath. 2007. 'Current Status of National Rural Health Mission', *Indian Journal of Community Medicine*, 32(3): 171–2.

Gautam, Meenakshi and K.M. Shyam Prasad. 2010. 'The Basic Doctor for Rural India: A Failed Promise', *Economic & Political Weekly*, 45(38): 25–9.

Ghose, Toorjo, Dallas Swendeman, Sheba George, and Debasish Chowdhury. 2008. 'Mobilizing Collective Identity to Reduce HIV Risk among Sex Workers in Sonagachi, India: The Boundaries, Consciousness, Negotiation Framework', *Social Science & Medicine*, 67: 311–20.

Gill, Kaveri. 2012. 'Promoting "Inclusiveness": A Framework for Assessing India's Flagship Social Welfare Programmes', Social Policy Working Paper Series 2, UNICEF India, New Delhi.

Global Health Watch: An Alternative World Health Report. 2014. New York: Zed Books.

GOI. 2011. *Working Group Report for 12th Five Year Plan of the Department of Drinking Water and Sanitation*.

Grindle, Merilee S. and John W. Thomas. 1991. *Public Choices and Policy Change: The Political Economy of Reform in Developing Countries*. Baltimore: John Hopkins University Press.

Gulati, S.C., Raghubansh M. Singh, Rajesh Raushan, and Arundhati. 2011. 'Evaluation Study of NRHM', Institute of Economic Growth, University of Delhi.

Gupta, A. 1962. 'State of the Nation's Health', *Economic & Political Weekly*, 14(20).

'Health and Family Welfare Statistics in India', 2013, MOHFW, GOI.

Haacker, Markus and Mariam Claeson. 2009. *HIV and AIDS in South Asia: An Economic Development Risk*. Washington D.C.: IBRD, World Bank.

Harvard Medical School and Brigham and Women's Hospital. 2011. 'The Avahan India AIDS Initiative: Managing Targeted HIV Prevention at Scale', Cases in Global Health Delivery, available at https://cb.hbsp. harvard.edu/resources/marketing/docs/GHD020p2.pdf (accessed on 27 September 2016).

Heifetz, Ronald A. and Marty Linsky. 2002. *Leadership on the Line: Staying Alive through the Dangers of Leading*. Cambridge: Harvard Business Review Press.

Horton, Richard and Pam Das. 2011. 'Indian Health: The Path from Crisis to Progress', *The Lancet*, 377(9761): 181–3, DOI:10.1016/S0140-6736(10)62179-4.

Human Rights Watch. 2009. *No Tally of the Anguish: Accountability in Maternal Health in India*. New York: Human Rights Watch.

Hunter, Susan. 2005. *AIDS in ASIA: A Continent in Peril*. New York: Palgrave Macmillan.

IDFC. 2014. *India Infrastructure Report 2013–14: The Road to Universal Health Coverage*. New Delhi: Orient Blackswan.

'Indian Public Finance Statistics 2013–14', Ministry of Finance, GOI.

Jha, Prabhat. 2011. 'Million Death Study'.

'Journey of ART Programme in India: Story of a Decade', 2014, NACO, GOI.

John, Jacob and Jr Sankaran. 1993. 'The Epidemiology of HIV/AIDS', in B. Rajan (ed.), *AIDS*. Chennai: Tamil Nadu Dr M.G.R. Medical University.

Joshi, Sujay and George Mathew. 2012. 'Healthcare through Community Participation: Role of ASHAs', *Economic & Political Weekly*, 47(10).

Kapoor, Radhika. 2013. 'Inequality Matters', *Economic & Political Weekly*, 48(4).

Karan A., S. Selvaraj, and A. Mahal. 2014. 'Moving to Universal Coverage? Trends in the Burden of Out-of-Pocket Payments for Health Care across Social Groups in India, 1999–2000 to 2011–12', *PLoS ONE*, 9(8): e105162. DOI:10.1371/journal.pone.0105162.

Khanna, Renu and Anagha Pradhan. 2013. *Evaluation of the Process of Community Based Monitoring and Planning of Health Services in Maharashtra*. Pune: Support for Advocacy and Training to Health Initiatives (SATHI).

Khera, Ajay, Anuradha Gupta, Hema Gogia, and Sujatha Rao. 2012. 'India's National Immunization Programme', seminar vol. 631, available at http://www.india-seminar.com/2012/631/631_ajay_khera_et_at.htm (accessed on 27 September 2016).

Khilnani, Sunil. 1997. *The Idea of India*. New York: Farrar, Straus and Giroux.

Kohli, Atul. 2012. *Poverty amid Plenty in the New India*. Cambridge: Cambridge University Press.

Mahal, Ajay, Bibek Debroy, and Laveesh Bhandari (eds). 2010. *India Health Report 2010*. New Delhi: Business Standard Books.

Mathew, George. 2014. 'Viewpoint: Re-instating a "Public Health" System under Universal Health Care in India', *Journal of Public Health Policy*, 36(1): 15–23.

Mazumdar, Sumit. 2015. 'The Murky Waters of Medical Practice in India: Ethics, Economics and Politics of Healthcare', *Economic & Political Weekly*, 50(29).

McDonald, David A. and Greg Ruiters (eds). 2012. *Alternative to Privatization: Public Options for Essential Services in the Global South.* New York: Routledge.

McKinsey & Company. 2009. 'NACO Organizational Assessment', New Delhi.

McKinsey and Company. 2009. 'Organizational Diagnostic of NACO and selected SACS', New Delhi.

Meadows, Donella H. 2008. *Thinking in Systems.* Burlington: Chelsea Green Publishing.

Misra, J.P. 2011. *Draft Report on Evaluation of Community Health Worker (Mitanin) Programme,* European Union State Partnership Programme. Raipur: Department of Health.

MOHFW. 2005. *Report of the National Commission on Macroeconomics and Health.* New Delhi: GOI.

MOHFW. 2007. *A Comparative Analysis across the National Sample Survey Organization, 42nd, 52nd, and 60th Rounds.* New Delhi: GOI.

MOHFW. 2011. *Report of the Working Group on National Rural Health Mission (NRHM) for the Twelfth Five Year Plan (2012–2017).* New Delhi: GOI.

MOSPI. 2014. *Key Indicators of Social Consumption in India Health.* NSSO 71st Round. New Delhi: GOI.

Mudur, Ganapati. 2012. 'Experts Question Proposals to Use Private Sector in India's Health Reforms', *BMJ,* DOI: 10.1136/bmj.e5489

NACO. 2007. *NACP III: To Halt and Reverse the HIV Epidemic in India,* available at http://osacs.nic.in/sites/default/files/NACP%20III%20-%20To%20Halt%20and%20Reverse%20the%20HIV%20Epidemic%20in%20India.pdf (accessed on 27 September 2016).

Nandraj, Sunil, Jaison Joseph, Mannethodi Kamaruddeen, Yamini Thankachy, Rahul Shastri, Devaki Nambiar, and Prathibha Ganeshan. 2016. *God's Own Country: Moving Towards Universal Health Coverage in Kerala.* New Delhi: PHFI.

National AIDS Control Organization. 2011. *Annual Report 2010–11.* New Delhi: Department of Aids Control, MOHFW, GOI.

'National Health Policy', 1983 and 2002, MOHFW, GOI.

'National Health Profile', 2010, CBHI, DGHS, GOI.

National Institute of Urban Affairs. 2005. *Study of Water Supply, Sanitation and Solid Waste Management in Urban Areas.* New Delhi: Ministry of Urban Development, GOI.

'National Sample Registration Survey', 60th and 71st rounds.

'NRHM Framework for Implementation', 2005, GOI, available at http://www.mohfw.nic.in/NRHM/Documents/NRHM_Framework_Latest.pdf

'NRHM in the Eleventh Five Year Plan (2007–2012)', NHSRC, New Delhi.

Over, Mead. 2009. 'AIDS Treatment in South Asia: Equity and Efficiency Arguments for Shouldering the Fiscal Burden When Prevalence Rates are Low', Working Paper No. 161, Center for Global Development, Washington.

Over, Mead, Peter Heywood, Julian Gold, Indrani Gupta, Subhash Hira, and Elliot Marseille. 2004. *HIV/AIDS Treatment and Prevention in India: Modeling the Costs and Consequences.* Washington, D.C.: World Bank.

Panda, Samiran, Anindya Chatterjee, and Abu S. Abdul-Quader. 2002. *Living with the AIDS Virus: The Epidemic and the Response in India.* New Delhi: SAGE Publications.

Patel, Vikram, Rachana Parikh, Sunil Nandraj, Priya Balasubramaniam, Kavita Narayan, Vinod K. Pau, A.K. Shiva Kumar, Mirai Chatterjee, and K. Srinath Reddy. 2015. 'Assuring Health Coverage for All in India', *The Lancet*, 386: 2422–35.

'Performance Audit of National Rural Health Mission', report of the Comptroller and Auditor General, Union Government (Civil), No. 8 of 2009–10.

Phadke, Anant. 2012. 'Polio Eradication, a Dubious Claim', *The Hindu Business Line*, available at http://www.thehindubusinessline.com/opinion/polio-eradication-a-dubious-claim/article2837352.ece (accessed on 27 September 2016).

PHFI and NHSRC. 2010. *Factors Influencing Decision of Doctors to Serve in Rural and Remote Areas of Chattisgarh State.*

Pisani, Elizabeth. 2008. *The Wisdom of Whores: Bureaucrats, Brothels and the Business of AIDS.* New York: W.W. Norton & Company.

Planning Commission of India. 2011. 'Executive Summary', in *High Level Expert Group Report on Universal Health Coverage for India*, pp. 1–39. New Delhi: Planning Commission, GOI.

Planning Commission of India. 2011. *High Level Expert Group Report on UHC.* New Delhi: GOI.

Planning Commission of India. 2011. *Evaluation Study of National Rural Health Mission (NRHM) in 7 States.* New Delhi: Programme Evaluation Organisation, GOI.

Powell-Jackson, Timothy, Arnab Acharya, and Anne Mills. 2013. 'An Assessment of the Quality of Primary Health Care in India', *Economic & Political Weekly*, 48(19).

PHFI. 2012. *Why Some Doctors Serve in Rural Areas: An Assessment from Chhattisgarh State.* Geneva and Chattisgarh: World Health Organization and State Health Resource Centre.

'Project Appraisal Document for Second National HIV/AIDS Control Project', 1999, World Bank.

Rajya Sabha. 2011. *Department-related Parliamentary Standing Committee on Health and Family Welfare Sixtieth Report on NCHRH Bill.* New Delhi: MOHFW, GOI.

Ram, Usha, Prabhat Jha, Faujdar Ram, Kaushalendra Kumar, Shally Awasthi, Anita Shet, Joy Pader, Stella Nansukusa, and Rajesh Kumar. 2013. 'Neonatal, 1–59 Month, and Under-5 Mortality in 597 Indian Districts, 2001 to 2012: Estimates from National Demographic and Mortality Surveys', *The Lancet*, 1(4): e219–e226.

Ramachandran, Vimala, and Kameshwari Jandhyala (eds). 2012. *Cartographies of Empowerment: The Mahila Samakhya Story—Biography of a Programme and a Movement.* New Delhi: Zubaan.

Rao, Govinda M. 'Chapter V', in *States' Development Expenditures and Implications for Regional Development* (forthcoming).

Rao, Govinda M. and Mita Choudhury. 2008. *Inter-State Equalization of Health Expenditures in Indian Union.* New Delhi: NIPFP.

Rao, Govinda M. and Nirvikar Singh. 2005. *Political Economy of Federalism in India.* New Delhi: Oxford University Press.

Rao, M. Govinda. 2015. 'Political Economy of Government Finance in India', *India Review*, 14(1): 58–72.

Rao, Sujatha K. 2012. 'Long on Aspiration, Short on Detail', *Economic & Political Weekly*, 47(6).

———. 2015. 'When Corruption becomes the Norm and Ethical Conduct an Exception', *Indian Journal of Medical Ethics*, available at file:///C:/Users/Dimris/Downloads/2306-5160-4-PB.pdf (accessed on 26 September 2016).

RBI. 2012. 'Statistical Abstract of India', in *Handbook of Statistics on India*, various issues. GOI.

RBI. 2012. *Report on Currency & Finance.* Various Issues. New Delhi: GOI.

Reddy, G.R. 2013. 'Paper submitted to 14th Finance Commission'.

Registrar General of India. 2013. 'Annual Health Survey'.

Reza-Paul, Sushena, Rob Lorway, Nadia O'Brien, Lisa Lazarus et al. 2012. 'Sex Worker-led Structural Interventions in India: A Case Study on Addressing Violence in HIV Prevention through the *Ashodaya Samithi* Collective in Mysore', *The Indian Journal of Medical Research*, 135(1): 98–106, DOI: 10.4103/0971-5916.93431.

Sathyamala, C., N.J. Kurian, Anuradha De, K.B. Saxena, Ritu Priya, Rama Baru, Ravi Srivastava, Onkar Mittal, Jacob Puliyel, Claire Noronha, and Meera Samson. 2012. 'Public Report on Health: Some Key Findings and Policy Recommendations', *Economic & Political Weekly*, 47(21): 43–54.

Sen, Gita. 2012. 'Universal Health Coverage in India: A Long and Winding Road', *Economic & Political Weekly*, 47(8).

Sharma, Aradhana. 2006. 'Globalization and Postcolonial States', Division II Faculty Publications, Paper 41, available at http://wesscholar.wesleyan.edu/div2facpubs/41 (accessed on 29 July 2016).

———. 2006. 'Introduction: Rethinking Theory of the State in an Age of Globalization', in Aradhana Sharma and Anil Gupta (eds), *An Anthropology of the State: A Reader.* Malden: Blackwell Publishing.

Sharma, Arun Kumar. 2009. 'National Rural Health Mission: Time to Take Stock', *Indian Journal of Community Medicine*, 34(3): 175–82, available at http://www.ijcm.org.in/text.asp?2009/34/3/175/55268 (accessed on 29 July 2016).

Sheikh, Kabir, Lynn Freedman, Abdul Ghaffar, Bruno Marchal, Fadi el-Jardali, Jim McCaffery, Jean-Pierre Olivier de Sardan, Mario Dal Poz, Walter Flores, Surekha Garimella, and Marta Schaaf. 2015. 'Posting and Transfer: Key to Fostering Trust in Government Health Services', *Human Resources for Health*, 13(82), DOI: 10.1186/s12960-015-0080-9.

Shukla, Abhay, Renu Khanna, and Nitin Jadhav. 2014. 'Using Community-based Evidence for Decentralized Health Planning: Insights from Maharashtra, India', *Health Policy and Planning*, DOI:10.1093/heapol/czu099.

Shukla, Abhay. 2005. 'National Rural Health Mission: Hope or Disappointment?', *Indian Journal of Public Health*, 49(3).

'Six Years of NRHM (2005–2011): Achievements and Challenges—the Reform and Strategies for Strengthening of Health Systems', MOHFW, GOI, available at http://nhsrcindia.org.

'Sixth Five Year Plan (1980–85)', Planning Commission, GOI.

Smith, Jean Clare. 2010. 'The Structure, Role, and Procedures of the U.S. Advisory Committee on Immunization Practices (ACIP)', DOI: 10.1016/j.vaccine.2010.02.037.

Sood, Neeraj, Eran Bendavid, Arnab Mukherji, Zachary Wagner, Somil Nagpal, and Patrick Mullen. 2014. 'Government Health Insurance for People below Poverty Line in India: Quasi-experimental Evaluation of Insurance and Health Outcomes', *BMJ*, 349: g5114, DOI: http://dx.doi.org/10.1136/bmj.g5114.

Srivatsan, R. and Veena Shatruguna. 2012. 'Political Challenges to Universal Access to Health Care', *Economic & Political Weekly*, 47(8).

Standing, Guy. 2012. 'Cash Transfers: A Review of the Issues in India', Social Policy Working Paper Series 1, UNICEF India, New Delhi.

Sundararaman, T., Shomikho Raha, Garima Gupta, Kamlesh Jain, K.R. Antony, and Krishna Rao. 'The Chhattisgarh Experience with 3-Year Course for Rural Health Care Practitioners: A Case Study', Chhattisgarh, available at http://cghealth.nic.in/ehealth/studyreports/chhattisgarh%20experience%20with%203-year.pdf (accessed on 27 September).

Sundari, T., Kamlesh Jain, and V.K. Raman. 2005. 'National Rural Health Mission: Hopes and Fears—Retreat of the States and Prioritization', *Indian Journal of Public Health*.

'Survey in Morbidity and Health Care', 2004–5, National Sample Survey 60th Round, NSSO, Ministry of Statistics and Programme Implementation, GOI.

Thresia, C.U. 2015. 'Social Inequities and Exclusion in Kerala's Egalitarian Development', *Monthly Review*, 65(9).
'Twelfth Five Year Plan', 2012, vols 1 and 2, Planning Commission, GOI,
'Twelfth Five Year Plan', Vol II, Chapter on Health, Planning Commission, GOI.
UNDP. 2013. *The Rise of the South: Human Progress in a Diverse World*. HDI Report.
Ved Rajani, R. and A.S. Dua. 2005. 'Review of Women and Children's Health in India: Focus on Safe Motherhood', background paper for 'Burden of Diseases in India', National Commission for Macroeconomics and Health, pp. 103–69.
Vithal, B.P.R. and L. Sastry. 'Xth Finance Commission' (unpublished).
WHO. 2011 and 2013. 'Health Statistics'.
World Bank. 1992. *Staff Appraisal Report of India National AIDS Control Project*.
———. 2013. 'Country Statistics'.

Index

Access International 92
accounting–auditing model xiv
accredited social health activists
   (ASHAs) 155, 177, 180,
   308, 312, 316, 319, 324, 326,
   329–30, 332, 338, 340–52, 355,
   376, 397
   design of 340–3
   earnings of 342
   eligibility criteria for 340
   initiatives 312
   remuneration of 326
   role of 309
Adolescence Education
   Programme (AEP) 230
Advisory Group on Community
   Action (AGCA) 316, 351
Affordable Care Act (2010,
   Obamacare) 39
Ahluwalia, Isher 302
Ahluwalia, Montek Singh 309
AIIMS 12, 56, 77, 104, 124, 130,
   134, 157, 182, 190, 192, 209,
   272, 362, 401
Ainsworth, Martha 255
All India Institute of Hygiene
   and Public Health (AIIHPH)
   209
All India Pre-Medical
   Test (AIPMT) 130. *See
   also* National Entrance
   Examination Test (NEET)

Alma-Ata Declaration 14–15, 115,
   189n. 6, 307, 395
ambulatory care 31, 38
Andhra Pradesh
   HIV/AIDS prevalence in 210
   HIV testing mandatory before
     marriage 284
   injecting drug users (IDUs)
     272
   MNREGS 416
   NRHM spending in 59
   primary care budget of 67
   RAS 91
   SACS 218
anganwadi worker (AWWs) 120,
   341, 354, 397
ANM 120, 160, 177, 181, 225,
   235, 324, 327, 329, 341, 343,
   349, 356
   training and monitoring
     of 235
Anti Corruption Bureau (ACB)
   182
antiretroviral treatment (ART)
   204, 206
Apollo group 16, 29, 169
Aravind Eye 193n. 49
architectural corrections 25, 331,
   364, 370, 372, 393
ART centres 213, 235–9, 243, 376
ASHA Mentoring Group (AMG)
   343–4

Ashodaya 206, 257–61, 275, 279–80
Ashraya 258
Avahan 205–6, 224, 266–8, 274–82
  implementation processes of 276
  internal contradictions of 277
  learnings of DFID experiments 274
  reports and feedback 276
  rights-based approach 279–80
Ayush practitioners 181

BCG vaccination programme 12
behaviour change communication (BCC) 230
Beveridge, William xviii
Bhore Committee 9, 12, 114, 339
Bihar
  blood-transfusion services 226
  injecting drug users (IDUs) 272
  primary care in 67
Bill & Melinda Gates Foundation (BMGF) 36n. 28, 115, 179, 205, 257, 260, 274, 278, 284, 377
Biocon 359
blindness control programme 193n. 49
Brazil
  predicated universal insurance 99
  tax-based financing accounts 39
British Medical Association (BMA) 28
British Medical Council 151, 192, 348

Canada
  commercialization of healthcare 28
  free healthcare to every citizen 39
CARE 279

CASAM 294n. 37
case-based payment 3
cashless treatment 23, 100, 397, 406
cash-transfer scheme 85. *See also* Janani Suraksha Yojana (JSY)
Centers for Disease Control and Prevention (CDC) 206
Central Bureau of Investigation (CBI) 182
Central Council of Health and Family Welfare (CCHFW) 115, 123, 159n. 5, 189, 316, 369
Central Drugs Standard Control Organization (CDSCO) 171–2, 174
Central Government Health Scheme (CGHS) 86, 91, 95, 128, 185, 403
centralized policymaking 136–41
centrally sponsored schemes 27, 50–1
Central Vigilance Commissioner (CVC) 119
Centre for Enquiry into Health and Allied Themes (CEHAT) 313, 382n. 11
Chadha Committee (1963) 13
Chaturvedi, Girish 317
Chaudhary, Vineet 138, 191
Chauhan, Shivraj 48
Chhattisgarh
  blood-transfusion services 226
  injecting drug users (IDUs) 272
  NRHM spending in 59–60
childhood immunizations 394
childhood mortality 27
child morbidity 118
Child Survival and Safe Motherhood Programme 345
China
  decline in waterborne diseases 42

GDP loss due to SARS 420n. 1
increased life expectancy 42
tax-based financing accounts 39
chronic underfunding 40
civil society, alternative narrative of 29
Clinical Establishment Act 164, 195n. 61
clinical trials
    compensation 175
    regulation of 124, 175
    unethical conduct of 174
closed-door system 348
clustered disadvantage x
commercial sex workers (CSWs) 249–59
    Ashodaya (Mysore) 257–9
    collectivization approach of 253, 255, 256
    Kamathipura 249–50
    leadership-dependent model 256
    rights-based approach 255
    Sangli 254–7
    Sonagachi 251–4
    See also sex worker
Commission on Macroeconomics and Health (CMH) x, 302
Common Review Missions (CRMs) 319
communitization 337–40
    civil-society agenda 337
    components of 338–9
community-based initiatives 22, 306, 339, 352
community-based organizations (CBOs) 206
community health centres (CHCs) 30, 55, 148–9, 231, 324, 327–8
community health workers (CHWs) 14
Community-led Structural Intervention (CLSI) 252, 294n.33

Comprehensive Rural Health Project (CRPH) 339
Comptroller and Auditor General (CAG) 112, 119, 182, 301
condom marketing 218, 226–9
    administration of condom promotion 227
    donor-funded social marketing 228
    female condoms 229
    government's role in 227
    monitoring mechanism 228
    NACO's role in 227–8
    programme-based funding 228
    Red Ribbon Express (RRE) campaign 230
    sex-worker interventions 229
Constitutional 73rd and 74th amendments 140
Contagious Diseases Act 8
Cooperative Act 254
cooperative federalism 32, 44, 133, 187, 389–93
corruption 183–6
    absenteeism in doctors 184
    bribes 184
    conflicts of interest 186
    corruption in procurement of services 185
    fraudulent billing by corporate hospitals 185
    intellectual and moral corruption 184
counsellors 135, 143, 217, 219, 221, 226, 230–3, 238, 377

Danish International Development Agency (DANIDA) 323
data management and evaluation systems 187
decentralization 389–93
demand-side financing 85–101
    cross-subsidization principle 85
    FDI cap for insurance 95

financialization of the private medical industry 95
reimbursement rates 91
dengue outbreak (Delhi, 2015) 141
Dental Council of India 192n. 37
Department for International Development (DFID) 205, 216–18, 269, 274, 277, 281
Desai, Ketan 111–2
Disability-Adjusted Life Years (DALYs) 17
disease burden 10, 32, 38, 40, 49, 55, 60, 103, 139, 141, 149, 151, 159, 217, 367, 392, 405
doctor-assistants, cadre of 123
donor-funded projects 424n. 34
DOTS strategy 189n. 7
Drucker, Peter 195n. 62
Drug Control Authority 411
drug mafias 423n. 28
Drug (Price Control) Order 173
Drugs and Cosmetics Act (1940) 171–2
Drugs and Cosmetics (Amendment) Bill 172
Drugs Controller General (India) 175

Ebola xxi, 145–6, 419
Economic Advisory Council 119
economic liberalization (1990s) 15–17
empanelled hospitals 23
Employees State Insurance Scheme (ESIS) 95
Empowered Action Group (EAG) states 304
Empowered Programme Committee (EPC) 316
Epidemics Control Act 8
Ernst & Young 115, 134
Essential Commodities Act 172
ethics 183–6. *See also* corruption
Ethiopia, health workers in 347

Evans, Timothy xi
evidence-based gap analysis 375
evidence-based goal-setting 392
evidence-based policymaking 409
Expenditure Finance Committee (EFC) 77, 272

Fabian socialism xii
faith-based organizations 245, 314
Federation of Indian Chambers of Commerce and Industry (FICCI) 115, 403
fee-for-service systems of payment 3, 101
female sex workers (FSWs) 251. *See also* sex worker
financialization 28, 36n. 34, 95
fiscal deficit 16–17, 54, 62, 108n. 42, 193n. 42, 350
Food Safety and Standards Authority of India (FSSAI) 411, 413
Foundation for Research in Community Health (FRCH) 382n. 11

Gadgil formula 45, 49
Gandhi, Rajiv 115
Gandhi, Sonia 300, 362
gender violence 263–4
Germany 28, 405
  doctor–patient relationship 28
Gilada, I.S. 249–50
Global Fund 233, 235–7, 268, 274, 284
Gopalakrishnan 306–7, 340
government-sponsored insurance schemes 23, 87t–90t, 411
grants-in-aid 46, 57
grievance redressal mechanisms 31, 164, 183, 186
  absence of 31
Guinea worm eradication 141
Gujarat
  NRHM spending in 60

primary care spending in 67
spent on drugs 68
SACS 218

hakims 7
Hart, Julian 105
health and social determinants 49, 52, 103, 410
health insurance 21, 23–4, 38–9, 41, 69, 85–6, 95, 97–9, 125, 134, 302–3, 309, 358, 360, 405, 408–9
  cost-effectiveness 100
  supply-side deficiencies 101
  tax-based insurance models 99–100
Health Management Information System (HMIS) 176
Health Springs 156
highly active antiretroviral therapy (HAART) 204
Hindustan Latex Family Planning Promotion Trust (HLFPPT) 227
Hindustan Latex Limited (HLL) 227–8
HIV/AIDS 17, 19, 21, 27, 29, 77, 116–17, 145, 198, 201–2, 205–6, 229, 231, 240, 251, 253, 274, 279, 284–5, 287, 289–90, 323, 368, 373, 376, 379, 409, 416–17
  AIDS-related mortality 201
  budget reduction 27
  condom marketing 218–19, 226–9
  District AIDS Prevention and Control Unit (DAPCU) 219
  funds released for 285t
  high-prevalence states 210, 218
  HIV Sentinel Surveillance (HSS) 208
  implementation of the strategy 219–59
  integrated bio-behavioural assessments (IBBA) 211
  multipartner sexual relations 202
  NACP I 202
  NACP II 202–3
  NACP III 204–5
  scaling up ART 240f
  sentinel surveillance 207
  State AIDS Control Societies (SACS) 217–18
  treatment, care, and support 235–46
  trucker interventions 218–19
  Voluntary Counselling and Testing Centres (VCTCs) 212
  pregnant women 235
HIV Alliance 279
HLEG 26, 96–7, 134, 188, 358–66, 395, 402, 404, 408
HMIS 177, 180
H1N1 xxi, 102, 145, 419
home-based neonatal care (HBNC) model 345
Hsiao, William C. 1, 4, 163
human development index ix, x
human resources 150–62
Human Rights Law Network 242

immunization agenda 349
impoverishment 22, 38, 86, 92, 162, 402, 404, 408
India Health Report 302
Indian Academy of Pediatrics (IAP) 240, 345
Indian Council for Research on International Economic Relations (ICRIER) 302
Indian Council of Medical Research (ICMR) 21, 208
Indian Council of Social Science Research (ICSSR) 21
Indian Health Organisation (IHO) 250

Indian Institute of Health
    Management Research
    (IIHMR) 215
Indian Institute of Population
    Sciences (IIPS) 147
Indian Medical Association (IMA)
    29, 120, 123
Indian Medical Service 9–10, 128
    revival of 128
Indian Nursing Council 192n. 37
Indian Public Health Standards
    (IPHS) 55, 139, 191n. 24,
    326–8, 330
infant mortality 10, 21, 47, 177,
    179, 299, 332, 339, 344–5, 356,
    391
injecting drug users (IDUs)
    268–74
Institute of Rural Management
    (IRM) 215
institutional mechanisms 40, 44,
    95, 134, 144, 214, 319, 399,
    419
institutional reform 33, 132–4,
    188, 309, 410–14
Insurance Regulatory
    Development Authority
    (IRDA) 19, 86
Integrated Bio-Behavioural
    Assessments (IBBA) 210–1
Integrated Child Development
    Scheme (ICDS) 50, 108n. 135
    shortcomings of 143
Integrated Management of
    Neonatal and Childhood
    Illness (IMNCI) protocol 345
Integrated Testing and
    Counselling Centre (ICTC)
    210
intergenerational poverty 39
International Development
    Association (IDA) 202
International Labour
    Organization (ILO) 23

International Monetary Fund
    (IMF) 17
interstate disparities xiii, 40, 45,
    58
intra-state differentials xiii
IT-enabled data flows 188

Jamkhed experiment 14
Janani Shishu Suraksha Karyakram
    (JSSK) 179
Janani Suraksha Yojana (JSY)
    68–9, 85, 312, 317, 326–7,
    332–4
Jan Swasthya Abhiyan (JSA) 22,
    29, 307, 313–15, 318
Jan Swasthya Rakshak (JSR) 306,
    386n. 58
Jawaharlal Nehru National Urban
    Renewal Mission (JNNURM)
    415
Jayaprakash Narayan 309, 340
Jha, Prabhat 191, 255

kala-azar (black fever) 26, 368,
    375
Karnataka Health Promotion
    Trust (KHPT) 257
Kartar Singh Committee 13, 155,
    159
Kavi, Ashok Rao 206, 265
Kerala 21, 30, 53, 60, 69, 85, 94,
    140, 147, 218, 260, 273, 283–4,
    317, 335, 340, 351, 391, 404, 415
    better health indicators in 147
    finances available under the
        RSBY in 351
    maternal mortality rate in 21
    public health spending in 60
    SACS 218

laissez-faire 5, 113, 189n. 4, 393
life expectancy 10, 42
LifeSpring 182
lifestyle diseases 141, 149

macro and micro-level health system 2
Mahatma Gandhi National Rural Employment Guarantee Scheme (MNREGS) 144
Make in India policy 369
Malaria 12, 145, 191
malnutrition 105, 142–3
Mann, Jonathan 208
market failures 3, 5, 32, 39, 105, 114, 183, 381
maternal mortality rate (MMR) 21, 179, 332–6, 344
　impact of institutional deliveries on 334–7
　indicators impacting 336, 336
Maternity Benefit Scheme 332
McKinsey 25, 115, 320
Medanta 359
Medical Council Act 150, 165, 167, 169
Medical Council of India (MCI) 9, 29, 111–13, 119, 122–4, 126, 129–30, 132, 150–1, 165–70, 182–3, 189–90, 365, 411–13
　architecture of 126, 167
　reform process of 112, 413
　revamping of xix, 112–13, 122
　shortcomings of 412
medical education, reform of 368
medical records, computerization of 31
Medico Friend Circle 30
men having sex with men (MSM/homosexuals)
　epidemiological modelling 265
　family disapproval and social approbation of 265
　media attention to 268
　Section 377 of IPC 264–8
Middle East respiratory syndrome (MERS) xxi
Minimum Needs Programme 16
Mission Steering Group (MSG) 42, 143, 316, 342, 376

Mother and Child Tracking System (MCTS) 176–80, 333
Mudaliar Committee 13
Mukherjee Committee 13

NAC 119, 167, 300–1, 308–10, 316, 340, 352, 362–3
NACO
　achievements under 291t
　approach to CSW issues 259–68
　demoralization and fatigue 289
　empowerment process of the marginalized 282
　financial support 238
　organizational capabilities of 216
　replication of finances in 81
　scrutiny of the media and Parliament 262
　tight budgets 260
NACP III, financing of 284–6
Nadar, Shiv 182
Narayana Hrudayalaya 109n. 49, 359
Narcotic Drugs and Psychotropic Substances (NDPS) Act 270
Narcotics Control Bureau (NCB) 270
National Accreditation Board for Hospitals and Healthcare Providers (NABH) 93
National Accreditation Board for Testing and Calibration Laboratories (NABL) 234
National AIDS Control Project (NACP III) 197, 204–7, 209, 214–15, 218, 220, 227, 229, 246, 259, 261, 266, 272, 275, 278, 282, 284, 286–7, 290, 372–4, 380
National AIDS Research Institute (NARI) 209
National Bank for Agriculture and Rural Development (NABARD) 96

National Blood Transfusion
Council (NBTC) 225
National Commission for
Human Resources in Health
(NCHRH) 166
National Commission on
Macroeconomics and Health
(NCMH) 20, 53, 95–7, 128, 134,
188, 302, 314, 340, 364, 371, 402
National Common Minimum
Programme (NCMP) 300–4
National Development Council
(NDC) 50
National Dialysis Programme
(NDP) 369
National Dialysis Services
Programme 389
National Entrance Examination
Test (NEET) 129–31, 190n. 13
National Health Assurance
Mission (NHAM) 97
National Health Assurance
(NHA) 38, 53, 55, 367–9, 397,
406–8
National Health Mission (NHM)
26, 226, 369
National Health Policy (NHP) 14,
20, 57, 137, 302, 337, 340, 368
National Health Scheme in 1947
11
National Health Service (NHS)
xviii
National Health Systems
Resource Centre (NHSRC)
154, 318–22
National Institute of Cholera and
Enteric Diseases (NICED) 208
National Institute of
Communicable Diseases
(NICD) 128, 144
National Institute of
Epidemiology (NIE) 144, 209
National Institute of Health and
Family Welfare (NIHFW) 144,
318

National Institute of Medical
Science (NIMS) 209
National Institute of Nutrition
(NIN) 144
National Institute of Virology
(NIV) 208
National List of Essential
Medicines (NLEM) 174
National Malaria Control
Programme (NMCP) 12
National Medical Commission
(NMC) 167, 412
National Pharmaceutical Pricing
Authority (NPPA) 171, 190n. 10
National Programme for Control
of Blindness (NPCB) 117, 323
National Rural Health Mission
(NRHM)
abandoning of 25
allocative efficiencies of 62–8
analysis of major states 59
architectural reforms 331
birth of 304–7
broad goals of 358
budget allocations for 26, 323,
370*t*
evolution of policy 300
expenditure management 75,
82
expenditure patterns of 58
formation of societies 82–3
framers of 314
funding to high-focus states
58–9
funds for disease control
programmes 57
implementation of initiatives
309–10
increase in central funding 59
institutional innovation 299,
316–18
inter-sectoral convergence 312
interstate disparities 58
interstate per capita spending
61*t*

main objective 22
political context of 2005 300–1
pool 57, 69, 356
primary goals of 375
principles of 322–54
public–private partnerships (PPPs) 83–4
RCH pool 323
recruitment 330
reduction in childhood mortality 61
release of funds 77–80
release of grants 325–6
reproductive and child health 57, 332–7
resource allocation and utilization 75–7
rural primary healthcare 305
National Sample Survey Office (NSSO) xv, 20
National Technical Support Unit (NTSU) 216
National Technical Working Group (NTWG) 241
National Tuberculosis Institute 128
National Urban Health Mission (NUHM) 317
NationWide 156, 182
neonatal care, public policy for 344
neonatal mortality 309, 344–5
NITI Aayog 16, 51–2, 75, 112, 126, 132, 366, 368, 406, 412. *See also* Planning Commission
no-conflict-of-interest policy 118
non-communicable diseases (NCDs) 410
nursing homes 13, 30, 96, 184, 186, 402, 404

ombudsman 113, 183, 194n. 58, 309
Operations Research Group (ORG) 229
organizational capacity 199, 205

out-of-pocket expenses 2, 39, 303, 360, 407

panchayati raj 191n. 26, 304, 310, 314, 342
pandemic flu 145
Partnerships of Sexual Health (PSH) Project 217
Patent Act (2005) 173
Pathfinders 279
patient-redressal systems 403
Pay Commission
  Fifth 52
  Sixth 68, 152, 157, 330
pay-for-performance 104
People's Health in People's Hands 21
performance-based payments 342
PGI 182, 209, 333, 407
PHC 30, 55, 148–9, 231–2, 326–8, 341, 350
Planning Commission 16, 25–6, 40, 44–5, 49–51, 62, 75–6, 119–20, 124, 137, 142–3, 154, 190, 289, 308–11, 316, 326, 352, 358–63, 366, 368, 405
polio pulse campaign 115, 323
Population Foundation of India (PFI) 351
Population Service International (PSI) 227, 250
population stabilization 304
President's Emergency Plan for AIDS Relief (PEPFAR) 236
price inflation 31, 407
The Price of Inequality xx
PricewaterhouseCoopers (PWC) 115, 134
primary healthcare
  current status of 396
  importance of 395
primary health centres (PHCs) 30, 55, 148–9, 231–2, 326–7, 328, 341, 347, 350
prioritization, politics of 392
prioritizing immunization 117

private sector, role of 105
 misrepresentations and
  conflicts 105
 political and economic
  compulsions 105
profiteering from healthcare 28
Programme Management Unit
 (PMU) 317
public delivery structure 398–410
 institutional design of primary
  care 398
 mapping of facilities 399
 remodelling of 398
 secondary and tertiary care
  399–410
 supervisory–mentoring
  structures 399
public health capacity 144–6
 budgetary constraints 145
 community surveillance 145
 scaling up of interventions 145
Public Health Commissionerate
 10
public health emergencies 102
Public Health Foundation of
 India (PHFI) 25–6, 359, 377
public–private partnerships (PPPs)
 17–19, 23, 31–2, 83–4, 116,
 183, 232, 313, 360, 362, 369,
 389, 403, 419
public-sector insurance
 companies 19
public spending on health 52–6,
 102
 central government's share 52–3
 centralization of financing 53
 expenditure compression 52
 IMF conditionalities 54
 interstate variations 53
 low capital spending 55–6

quacks 7, 16, 140, 155, 402

Rajasthan
 primary care expenditure in 67

spent on drugs 68
Rajiv Aarogyasri Scheme (RAS)
 23, 67, 91–3, 95, 358, 406, 419
 Aarogyasri Trust 109n. 43
 impact of 92
 IT platforms, 93
 reimbursement rates 93
Ramadoss, Anbumani 124, 266–7,
 283, 301
Ranjit Roy Chaudhury
 Committee 167, 412
Rao, P.V. Narasimha 150
Rashtriya Krishi Vikas Yojana
 (RKVY) 360
Rashtriya Swasthya Bima Yojana
 (RSBY) 23–4, 30, 59, 85–6, 94,
 97, 108n. 135, 134, 351, 358,
 360, 368–9, 389–90, 403, 407,
 419
Reddy, Y. Rajasekhara 91
Red Ribbon Express (RRE)
 campaign 230. *See also* condom
 marketing
registered medical practitioners
 (RMPs) 309
regulations 4, 163, 414
regulatory architecture 402
reproductive and child health
 (RCH) 18, 116
resource gap 392, 399
resource-intensive projects 42
resource mobilization 43–52
 Finance Commission 45–9
 institutional mechanisms for
  resource-sharing 44–5
 Planning Commission 49–52
 rights-based approach 33, 255,
  262, 264, 279–80, 346
Right to Education Act (2010)
 xviii, 381n. 1
Right to Food 381n. 1
Right to Information (RTI) xix,
 301, 418
Right to Work (RTW) 301
RMNCH+A programme 179

Rockefeller Foundation 12, 26, 115, 358–9
Rogi Kalyan Samiti (RKS) 339, 350–1
rule of law 162–76, 410–14
    drugs and medical devices 170–6
    regulating medical education 165–70
    regulation 162–5

Sample Registration System (SRS) 47, 177
Samraksha 258, 260
Sangram 254, 294n. 37
School AIDS Education Programme (SAEP) 230
Section 377 of IPC 247. *See also* men having sex with men (MSM/homosexuals)
self-help groups 19–20, 144, 162
Sen, Amartya 41
sentinel surveillance 202, 207, 210, 212
serious adverse events (SAEs) 175
service delivery 1–3, 15, 17, 44, 67, 124, 139, 180, 213, 278, 304, 308, 322, 324, 360
severe acute respiratory syndrome (SARS) xxi, 146, 419
sexual abuse 263–4
Sexual Health Intervention Project (SHIP) 251
sexual networks, remapping of 287
sex worker
    brothel-based 287
    protest against the anti-trafficking bill 264
    rehabilitation of 263
    rights and aspirations of 264
    vulnerability of 264
Shah Bano case 248
Shetty, Devi 22, 359
Shrivastava Committee 13

Shrivastava Report 339–40, 360, 363
Shukla, Abhay 306, 313
Singh, Kartar 13, 155, 159–60, 193
Singh, Manmohan 300, 302
skilled birth attendants (SBAs) 334
social audit 135, 141, 321, 339, 353–4, 416
social determinants 141–4
Social Health Insurance Corporation 96
social media 188, 418
social-sector schemes 27
social solidarity 4, 39, 341, 347, 405
Societies Act 204
Societies Registration Act (1860) 35n. 17
Society for Community Intervention and Rehabilitation (SCIR), 269
Sokhey Committee 339
South India Action AIDS Programme (SIAAP) 260
Sri Lanka
    child health strategy 116
Srinivasan, R. 18
stakeholder involvement 376
stand-alone diagnostic clinics 13
standard formulation 408
State AIDS Clinical Expert Panel (SACEP) 243
State Health Systems Resource Centre (SHSRC) 318
State Institute of Health and Family Welfare (SIHFW) 144
Stiglitz, Joseph xx
structural adjustment loan 52
structures of governance 121–32
supply-side deficiencies 69, 98, 101, 149
Suraksha Clinics 225
surveillance 118, 134–5, 145–6, 155, 188, 202, 207–10, 212–13,

215, 217, 221, 268, 292n. 2, 396, 398
Sustainable Development Goal (SDG) 395, 410
Swaraj, Sushma 204, 235, 283
swine flu 145
systemic inequities xii

Tamil Nadu
 maternal deaths in 335
 prevalence of HIV/AIDS in 210
 primary care spending in 67
 spending on district hospitals 68
Tamil Nadu Medical Supplies Corporation (TNMSC) 161
Tamil Nadu State AIDS Control Society (TANSACS) 206
Tata Institute of Social Sciences (TISS) 215
Tata, J.R.D. 351
tax-based tertiary insurance schemes 24
tax-to-GDP ratio xiii, 103, 410
TB 12, 18–19, 21, 26, 92, 139, 145, 189, 208, 232, 235, 238, 240–1, 243, 283, 323, 342, 396, 420
Thailand
 child health strategy 116
 government doctors and private practice 193n. 46
 nutrition counsellors 143
 100 per cent condom use by prostitutes (CUP) policy 250
 predicated universal insurance 99
 tax-based financing accounts 39
 UHC policy 56
Thapar, Romesh 312
Thatcher, Margaret 15
TI programme 282–3, 354
total fertility rate (TFR) 179
trade-offs 4–5, 77, 84, 342

Transgender Persons (Protection of Rights) Bill, 2016 246
transgenders 211, 246–8, 256, 264–5, 267–8, 288
Transparency International 183, 194
treatment protocols 19, 31, 321–2
Trehan, Naresh 359
Tuberculosis Research Centre (TRC) 144
Turkey
 drug-prescription powers to nurses 331
 health transition reform programme of 406

UK
 commercialization of healthcare 28
 decriminalized gay behaviour 247
 free healthcare to every citizen 39
 National Health Service privatization 113
under five mortality rate (U5MR) x, 142, 179
UNICEF 12, 206, 230–1, 240, 345–6
Union Public Service Commission (UPSC) 76, 152
United Nations Development Programme (UNDP) 205
United Nations Office on Drugs and Crime (UNODC) 271
United Nations Population Fund (UNFPA) 205
United Progressive Alliance (UPA) 22, 33, 119, 124, 298, 300–3, 358, 413
United States Agency for International Development (USAID) 19, 211
universal health coverage (UHC)

aspirational goal of 26
global movement for 28
universal health insurance
  scheme 19, 86
universal immunization
  programme 115, 136, 146, 229
universal primary healthcare 407
USA 4, 10, 15, 27–8, 39, 62, 96,
  98–100, 113, 118, 186, 194,
  208, 236, 262–64, 271, 274,
  360, 394, 400, 404, 408, 414
  anti-trafficking bill 262
  budget on health 10
  childhood mortality 27
  commercialization of
    healthcare 28
  focus on primary care 394
  fragmented health system 3
  mandatory health insurance 39
  Technical Cooperation
    Mission 12
  total health spending in 400
USAID 19, 211, 217, 221, 274, 281
Uttarakhand
  blood-transfusion services 226
  NRHM spending in, 59–60
  secondary care expenditure
    in 68
  spent on drugs 68
Uttar Pradesh
  blood-transfusion services 226
  injecting drug users (IDUs)
    272
  NRHM spending in 59
  secondary care expenditure
    in 68

Vajpayee, Atal Bihari 204
Veshya Anyay Mukti Parishad
  (VAMP) 254

Village Health and Sanitation
  Committees (VHSCs) 338
Village Health Sanitation and
  Nutrition Committee 349–50
village health worker (VHW)
  scheme 14
Village Sanitation Act 8
Voluntary Health Association of
  India (VHAI) 21
Vyapam (Vyavsayik Pareeksha
  Mandal) 169, 194n. 51

welfare state ix
West Bengal
  NRHM spending in 59
  spending composition 68
Western-oriented medical
  system 11
Women's Initiatives (WINS) 260
Workers' Social Security Act 23
World AIDS Day 204
World Bank 17–23, 54, 56, 114,
  117, 137, 146, 160, 202, 204,
  206, 216, 255, 284, 306, 323,
  359, 403
  funding of NGOs 19
  IMF-inspired policy 20
  loans for family planning
    programmes 17
  loans for HIV/AIDS
    control 17
World Health Organization
  (WHO) x, 12, 21, 29, 101,
  114–15, 189, 202, 206, 208,
  210, 216, 236, 241, 243, 249–1,
  253, 303, 377, 393, 410
World Health Report 1

Yadav, Raghuvansh 342
Yeshasvini 22–3, 86–7, 91, 403

About the Author

K. Sujatha Rao is a former union secretary of the Ministry of Health and Family Welfare, Government of India. Of her 36-year-long service as a civil servant, she spent close to 20 years in the health sector in different capacities at both state and federal levels.

Rao was the chairperson of the portfolio committee of the Global Fund to fight AIDS, TB and Malaria (GFATM), member of the global advisory panel of the Bill & Melinda Gates Foundation, founding member of the Public Health Foundation of India, member of the advisory board of the Ministerial Leadership Program of the Harvard School of Public Health (HSPH), Harvard University, Boston, USA, and member of the high-level panel on Global Risk Framework of the National Academy of Sciences, Washington, D.C., USA.

She did her master's in history from the University of Delhi, India, and in public administration from Harvard University (1991–2). She was a Takemi Fellow (2001–2) and a Gro Harlem Brundtland Senior Leadership Fellow (2012) at the HSPH.